THE TURTLE
AND THE CADUCEUS

THE TURTLE AND THE CADUCEUS

How Pacific Politics and Modern Medicine Shaped the Medical School in Fiji, 1885-2010

Professor David Brewster, AM

BA Honours, MD, MPH, FRACP, PhD
James Cook University School of Medicine,

Former Dean of Fiji School of Medicine

david.brewster48@gmail.com
Current address: School of Medicine, University of Botswana
Private Bag 0022, Gaborone, Botswana

Copyright © 2010 by Professor David Brewster, AM.

Library of Congress Control Number: 2009914211
ISBN: Hardcover   978-1-4500-2262-0
         Softcover   978-1-4500-2261-3
         Ebook   978-1-4500-2263-7

All rights reserved. No part of this book may be reproduced or transmitted in any form or by any means, electronic or mechanical, including photocopying, recording, or by any information storage and retrieval system, without permission in writing from the copyright owner.

This book was printed in the United States of America.

To order additional copies of this book, contact:
Xlibris Corporation
1-888-795-4274
www.Xlibris.com
Orders@Xlibris.com
73232

CONTENTS

Abbreviations 13

Figures & Tables 15

Introduction 21
    The Tale 21
    Medical Historians 23
    The Book's Thesis 25
    The Caduceus Symbol 26
    The Turtle (Pacific Islands) 28

PART I: THE SUVA MEDICAL SCHOOL, 1885-1928

Chapter 1—A Medical School for Natives 35
    Suva Medical School, 1885-1902 35
    William MacGregor 42
    Colonial Medical Officers 45
    Fiji Medical School, 1902-1928 47
    Influenza Pandemic, 1919 49
    First World War 50

Chapter 2—Epidemics and Depopulation 53
    The Scourge of Epidemics 53
    The Measles Epidemic, 1875 56
    Later Outbreaks 60
    Measles Epidemiology 61
    Population Decline 65
    Pre-Contact Populations 67
    Perspectives on Depopulation at the Time 71
    Anthropology Perspectives 75
    Public Health Perspectives 81

    Contemporary Perspectives 84
    Indian Demographic Dominance 87

Chapter 3—Colonialism with a Human Face 91
    Sir Arthur Gordon 91
    Indirect Rule 97
    Perspectives on Colonialism 99

Chapter 4—The Empirical Tradition 104
    Physicians, Surgeons and Apothecaries 104
    Medical Education in England 107
    Medical Education in Europe 108
    The London Hospitals 109
    Scottish Medical Education 111
    Regulation of Medical Practitioners 112
    British Empiricism 114
    Clinical Examination 116

Chapter 5—Labour and Land 121
    The 'Polynesian' Labour Trade ('Blackbirding') 121
    Indian Indentured Labour 123
    Indian Permanent Settlement 128

Chapter 6—Rockefeller Philanthropy 132
    Hookworm Campaigns 134
    The Queensland campaign 134
    Melanesian Campaigns 135
    Carbon Tetrachloride Treatment 137
    Other Pacific Campaigns 138

PART II: CENTRAL MEDICAL SCHOOL 1928-1961

Chapter 7—A Regional Medical School 143
    Sylvester Lambert 143
    Origins of the New School..146
    Rockefeller Opposition 148
    Critiques of Rockefeller Philanthropy 149
    Final Preparations 151
    Central Medical School Opening, 1928...............................153
    David Hoodless 158
    The Curriculum..161
    Pathology Laboratory...164
    Conclusions..167

Chapter 8—New Guinea and Micronesia 169
    Papua New Guinea..169
    Papua and New Guinea Medical Students 170
    League of Nations Report, 1929..172
    The PNG 'Medical Orderly' Model 177
    John Gunther..178
    Sir Raphael Cilento 180
    John Cumpston 184
    A Critique of Tropical Medicine..185
    University of PNG 191
    The Pacific Basin Medical Officers Training Program 197
    'Off-Shore' Medical Schools 199

Chapter 9—The School and its Graduates................................ 201
    Central Medical School after the War.................................201
    Stories of School Graduates...204
    The Burden of Disease...209
    A Unified Medical Service 213
    South Pacific Commission...217

Chapter 10—The Biomedical Model... 219
    Scientific Laboratory Medicine 220
    Flexner Reports on Medical Education, 1910-12 223

PART III: FIJI SCHOOL OF MEDICINE 1961-2010

Chapter 11—The Politics of Transition to a Degree 229
    Fiji School of Medicine 229
    Assistant Medical Officers (AMOs) 233
    New Programmes at FSMed 235
    The USP Fiasco 238
    Poor Management at Ministry of Health 249
    The School Centenary 250
    1987 Coup 253
    Autonomy at Last 261
    2000 Coup 262
    Research 265

Chapter 12—Problem-Based Learning 269
    PBL at McMaster 269
    Clinical Reasoning 272
    My McMaster Experience 276
    Focus on Learning 280
    Cognitive Errors 283
    Assessment 286
    The Hidden Curriculum 290
    Medical Professionalism 291
    Medical Ethics 293
    Evidence-Based Medicine (EBM) 297

Chapter 13—The Aid Racket 300
    Aims of Aid 300
    Official Developmental Assistance (ODA) 303
    New Paradigm for Aid 306
    Migration of Health Workers 308
    Australian Aid 313
    The Pacific Paradox 316
    Conclusions 321

Chapter 14—The Coup Culture 324
    Ratu Sir Kamisese Mara 325
    Indigenous Fijian Disadvantage..328
    Lead-up to the Coup..331
    Taukei Movement 338
    Reactions to the Coup 340
    Second 1987 Coup 344
    New Constitutions...346
    2000 Coup 348
    The 2006 Coup 350
    Conclusions...352

Chapter 15—A Poisoned Chalice 354
    Appointment as Dean..355
    The Corporate Review 358
    School Fees 364
    New Pasifika Campus...366
    Dental School Nightmares 367
    Project Funding...372
    Research Challenges 374
    Graduate Entry Proposal...377
    A Dreadful Monday 380
    Another Coup..383
    Loss of Lautoka Clinical School...384
    Resignation 389
    Conclusions...393

Annex 1—Heads of the School of Medicine in Fiji, 1885-2010 405

Annex 2—Chronology of the School... 408

References 413

Index 445

Dedication

À Catherine, ma compagne de 40 ans

ABBREVIATIONS

AMO/AMP	Assistant Medical Officer/Practitioner
ANU	Australian National University, Canberra
AusAID	Australian aid, formerly AIDAB
BDS	the dental degree
CEO	Chief Executive Officer
CMO	Chief Medical Officer
CROP	Council of Regional Organisations of the Pacific
CWM	Colonial War Memorial Hospital, Suva
DALY	Disability-Adjusted Life Years (health outcomes)
DDT	an insecticide
DFL	Distance and Flexible Learning
DSM	Diploma of Surgery and Medicine
EBM	Evidence-Based Medicine
ENT	Ear, Nose and Throat speciality
FSMEA	Fiji School of Medicine Employees Association (union)
FSMed	Fiji School of Medicine
FSM	Federated States of Micronesia
GNP/GNI	Gross National Product/Income of a nation
HEO	Health Extension Officer (PNG)
HRH	Human Resources for Heath (health manpower)
MBBS	the medical degree
MCQ	multiple choice questions
MMed	Master of Medicine (like a specialist Fellowship)
MoH	Ministry of Health
MoU	Memorandum of Understanding
NAB	arsenical injection for yaws
NCD	Non-Communicable Diseases
NHMRC/HRC	Australian/NZ national health research councils

NMP	Native Medical Practitioner
NSW	New South Wales, State of Australia
NZ/NZAID	New Zealand / aid
ODA	Overseas Development Assistance
OSCE	Objective Structured Clinical Examination
PBL	Problem-Based Learning
PCP	Primary Care Practitioner
PIM	Pacific Island Monthly magazine
PNG	Papua New Guinea
PHRC	Pacific Health Research Council
SPC	Secretariat of the Pacific Community
School	Refers to the medical school in Fiji, 1885-2010
TB	Tuberculosis
UWA	University of Western Australia
USP	University of the South Pacific
UPNG	University of Papua New Guinea
VC	Vice-Chancellor of a university
WHO	World Health Organization

FIGURES

Fig. 1:	Author's Postings for Education and Work Positions	18
Fig. 2:	Map of the Pacific Islands with numbers of doctors per 100,000 population	19
Fig. 3:	Staff of Hermes (Caduceus)	28
Fig. 4:	The Rod of Asklepios (Asclepius)	28
Fig. 6:	Map of Fiji	32
Fig. 7:	Class of 1885	39
Fig. 8:	Sir William MacGregor	43
Fig. 9:	NMP at a Rural Hospital	47
Fig. 10:	Hospital Dispensary	52
Fig. 11:	Tinea imbricata rash	55
Fig. 12:	Yaws	56
Fig. 13:	Severe Measles (TALC)	62
Fig. 14:	Population of Fiji, 1891-1927, modified from SM Lambert	66
Fig. 15:	WHR Rivers	75
Fig. 16:	George Pitt-Rivers	77
Fig. 17:	Thomas Nicholas	84
Fig. 18:	Prof Stephen Kunitz	86
Fig. 19:	Annual Population Growth Rates (%) by Decade for Fijians and Indians in Fiji, 1927-56	88
Fig. 20:	Sir Arthur Gordon	91
Fig. 21:	Victor Heiser	133
Fig. 22:	The Hookworm	134
Fig. 23:	CWM Hospital	154

Fig. 24:	Central Medical School Buildings	155
Fig. 25:	Hoodless and Lambert (right)	158
Fig. 26:	Sir Raphael Cilento	180
Fig. 27:	Abraham Flexner	223
Fig. 28:	Operating Theatre CWM Hospital.	232
Fig. 29:	Declared or Implied Migration from Fiji.	256
Fig. 30:	Prevalence of Obesity in the Western Pacific (WHO Database on Body Mass Index, 2006)	266
Fig. 31:	School Graduates by Discipline of Study	267
Fig. 32:	School Graduates, Regional & Total	268
Fig. 33:	Howard Barrows	271
Fig. 34:	Geoffrey Norman	272
Fig. 35:	Framework for Clinical Assessment	289
Fig. 36:	Prof David Sackett	298
Fig. 37:	Lester B Pearson	303
Fig. 38:	Willy Brandt	304
Fig. 39:	Official Developmental Assistance as a Percentage of Gross National Income, 2008.	305
Fig. 40:	Dambisa Moyo	307
Fig. 41:	William Easterly	308
Fig. 42:	Ratu Sir Kamisese Mara	325
Fig. 43:	Dr Timoci Bavadra	334
Fig. 44:	Sitiveni Rabuka	336
Fig. 45:	George Speight	348
Fig. 46:	Commodore Frank Bainimarama	350
Fig. 47:	FSMed Management Structure, 2005	359
Fig. 48:	The Teaching Block	367
Fig. 49:	Staff & Student Numbers 1998-2007	397

TABLES

Table 1:	Medical Graduates by Titles and Duration of Course	32
Table 2:	1883 Commission on Depopulation Report	72
Table 3:	Scottish Curriculum for a Medical Degree	111
Table 4:	FSMed Teaching Staff, 1972	237
Table 5:	MBBS 6-year Curriculum, 1987	241
Table 6:	Curriculum of the Primary Care Practitioner Programme	260
Table 7:	McMaster IV-Phase Curriculum in 3-Years (1970-73)	280

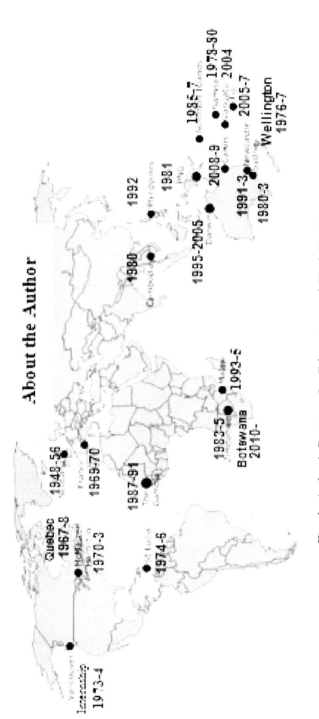

Fig. 1: Author's Postings for Education and Work Positions

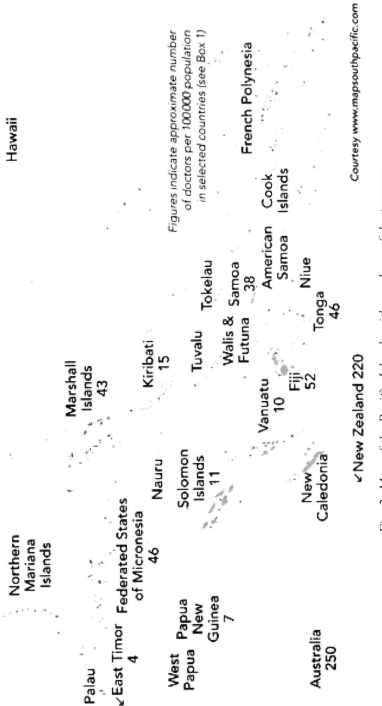

Fig. 2: Map of the Pacific Islands with numbers of doctors per 100,000 population

Introduction

The Tale

Once upon a time, in a distant group of islands in the Pacific Ocean, there was a King named Cakobau who decided to cede his kingdom to the British Queen Victoria, in order to circumvent a debt and a rival chief. As part of the celebrations, he went on a voyage to Sydney, where he and his party contracted measles. Upon his return home, measles was transmitted to the islands resulting in the death of over a quarter of his subjects.

The new Scottish Governor of the colony, named Gordon, wanted to protect the natives from further depopulation and the destructive effects of plantation labour, so he imported indentured labourers from India to work on the sugar cane plantations. His Chief Medical Officer, another Scot by the name of MacGregor, was also concerned about the welfare of the native population as well as the severe shortage of colonial medical officers, so he commenced a School to train native practitioners. Thus began the medical school in Fiji in 1885.

But many of the Indian indentured labourers and their offspring remained in the colony, increasing in numbers until they outnumbered the native population. The *dénouement* of these political events greatly affected the medical school.

This book tells the tale of the School, as we must learn from the past or we are doomed to repeat past mistakes. It also examines the background to the story, such as:

1) an apparently benign form of British colonialism favouring native Fijians

the population changes: on the one hand, the decline in Fijians from epidemics and malaise; on the other hand, the demographic rise in Indians due to high fertility and an inclination to remain in Fiji after completing their labour contract
3) the resulting ethnic tension
4) the impact of new developments in medicine and medical education on the School
5) the importance of philanthropy and foreign aid, and above all
6) the political, economic and migration developments following from the four *coups d'état* between 1987 and 2006.

Fiji and the School are still struggling from the consequences of these momentous events.

The Western tradition of biomedical science (the caduceus) was introduced into traditional Pacific Island cultures (the turtle), and the native practitioners who graduated from the School were the intermediaries. It was not an easy role, and some fell by the wayside. But the battle was ultimately won, and the School was strengthened and regionalised by Rockefeller philanthropy in the 1920s. Finally, however, in the transition to a modern university medical school, the School faltered and lost its way due to political events beyond its control. Only time will tell whether it can rise from the ashes to triumph over 'an uncertain future' and assume once again the role it had occupied for a hundred years.

This book has been written for the general reader with an interest in Pacific Islands politics, history, health and medical education. It is not a dry academic history—as it is not based on a systematic search of all primary sources, and is not written by an academic historian. Nor is it a conventional institutional history—as it does not just aim to celebrate the School's accomplishments, indeed is often critical of some aspects of its history, and is also very selective of the interesting parts of the story. Nevertheless, it is a work of academic scholarship which tells an interesting tale, a 'narrative', as historians prefer to call it, from which lessons can be drawn. I agree with the distinguished medical historian, John Burnham, that "within the realm of scholarship, medical history ... [is] the most fascinating subject of all."[1] It is also generally acknowledged that there has been a relative neglect of historical scholarship of the Pacific Islands.

Medical Historians

It is not uncommon for an older medical practitioner, like myself, to develop an interest in medical history. Indeed, the story is told of a discussion between an aging doctor and a historian, in which the medical practitioner tells the historian that he plans to become a medical historian on his retirement, to which the historian replies that he is going to become a neurosurgeon. The doctor did not see the joke and pointed out the need for proper training, which was, of course, the historian's point that many doctors write about the past without any training in academic history. Indeed, much of clinician history has been dismissed as bad history.

Although I have no pretensions as an academic historian, one of the advantages of McMaster University, where I studied medicine, was that it allowed humanities students into medicine without the need for having studied sciences as an undergraduate. Thus, I studied history and the history of philosophy for 10 semesters at 3 universities prior to commencing medicine. I have also read widely in history, the social sciences and public health since 2005 for this book.

To cite Burnham again: "another special character of medical historians of the twentieth century ... [is] the openness of physicians, who for so long monopolized interest in the subject of the history of medicine, to other scholars who began to come into the field."[1] It is in the spirit of this tradition in which this book is written. But it would be a mistake to assume that medical history is only the concern of historians. It is certainly true that their interest in the subject and rigour in consulting primary sources has contributed greatly to the field. Nevertheless, there is more than ever the need for an insider's medical interpretation and perspective on medicine's past, which takes into account work in other disciplines and the political background of events.

In my reading in medical history, I discovered that there were quite different traditions of writing between medical practitioners as amateur historians and medical historians. The former tend to tell the story of:

> disease discoveries, diagnosis, and treatment from the perspective of medical practice and science, but insulated from wider cultural influences. By contrast, academic historians view history as a contextual enterprise ... Historians of medicine study institutions, classification systems, and the social and cultural values that physicians, patients, and their families bring to the clinical encounter.[2]

In the USA, there are even distinct professional organisations for the two groups, with doctors belonging to the exclusive American Osler Society and medical historians to the American Association of the History of Medicine. They even use footnotes and references differently with doctors tending to use *Reference Manager* to give the sources of information whereas historians are more likely to rely on *Endnote* with extensive footnotes to accompany the text. Whereas medical practitioners as historians have tended to tell stories of conquering diseases, medical historians and sociologists have focussed more on the professionalization of medicine and medicalization of society, including many critics of these trends. There is even a recent collection of 'clinician-historian' stories of how history had an impact on clinical activities.[3] In this book, however, we focus more on the impact of political developments and the history of medicine upon an institution. We also lament the detrimental effects of 'Politics'—as opposed to state regulation of the profession—on a medical institution; its politicization as part of partisan agendas and military coups.

In his *Lancet* paper, Kushner throws down the challenge to create a collaborative environment to bring these two strands together.[2] He calls for an educational effort, on one hand, to expose academic historians to patient care and medical science, and on the other hand, to provide doctor 'historians' with the training to appreciate the extent to which medical practice and research take place within a broad social context, which must be understood and critiqued, even deconstructed. I have attempted to follow this advice, by telling the story of the medical school in Fiji in its historical and cultural context. Ten of the 15 chapters cover the political and medical education background to events at the School. The title is analogous to a *La Fontaine* fable; here is a tale, which I have tried to tell it in an interesting and accessible way for the general reader.

The Book's Thesis

The thesis of the book is that the first hundred years of the medical school in Suva (1885-1987, to be exact) were its glorious days, and its downfall was intimately linked to the political instability of the military coups, which were in turn largely dictated by the unique mixture of Polynesian and Melanesian cultures in Fiji and by the majority of inhabitants of Fiji being of Indian descent at independence in 1970. But there were other key factors in the decline, such as its failure to become part of the regional university, the dominance within the school of Fijian nationalists and an old boys' network and the exponential rise in student numbers (Figs 31-2 & 49) without the administrative competence and structures to cope with them. So rather than a story of conquering diseases or the professionalization of medicine, this book is about how medical education and its institutions were affected by the political context—the politicization of medical education.

This is certainly not unique to Fiji, as Australia saw much the same during the Howard era in an attempt to get more rural doctors for the National Party's election campaign against the onslaughts of Pauline Hansen (e.g. University Departments of Rural Health, rural clinical schools, massive increases in medical school places, bonded scholarships, rural placements, etc.). Medical deans now have more of a political than educational or medical role in their institutions. The moral of the story is that we need to fight the encroaching politicization of our medical institutions, so they can get on with the important business of training future doctors—a role too important to be left entirely to politicians, or to professors either for that matter.

The first Professor of Pacific History, James W Davidson, observed in 1953 that:

> The writing of valid history requires not merely technical training but also mature understanding of the human mind. The historian has to understand the ways of thought and action of a whole society; and to gain this understanding he cannot go to the actors themselves but has to rely on the desiccated residue which they left behind—a pile of documents . . . The historian's training comes as much from an understanding of men as from an understanding of books.[4] (p99)

The danger of the contemporary participant history favoured by Davidson, in his book *Samoa mo Samoa*, is the loss of objectivity, detachment and critical distance which is required for history.[5] As Dean of the Fiji School of Medicine from 2005-7, the author was a brief participant in the story, and the last chapter tells his version of events. In one sense, this book is an attempt to understand those years with the benefit of hindsight and in a larger historical perspective. I have tried to tell this personal story with reasoned fairness, as a cautionary tale from which there are lessons of general interest to medical education, institutional management and the Pacific Islands. The past can teach us a lot about what is going on in the present, and this is a story which I felt compelled to tell.

The Caduceus Symbol

The title of this book is taken from the two symbols on the School insignias of both Central Medical School (Fig 5) and Fiji School of

Medicine (front cover), in which the caduceus stands for medicine and the turtle represents the Pacific Islands. The title was chosen to symbolise the result of the introduction of Western medicine (the caduceus) into traditional Pacific island societies (the turtle). It was likely to have been the American, Dr Sylvester Lambert of the Rockefeller Foundation, who chose the caduceus symbol (staff of Hermes in Fig 3) for the insignia of the new Central Medical School in 1928, presumably following the US Army Medical Corps.

The caduceus is a symbol of Greco-Roman origin, but there is an interesting twist which is relevant to our story. The School chose to use the double serpent entwined staff with wings from the Greek messenger Hermes (or his Roman counterpart Mercury), which it superimposed on the shell of a turtle to represent the Pacific islands. However, the correct Greco-Roman symbol for medicine is the rod of Asklepios (or Roman Aesculapius or Asclepius), which has a single snake and rough hewn staff without wings (Fig 4). Asklepios was the mythical son of Apollo and was trained in the arts of healing by Chiron, the centaur. Asklepios is mentioned in both Homer's *Iliad* and the Hippocratic oath. The Asklepian cult built hundreds of health-related temples during the Roman Empire, where healing was practiced by the magical intervention of the gods during sleep. This heathen symbol of healing was suppressed by Christianity from about the 6th century, when the urine flask became the favoured medical symbol.

The reintroduction of the staff of Asclepius as the symbol of medicine commenced after the Protestant reformation in northern Europe. It was used by the US Army Medical Department as early as 1818, but the influential US Army Medical Corps adopted the caduceus as a medical symbol in 1902. Although this was later claimed to be a symbol of non-combatants in war, it is clear that it was used in ignorance of its Greco-Roman origins. It was not used as the staff of Hermes but copied from a London publisher, John Churchill, who used it as a printers mark on scientific books, with the twin serpents signifying the bond between medicine and literature. Churchill understood the distinction in staffs, as he still used the Asklepian staff as a specific symbol of medicine on his medical publications. The staff of Hermes was perhaps an unfortunate choice of symbol for medicine as Hermes was the god of thieves, games, travellers, merchants and commerce.[6,7]

Fig. 3: Staff of Hermes (Caduceus) *Fig. 4: The Rod of Asklepios (Asclepius)*

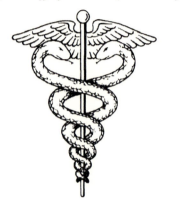 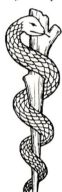

Perhaps Lambert's use of this insignia was anticipating the commercial nature of medicine as it would develop in America and elsewhere. Many medical organisations use the correct Asklepian staff as their symbol, but still refer to it as the caduceus (or *la caducée* in French). However, the use of the incorrect insignia, at least from a Greco-Roman perspective, is widespread. With the name change of Central Medical School to Fiji School of Medicine in 1961, the logo was changed with the caduceus and turtle depicted separately, but the erroneous symbol for medicine was retained.

The Turtle (Pacific Islands)

The setting for this story is Fiji and the Pacific Islands, symbolised by the turtle on the School's insignia. For those unfamiliar with the region, we will attempt very briefly to set the scene. The Figure 2 map illustrates the vast array of islands over a larger area than any continent, but the population of the region is small at 9.2 million (including 6.2 million in PNG). The islands were populated by at least two distinct waves of migrations: the first some 50,000 years ago brought settlers on foot to the New Guinea region who now speak some 800 languages; the second wave only arrived some 3,500 years ago as Austronesian speakers and voyageurs by canoe to the smaller distant islands of Polynesia and Micronesia. One can hardly exaggerate the diversity and variability of the populations in the region. The Pacific Islands have often been portrayed as 'paradise', which is a highly misleading myth—nor was the region inhabited by either 'noble savages' or 'savage brutes', although there was cannibalism in the past. But such stereotypes are unhelpful.

The region is also experiencing rapid social change with globalisation, one aspect of which is epidemic levels of obesity with most of the adult morbidity and mortality due to non-communicable diseases (over 70%). Issues of land tenure are also central concerns of Pacific islander's lives, as are increasingly global warming for the coral atolls and HIV/AIDS for PNG. The experience of colonialism, philanthropy, foreign aid and migration will be dealt with in the book. Finally, the issue of political unrest and instability have emerged in recent decades, and its impact on the regional medical school in Fiji is the subject of this book.

Fig. 5: Insignia of Central Medical School

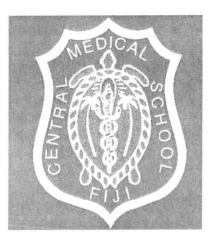

Acknowledgments

The author would like to thank the following people for their kind assistance: Niraj Swami of Fiji School of Medicine, Graeme Maguire of James Cook University, Brian Cameron of McMaster University and Ian Lewis of Tasmania.

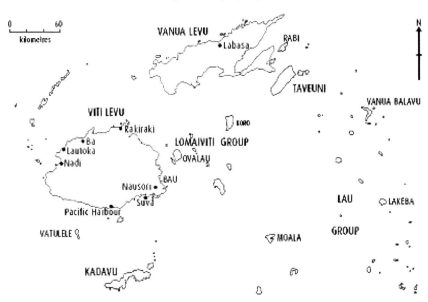

Fig. 6: Map of Fiji.[8]

Table 1: Medical Graduates by Titles and Duration of Course

YEARS	TITLES OF GRADUATES	NO. GRADUATES Total (Mean/Year)	DURATION OF COURSE
1885-1902	Native Practitioner	168 (3-4/yr)	3 years
1902-33	Native Medical Practitioners		
1934-51	NMPs	261 (12-13/yr)	4 years
1951-55	Assistant Medical Practitioners		
1956-64	Assistant Medical Officers	383 (12-13/yr)	5 years
1964-87	Medical Officers		
1987-2010	Doctors (MBBS)	816 (35-40/yr)	6 years

PART I

THE SUVA MEDICAL SCHOOL, 1885-1928

Chapter 1

A Medical School for Natives

Suva Medical School, 1885-1902

In 1885, a medical school for native Fijian boys was initiated at the Colonial Hospital in Suva by the Chief Medical Officer (CMO) of the colony, Dr William MacGregor. The background to this initiative included factors such as:

1. the devastating measles epidemic in 1875,
2. the fear of smallpox and cholera among indentured labourers aboard the first ship from India in 1879,
3. the acute shortage and high cost of European medical officers, and undoubtedly
4. the favourable but patronising attitude of the British Colonial administration of Sir Arthur Gordon towards the native Fijian population.

Each of these factors will be explored over the next few chapters.

One of MacGregor's chief concerns as CMO was the chronic shortage of colonial medical officers in Fiji. In 1876, he instituted an initiative to train Wesleyan mission teachers as medical assistants, intending personally to supervise their purely practical course at Levuka Hospital in Fiji's capital at that time. Although aware of the limitations of such a rudimentary apprenticeship, he felt it would be adequate for training them to treat common diseases such as dysentery, bronchitis, worms, wounds, burns, and skin and eye infections. He urged all Christian missions in the Pacific Islands to have "every missionary and teacher, white or coloured, man or woman, put through a course of medical instruction that would enable them to alleviate and mitigate the maladies that now menace the different races of the islanders."[9] The Methodist, Wesleyan and Catholic Christian Missions had already begun training natives as assistant missionaries, ministers or catechists by the 1850s, so MacGregor had a model which could be equally applied to health in order to save lives as well as 'saving souls'.[10]

Prior to Fiji becoming a British colony in 1874, the major health threat to the settler population in the capital, Levuka, was environmental—as in Europe at the time.

> Anyone going through Levuka cannot fail to be struck with the filthiness and unwholesomeness of the place . . . Drains flushed with filthy refuse, . . . the effluvium of refuse from shambles which come floating down Totoga creek, the stinking refuse which is thrown out onto the beach . . . [11] (p231)

Although there were four doctors in practice in Levuka, they could do little to improve the health of settlers under such appalling sanitary conditions—which were arguably worse than for the indigenous population in their villages. The outcome of European settlement depended primarily on the price of cotton, security of land tenure, and the availability of cheap labour. The outbreak of the American Civil War in 1860 was followed by a steady rise in the price of cotton, attracting European adventurers from the Australian and New Zealand (NZ) frontier, who were looking to make a quick fortune and believed in their racial superiority. By 1871, their ranks had swelled to a population of 2,560, and they expected to be favoured by the new British colonial administration for which they had agitated.[11] Their hopes would soon be frustrated both by the pro-Fijian attitude of the colonial administration and by the fall in the price of cotton with the ending of the American civil war.

When the first ship of Indian labourers was found to have cholera and smallpox cases on board, the colonial administration imposed a three month quarantine. It heeded the lesson from the previous quarantine failure in the devastating 1875 measles epidemic (chapter 2), so prevented smallpox and cholera from affecting the population of Fiji. But such a long quarantine period was expensive and difficult to enforce, so the colonial administration looked to vaccination as better protection against smallpox. European vaccinators were costly, so MacGregor trained a team of young natives boys in vaccination technique. While working in Fijian villages, these vaccinators developed an interest in the illnesses affecting communities, and their reports disclosed the considerable burden of disease in the native population. Moreover, even after the measles epidemic, the native population continued to decline further, which greatly concerned the colonial administration. MacGregor proposed an expansion of the vaccination training program for natives so they could be trained to assist in healing the sick and arresting the spread of disease, similar to what he had suggested for missionaries previously.[12] This was one of the incentives for the initiative which led ultimately to the Suva Medical School, as it was later called.

The first official proposal by MacGregor to train natives was in 1879, following an outbreak of dysentery (bloody diarrhoea) at Kadavu in which over 60 people died without medical care. In getting approval for the proposal, MacGregor had to contend with considerable scepticism among colonial authorities and colonists about the inherent intelligence of the 'savage' and his ability to understand modern medical concepts. On the whole, Europeans at the time had little doubt that they were a biologically superior species, with little awareness of the importance of what are now recognised as social determinants of health—the non-medical context of disease, such as good nutrition and living conditions as the explanation for better European health status. Sir Charles Mitchell, who was Governor from 1877-88, expressed a common European perspective of the time that medical training would upset the equilibrium of the native's mind due to rapid promotion over other natives leading to 'the slothful life of petty chiefs'. He stressed the need for natives to be kept 'in due subjection to their chiefs'.

Nevertheless, an initial trial of medical training of natives started in 1884 when a few Fijians, mostly sons of chiefs, were given practical instruction on vaccination techniques and simple medical procedures at the new Colonial Hospital in Suva, the new capital of the colony. The training was carried out by MacGregor as CMO with the intention of them assisting European medical officers in providing basic health services to the indigenous population. Meanwhile, MacGregor persevered in his lobbying endeavours for a formal training programme, until funds were eventually officially approved by Governor Des Voeux.[12]

The official proposal to Fiji's Legislative Council in December 1883 explained the proposal in the following terms:

> It not infrequently happens that sickness of an epidemic form breaks out in a remote part of the Colony or at a spot which, while geographically near, is in consequence of the infrequency or difficulty of communication virtually remote and that tens and scores of natives are swept off before any confirmation can reach the seat of Government. Dr. McGregor proposes to form a class of students, carefully selected from among the most intelligent of the Fijian people, who, after completing a course of practical instruction in the hospital, including nursing, may be sent out to assist in healing the sick and arresting the progress of disease in those parts of the Colony These students will also be taught to vaccinate and it is probable that those among them who evince any aptitude or inclination for it may be taught to dispense the simpler form of medicines.[13] (p3)

Thus, following the successful initial trial, the Suva medical school project began in 1885 with a small group of young men who were given three years of instruction in the rudiments of human anatomy and physiology, and clinical experience in medicine and surgery at the Colonial hospital under the supervision of the CMO and Matron. Even in Europe at the time, medicine was an apprenticeship and did not involve any teaching of basic sciences, which in any case were rather rudimentary at the time (chapter 4). Incompetent or otherwise unacceptable candidates were eliminated from the class during the first year. After three years of satisfactory performance, students were granted the status of native practitioner.

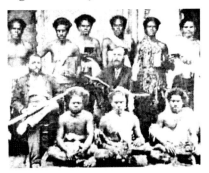

Fig. 7: Class of 1885.[13]

The first group of 10 students began the course in 1885, and three years later, three of the trainees had passed the oral examination in medicine and surgery, with six more the following year. This was the same year as the first University of Sydney medical school graduation for the MB ChM degree.[14]

In June 1888, the Native Practitioners Ordinance gave native practitioners legal status upon condition that they had been medical students at a public hospital for three years and passed an examination in medicine and surgery.

They were then granted a certificate as a Native Practitioner, which gave them the right to practice medicine and surgery in a district specified by the CMO, where they would be provided with a house and a garden. Although the CMO was their official chief, they still had to obey their native superiors, but their services as Native Practitioners were to take precedence over normal village duties. The salary was at least £5 a year from the province, and £2 10s a year from the Colony with the proviso that they were not allowed to demand any fees for their services, although they were allowed to accept gifts offered to them.[13] Thus, the cost of native practitioners (including training costs) was still only a fraction of the minimum salary of colonial medical officers (£350/year).

Although it was MacGregor who inaugurated the scheme, the credit for ensuring its success goes to his successor as CMO, Dr Glanville Corney, who was in charge of the Suva Medical School for its first graduation in 1888. He had studied at St. Thomas's Hospital and received the diploma of MRCS in 1874 without ever attending university, as was common at the time in England. According to David Hoodless, the first full-time Tutor of the School, it is:

> doubtful if any European official has ever been better known and more beloved by the Fijians than Dr Corney, and under his direction the training of Native Medical Practitioners (NMPs) developed steadily.[13]

Along with Sir Basil Thomson, Corney investigated the causes of the population decrease in Fiji (chapter 2). He also collected implements of traditional healers for the museum of the Royal College of Surgeons of England,[15] and wrote an English vocabulary of medical terms for the students with the assistance of Miss May Anderson, who was Matron from 1896 to 1919. Her knowledge of the Fijian language and customs was a great asset, and her authority over the students was remarkable, given Fijian males reluctance to be supervised by a woman at the time, yet she was obeyed 'like the CMO himself'.[13] In 1908, Corney retired after 31 years in Fiji and 20 years as CMO.

It is worth quoting at length from MacGregor's description of the establishment of the School, as he looked back 37 years later:

> In 1885 the Government of Fiji invited the chiefs to send forward eight or ten young men of proved intelligence, and of good character and family, with a view to them being given a course of instruction in the rudiments of human anatomy and physiology, supplemented by suitable teaching in the wards of the Colonial Hospital, with practice of minor surgery and domestic medicine. The proposal met with a willing response,

almost every province contributing at least one student; and these were housed near the Colonial Hospital, where they received technical and disciplinary training from the medical officers and the matron during a term of three years each. Particular attention was paid to such ailments as pneumonia, bronchitis, dysentery, conjunctivitis, and other diseases to which the natives are specially prone, and to the methods for arresting bleeding. General sanitation, both public and individual, and prophylaxis were, of course, included.

In course of time the most promising and careful of these students became useful adjuncts to the labours of the District Medical Officers; and even in parts of the islands out of reach of the latter. As a measure of their ability and precision it may be mentioned that three became in rotation dispensers and anaesthetists at the Hospital, and one of these served with unvarying success for more than a dozen years. Before very long their number reached fifty. Incompetent and otherwise undesirable candidates were generally detected and eliminated from the class long before entering upon a third year of study; but, when the sounder ones had completed the full term, they were subjected to a stiffish examination, written, oral, and practical, and those that passed satisfactorily were awarded a Certificate to that effect. They were then appointed to a provincial post, at first under the supervision of a European Medical Officer, but by degrees their usefulness was availed of, as I have said, for the benefit of the native population of remote islands where no European medical officer was ordinarily within reach, and after some natural hesitation and an occasional rebuff on the part of a biased and ignorant people, they became greatly appreciated, and no province deemed itself properly equipped without one or more of them, so that the total number of these "Native Practitioners," as

> they were officially called, has been maintained, and remains at present at more than fifty, year after year.[9] (pp81-2)

Native practitioners were meant to function like medical assistants to the native population, but their remote site and the shortage of doctors gave them considerable independence and a high degree of responsibility for the health of their communities, including often the dispensaries and district hospitals that opened between 1889 and 1904. Although supervision by European Medical Officers did not always happen as planned, the communal system in Fiji meant that any native practitioner who neglected his duties or mismanaged his cases would soon come to the notice of the chief and be reported to the Native Commissioner in Suva.[13] Many of them became skilled at treating diseases and carrying out simple surgical procedures, so they soon acquired a good reputation. Of course, some racist settlers attributed their surgical skills to familiarity with human anatomy from cannibalism so they could continue to deny their capacity to assimilate European education.[12]

William MacGregor

MacGregor served in the British Colonial Service for a total of 42 years. He was the son of an impoverished Scottish crofter, so it was a truly remarkable achievement not only to complete medical school but to end up a knighted colonial governor. He completed his medical training in Aberdeen and Glasgow in 1872, and immediately joined the Colonial Medical Service, first in Seychelles and then in Mauritius.

The story is told that, while completing his medical degree in Scotland, MacGregor survived on half a crown a week with a diet of porridge for breakfast, two fresh herrings or a kipper for lunch and another bowl of porridge for his supper. He was a bright and diligent student, winning the Gold Medal of the University at graduation. When only three years out of medical school, he was appointed Chief

Medical Officer (CMO) in Fiji, serving in that role from 1875 to 1888. MacGregor had more general intellectual interests apart from medicine: he was an autodidact, a multilingual scholar, and a student of the classics. But there was another side to this lonely dour Scot, according to his biographer, RB Joyce.[16] His correspondence reveals that he was often embittered and frustrated, feeling overlooked for promotion, convinced that his salary was inadequate and that he had been unfairly treated by the Colonial Office.

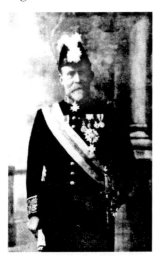

Fig. 8: Sir William MacGregor

After founding of the School, MacGregor went on to have a distinguished career in the region as Governor of Papua and later of Queensland. It is interesting to consider the appraisals of MacGregor by some of his contemporaries to convey both the nature of the man and the elegant writing of the time. Ronald Ross, who proved that malaria was transmitted by mosquitoes in 1897, formed a close acquaintance with MacGregor during his time as Governor of Nigeria, and wrote perceptively of him as:

> Wise, grave, but humorous, bearded, thick-set, with wrinkled forehead and a high and somewhat conical bald head, his low voice and kindly manner filled all with trust in him. He drank no wine and did not smoke, but was no fanatic in these respects, and kept a hospitable table. Every night he read from his Greek Testament, and was also skilled in French and Italian, and knew something of many barbarous tongues. He was a mathematician, a practised surveyor, a lapidary, and a master of many arts, but always proud of his medical upbringing and of his nationality. Simply dignified, he did not allow his dignity to obscure his personality, and he had

no trace of that meanest and most mischievous vice, jealousy. He was not a politician, but a genuine administrator careful of all the interests of the people entrusted to him—still more, a scientific administrator who added knowledge to his solicitude.[16]

Another prominent friend and New South Wales Government medical advisor described him in the following terms:

He was a great block of rough, unhewn granite, but recognized to be of sterling character and possessed of excellent, indeed unusual, ability, although I am sure no one could have predicted then that he would rise to the great position he ultimately occupied in the service of his country. As iron sharpeneth iron, so his intercourse with all sorts of men in so many parts of the Empire, hewed and polished his roughness of manner, until he became the polite and courteous man of later life. But even that did not remove all the angles. He maintained to the last an independent reticence and a stubborn opinionativeness, which were the result no doubt of a life which had fought its own way through a hard fight to a position of great eminence. . . . To bear loneliness and poverty in youth and to despise them and struggle on in spite of them, is to get an original impetus, which no obstacles in after years can wholly withstand. To the man who has conquered such initial difficulties, anything seems to be possible.[16]

However, not all of his colleagues saw him in such a positive light, as one felt that:

. . . he cannot be absolved from blame for the personal clashes of his governorship. Arguments are never one-sided, and this embittered, obstinate Scotsman had helped to destroy his own chances of happiness and his opportunities to influence British policy. The lessons of the need for tolerance and understanding of the ideas of others had proved hard to acquire ...[16]

Colonial Medical Officers

MacGregor was the first of five CMOs over the first 60 years of the colony of Fiji, all of whom played an important role in the School (Annex 1). The other four were:

a) BG Corney (1886-1908)
b) GWA Lynch (1909-18)
c) Aubrey Montague (1919-28), and
d) ABH Pearce (1930-37).

As mentioned, during his 11 years as CMO, MacGregor struggled with the shortage and poor quality of medical officers in Fiji. Just prior to his arrival, there were only four doctors in the colony for the measles epidemic of 1875. Initially, he tried to recruit young Scottish doctors, managing to increase the number of doctors to seven in 1882 and ten by 1884, but it dropped again to only four later that year for a population of 150,000 Fijians and 2,000 Europeans, as well as Islander and Indian labourers. In addition, MacGregor made it abundantly clear that he was very dissatisfied with both the quality of medical officers in the islands and also the poor health status of the native population. Following an initial survey carried out with two other doctors shortly after his arrival in the colony, MacGregor stated that:

> At present nine-tenths of the natives are allowed to die without medical attendance, scores of them lose their

eyesight for want of proper treatment, whilst hideous, raw, uncovered fly-eaten ulcers may be seen in every town. Dysentery and diseases of the chest, by no means rare, are allowed to take their own fatal way. Such a state of affairs will, I hope, not long exist.[16] (p24)

According to an 1891 Lancet advertisement for medical officers, there were eight established positions in Fiji, with the senior medical officer paid £600 per annum, and others receiving £300 and £50 for house allowance, along with the right of private practice. All applicants for medical employment in the colonies had to be 23-30 years of age and be doubly qualified in medicine and surgery, with preference given to those who had held hospital appointments as house physicians and surgeons. Certificates of moral character and of sobriety were also demanded, along with a medical examination of good health. In 1889-1890, there were 12 medical officer vacancies in the following colonies: Fiji, British Guiana, Gibraltar, Gold Coast, Hong Kong, Lagos, and St Helena, for which there were about fifty applicants.[17]

One of the doctors who responded to the advertisement was Charles Wilberforce Daniels, who joined the Colonial Medical Service in 1889, and his initial appointment from 1890-4 was to the Fiji Islands. In addition to his routine medical duties, he studied the annual epidemics of dysentery in labourers on the sugar plantations. One epidemic which he reported was among 120 migrant labourers from New Hebrides (Vanuatu) and Solomon Islands on board ship which had a case-fatality rate of 48%. Although bacteriology was not available, from the clinical description it was probably caused by *Shigella dysenteriae*. Daniels went on to make an important research contribution in Calcutta by confirming Ronald Ross's 1898 discovery of the complete life-cycle of avian malaria.[18]

Fiji Medical School, 1902-1928

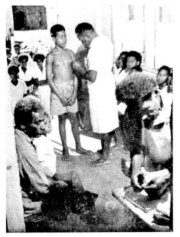

Fig. 9: NMP at a Rural Hospital.[13]

In 1902, the successful medical school project was expanded to accommodate 16 students for the three year course, and was formally named the Fiji Medical School, although it continued to be referred to as the Suva Medical School. The curriculum remained an apprenticeship but involved some lectures in Fijian by the CMO, whose fluency was limited, but most learning occurred from practical duties as medical dressers and dispensers at the hospital. However, there was no basic science or laboratory experience. Graduates were now called Native Medical Practitioners (NMPs).

Dr GWA Lynch was Corney's successor as CMO and Head of School from 1906 to 1919. Over that time, there were 43 NMP graduates. Lynch was described as a hard task-master, who worked hard and expected the same of his students and subordinates. With Lynch and Matron Anderson, the practical training of Fijian medical students continued in the same tradition as Corney. It was during this time that arsenical injections (NAB) for the treatment of yaws were introduced, which contributed significantly to the acceptance and success of NMP services to the native population since the disease was highly prevalent and responded well to NAB treatment.[13] It was one of the first successes of European curative medicine in the Pacific, despite being administered as a painful injection.

By 1911, there were 37 NMPs working in the districts or as hospital dispensers in Fiji, most of whom were performing well except for a few of the older ones.[19] However, three NMPs had to be dismissed and their qualification certificates cancelled due to "constant disobedience and general bad conduct."[20] District NMPs sent quarterly reports to the provincial medical officer, but the regularity of supervision varied greatly.

The salary of NMPs was increased to £18-£50 in 1905 under Corney, and Lynch divided them into three grades in 1917 with salaries increasing to £45-75, £75-120, and £120-150 per annum.[13] The maximum salary for the top grade gave them parity with native clerks in government departments, but was still much less than the minimum of £350 for European doctors, who also had private practice income. Although many NMPs functioned similar to doctors, their low cost had been their main rationale for the colonial administration, which was always struggling with budget constraints. Although NMPs began as a response to the need for vaccinators, dressers and assistants for preventive measures for the indigenous population, they soon became very successful low cost rural practitioners, thus complementing the low staffing levels of the colonial medical services in Fiji.

From the outset, there were concerns about maintaining NMPs' cultural integrity without Europeanising them, while at the same time ensuring their subordinate role to medical officers lest they become unwilling to work in remote communities, like European medical officers. In addition to the indigenous population, NMPs also met the health needs of plantation labourers, who were largely ignored by the colonial health services at the time. In this way, they helped fulfil the colonial administration's responsibility to civilise the natives, promote economic development and provide both preventive and therapeutic health services.[12]

Although the medical school had been approved by Fijian Chiefs, villagers still tended to bypass NMPs for traditional healers who offered herbal remedies, massage and sorcery. Hospitals were a last resort for native patients, only considered after traditional remedies had failed. It is clear from the early writings of native practitioners that superstition and sorcery were major challenges for them in convincing the native population to comply with the limited effective European treatments and health advice available at the time. This is why the introduction of an effective treatment for yaws was such an important tool in the struggle to convince the native population of the value of European medicine.

In spite of these difficulties, it is clear that native practitioners gained the confidence of the local population in a way that European doctors never could, so the experiment of training natives was a great success. One illustration of this success was that Governor Sir Henry May proposed in 1911 to send the best NMPs to Australia for further training and to allow them to undertake private practice, although these suggestions were never implemented.

Influenza Pandemic, 1919

The worst epidemic after measles in 1875 was the pandemic influenza of 1918-9 which affected almost 80% of the population of 92,000 and resulted in some eight thousand deaths, including 5,154 indigenous Fijians (5.7% mortality). Most of the deaths were in young adults aged 15-44 years (12.5% mortality for that age group). There were also 2,553 death among Indians (4.2% mortality) and only 69 European deaths (1.4%). Usually, the highest mortality rates from influenza are in young children and the elderly population, but the 1918-9 epidemic affected fit young men and women in whom about half the deaths occurred.

The demographer Norma McArthur has suggested that the higher Fijian to Indian mortality was due to greater adiposity in Fijians, since influenza tends to be more severe in well-nourished young adults.[21] This may have been mediated by a stronger primary immune response to the virus, which actually harms the host, as also occurs in leprosy. The lower European mortality was presumably due to a degree of pre-existing immunity to influenza as well as better access to medical care, although the latter had little to offer at the time.

This pandemic influenza of 1918 with over 50 million deaths demonstrated a triple failure of the newly emerging Western scientific medicine. Biologically, it mistakenly identified the cause as 'Pfeiffer's influenza bacillus' (*Haemophilus influenzae*) which was only a secondary bacterial invader in many cases. Therapeutically, medicine had little if any impact on mortality as treatment was only supportive, since there were no effective drugs against either the virus or the secondary bronchopneumonia. And finally, politically, medicine failed to prevent or mitigate transmission through available effective measures and also through politicians lying about its risk so as not to alarm the population. There were effective measures to reduce transmission, such as quarantine, face masks, good hygiene with coughing and sneezing, and restrictions on overcrowding and travel. Yet, the American military, for example, continued putting potentially infected soldiers aboard overcrowded ships, and states failed to heed the warnings of the impending epidemic so as not to alarm the population (e.g. 'it is only a seasonal *grippe*').[22]

Like measles, influenza mortality was strongly related to the complication of pneumonia. However, influenza also mutates over time, so there was a first wave of mild influenza in America in April 1918 before the second—and much more lethal—wave emerged in August. It was this second wave which hit Fiji in February 1919, with many of the deaths occurring over a 2-3 week period, as had occurred with measles. The reputation of NMPs was significantly enhanced due to their courageous work during this epidemic. Sadly, out of 48 NMPs in practice at the time, eight of them died of influenza. Nevertheless, they all performed well at a time when most colonial medical officers had not yet returned from the war in Europe.

First World War

After the war, Dr Aubrey Montague continued the School's tradition as CMO from 1919 to 1930, during which time a further 50 NMPs graduated.[13] By 1922, there were a total of 97 NMPs in practice, with most in Fiji but a few working in other Territories of the Western Pacific High Commission.[23] Hoodless cites two examples of successful NMPs from the Suva School:

> Sowane Puamau who qualified in 1899 . . . served for a short time in Fiji and was then transferred to the Gilbert Islands. There he was a complete success. Even the Europeans in the Islands regarded Sowane as their doctor, and his medical knowledge and his conscientious performance of duties endeared him to all races alike. [. . .] Another example of these early native practitioners is given by N.M.P. Asaeli Tamanitoakula who qualified in October 1891, and was appointed dispenser at the Suva hospital where he remained until his retirement on pension on 1st September, 1913. As well as dispenser he was anaesthetist, and for some years he carried out the duties of Government Pharmacist, the Colony's stock of drugs being kept at the hospital. He was a remarkable man, and had everyone's respect for his close adherence to duty.[13]

Although the School had been in operation since 1885, it was in some ways a medical school in name only. It had no dedicated school buildings, no full-time teaching staff and no pre-medical courses in basic sciences. It involved only a training apprenticeship as 'dressers' in the hospital combined with five lectures per week in Fijian, which depended upon the language and lecturing skills of the part-time European teachers. Despite these limitations, a total of 138 NMPs had qualified and 55 were still in practice, forming a valuable auxiliary medical service.[13] But NMPs were not really just 'dressers' since even during their three years training, they assisted with autopsies, gave injections, assisted at operations, dispensed treatments and carried out ward duties in the hospital.

Fig. 10: Hospital Dispensary [13]

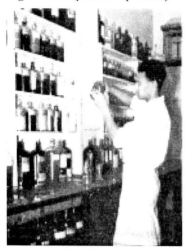

A SENIOR STUDENT IN THE HOSPITAL DISPENSARY

Above all, they were keen and enthusiastic learners and had established an excellent reputation in Fiji, and were even starting to establish a reputation in regional countries. There was no doubt that MacGregor's experiment in training natives in medical practice had proved a success. But medical science and practice had moved on over this time, and the School needed to catch up with advances in basic sciences, laboratory medicine and clinical skills. This was the challenge of the next phase of the School, when it also became a truly regional institution, as we shall see in part II. But in the meantime, we need to provide the background to the political and medical education developments which affected the School during this early phase of its development.

Chapter 2

Epidemics and Depopulation

As a prelude to understanding the later political developments in Fiji, we need to explain the demographic history of Fiji. On the indigenous Fijian side, the population was affected by epidemics which contributed to a marked demographic decline. As we have seen, both the 1875 measles epidemic and continuing concern by the colonial authorities about the declining Fijian population (as well as the shortage of colonial doctors) were important reasons for establishing the School. On the Indian side, the lower mortality and higher fertility rates along with the high settlement rate of indentured labourers after completing their contracts meant that the Indian population overtook the Fijian population by the Second World War. This would have momentous consequences for Fiji and the School. In this chapter, we examine the issue of epidemics and population dynamics during the early colonial period.

The Scourge of Epidemics

The earliest recorded epidemics in the Pacific Islands occurred in Tonga after Cook's visit in 1773 and in Tahiti after a Spanish visit in 1774-5. One of the earliest descriptions of an epidemic was that of dysentery (bloody diarrhoea) after the explorer Vancouver's visit to Tahiti, from where it spread to Fiji on the ship *Pandora* in 1791-2 with a further terrible outbreak in 1802-3, as described below. Influenza was first recognised in the islands in Tonga between the two Cook voyages of 1773 and 1777, and in Samoa in 1830—introduced ironically by the mission ship *Messenger of Peace*. Samoa also recorded epidemics of whooping cough in 1848 and mumps in 1850.[24]

Venereal diseases may have been present before Europeans arrived, although they are likely to have been transmitted in Tahiti by Bougainville's sailors and in the New Hebrides by sandalwood traders, but syphilis remained uncommon in Fiji due to cross-immunity from yaws, a non-venereal spirochaete infection (Fig 12).

The best contemporary account of the early epidemics in Fiji was by Basil Thomson, who worked in Fiji for a decade as a magistrate in the Native Department, including as a Commissioner of the 1893 report into depopulation of the natives. Although not a doctor, he relied heavily on resident doctors and Fijian oral history as his sources, including Dr Corney, who succeeded McGregor as CMO from 1888 to 1903. Thomson published his book *The Fijians* in 1908, which he described as "a study of the decay of custom in a race that is peculiarly tenacious of its institutions".[25] This is a prescient comment in view of the later issues at the School.

A terrible dysentery epidemic with bloody diarrhoea, dehydration and weight loss was recorded in February 1803 in Fiji, around the time of a total eclipse of the sun, following the arrival of shipwrecked sailors to one of the eastern islands of Lau. The natives called the illness *lila* or the wasting sickness. None of the sailors survived; some dying of the illness, and the rest killed for having brought the pestilence. The sailors were described by Fijians as spirits of the dead and had tobacco ('chew burning sticks') with them. The natives painted their faces and hair with the sailors' gunpowder, and as one stooped over the fire to dry his hair, there was a sudden flash of flame which left him bald.

This dysenteric illness spread rapidly and Banuve, the great chief of Bau, died of the introduced illness. The following poem was written in Fijian about this epidemic:

The great sickness sits aloft,	A lethargy has seized upon the chiefs,
Their voices sound hoarsely,	They fall prone; they fall with the sap still in them.[. . .]
They fall and lie helpless and pitiable,	How terrible is the sickness!
Our god Ndengei is put to shame,	We do not live, we do not die,
Our own sicknesses have been thrust aside,	Our body aches; our heads ache,
The strangling-cord is a noble thing,	The strangling-cord brings death to many, [. . .]
	The spirits run away like running water.[25]

The strangling-cord refers to the traditional custom of strangling the sick.

Influenza and probably other viral respiratory infections with coughing were also introduced around this time, with mortality from secondary bacterial infection (e.g. pneumococcal pneumonia), affecting mostly the young, the aged and those with underlying chronic ailments.[26] Skin diseases were also introduced from other Pacific islands through native passengers on European

Fig. 11: Tinea imbricata rash

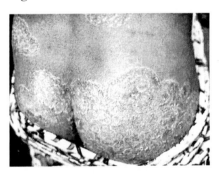

ships, such as the fungal infection Tinea imbricata (desquamans) (Fig 11), which came from Tokelau to Fiji and yaws (Fig 12) which spread from Fiji to neighbouring islands in 1864. Up to a quarter of children in Fiji were affected by the fungal rash, although it had no serious health complications.

Nowadays it responds well to potent new antifungal agents, which were unavailable at that time. Yaws, on the other hand, was also very common, but can lead in the tertiary phase to serious morbidity, similar to syphilis, such as destructive ulcerations of the nasopharynx, palate and nose (*gangosa*), painful skeletal deformities, especially in the legs (saber shins), and other soft-tissue changes (*gummas*).

Fig. 12: Yaws

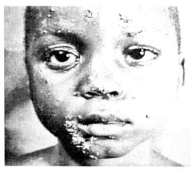

Yaws responds promptly to penicillin treatment nowadays, which only became available after the Second World War. Another non-fatal peeling skin disorder was introduced into Fiji in 1820, termed *vudicoro* (scalded banana), which might have been staphylococcal scalded skin syndrome. This condition is related to a dermal toxin produced by *Staphylococcus aureus* (golden staph), but the clinical description is insufficiently detailed to be sure about the diagnosis, so it might have been another form of cellulitis. It did not take long for islanders to grasp the association between white men and introduced illnesses, responding by killing or expelling missionaries in some cases.

Even after the devastating measles epidemic in 1875, Fiji experienced other epidemics, such as outbreaks of influenza and whooping cough in 1883-4 causing three thousand deaths, and dengue, dysentery and influenza in 1885-6 resulting in 1,500 deaths.[21] Despite frequent epidemics during the early period of European contact, none was as bad as the devastating measles epidemic of 1875 in Fiji, which will be discussed in some detail as it was a key factor in the origin of the School.

The Measles Epidemic, 1875

Measles was first introduced into Oceania by ships going to Sydney in 1834, with later Australian epidemics occurring in 1854, 1860 and the worst in 1867 which caused some 700 deaths. The 1834 epidemic also spread to New Zealand causing a high mortality amongst Maoris. Measles was also transmitted to Hawaii via California in 1848, and later caused devastating 'virgin soil' epidemics in New Caledonia and

New Hebrides with case fatality rates of 20-30%. In 1854 it was also introduced to Tahiti and the Cook Islands by ship.

The devastating 1875 epidemic in Fiji was introduced from Sydney on the ship *HMS Dido*, which continued on after Fiji to spread the virus to Norfolk Island, New Hebrides and Solomon Islands through taking islander labourers from Fiji back home. The missionary ship *Ellengowan* introduced measles to Papua in 1875, but Samoa and Tonga remained free of measles until 1893, when it was introduced from New Zealand. By this time, measles had become endemic in Australia and California, whereas Pacific Island populations were too small to sustain endemic infection.

The measles epidemic of 1875 in Fiji is considered catastrophic, a benchmark of Pacific history.[24,27-29b] Of course, this is not to ignore that the 1918 global pandemic of influenza killed more people worldwide (at least 50 million), and that the pneumonic form of bubonic plague in 14th century Europe had a higher case fatality rate (>90%). But our special interest in this particular epidemic relates to its contribution to the founding of the medical school for natives in Suva ten years later by Dr William MacGregor, as there had been only a few resident medical officers and a visiting ship's surgeon to cope with the epidemic.

Fiji had only recently become a British colony on October 10th 1874, once 'King' Cakobau had obtained the signatures of twelve other paramount chiefs with the assistance of Sir Hercules Robinson, Governor of New South Wales. As part of the celebrations, Robinson invited Cakobau to visit Sydney, so he travelled there by ship from December 1874 to January 1875. At the time, Sydney was experiencing a measles outbreak, and some of the Fijian retinue, including Cakobau himself, were exposed and became ill on the return voyage aboard *HMS Dido*. Although the ship's surgeon placed sick passengers on board ship in isolation, upon arrival in Levuka, the colony's capital at the time, the ship was not placed in quarantine. Great Britain did have quarantine regulations and public health provisions, but Fiji had not yet instituted a quarantine system as its new Governor, Sir Arthur Gordon, and CMO, Dr William MacGregor, had not yet arrived in Fiji.

Clearly, the danger of measles to the Fijian population was not fully appreciated. Measles is a highly contagious virus, and a non-immune population (immunity is lifelong), overcrowded conditions and travel are ideally suited to its spread. It might have been difficult to lock away the recovered King, his two infectious sons and other chiefs on the ship when thousands had gathered to welcome them back in true Fijian tradition. Yet the quarantine failure cannot be attributed to cultural factors alone as two other ships arrived in Levuka from Sydney a few weeks later with active measles cases, which were not quarantined either. The NSW quarantine laws were finally instituted 6 weeks after the start of the epidemic on February 25th 1875.[29] This was truly a case of 'shutting the gate after the horse had bolted'.

Over the next ten days (Jan 12-22), the King met with many of his chiefs, first in Draiba, near Levuka, then on the island of Bau, followed by Navuso on the Rewa River, where he met a crowd of 800 people to explain the implications of the cession of Fiji to Great Britain. Some of Cakobau's retinue and the crew of the *Dido* were still unwell with skin rashes. Thus, the combination of a highly contagious virus, a susceptible population, large numbers of people meeting in crowded conditions and then travelling back to all parts of the country, were all ideal conditions for spread of the infection.

Virtually the entire indigenous Fijian population was exposed and susceptible to measles ('virgin soil' or previously unexposed population), and reports of the time use 'case fatality' and 'population mortality' rates synonymously, implying exposure of virtually the entire population. The epidemic peaked in March-April in most sites and had subsided by May-June. Over these dreadful six months, an estimated 40,000 people died (range of estimates 27-50 thousand), out of an estimated total population of 150,000. This implies a case-fatality rate of 27%, which was consistent with reported death rates in areas where there was reliable data, which documented mean mortality rates of 27-29% of the population, with almost all of the deaths in Fijians.[30]

One can hardly imagine the impact this epidemic must have had on Fijians at the time. Fear, anguish and despair led to superstitious paranoia towards Christianity, missionaries, the white race and the recent cession to Great Britain. The epidemic was seen as punishment for abandoning their traditional way of life. Fiji had of course experienced previous epidemics since contact with Europeans, but nothing like the horror of this measles epidemic. We need to remember that in 1875, the cause of measles was unknown and very few Europeans or other races died from measles due to acquired immunity. Most deaths would have been related to pneumonia, either secondary bacterial pneumonia (*Haemophilus influenzae*, pneumococcus or *Staphylococcus aureus*) or the giant cell viral pneumonia of the measles virus. As with the later influenza epidemic, it may also have been complicated by Acute Respiratory Distress Syndrome (ARDS), but measles is a systemic disease involving multiple systems of the body (Fig 13).

Recently, the demographer Norma McArthur has suggested a lower number of deaths of 27,000, but the consensus is still closer to 36,000 deaths or at least 20% of the population.[21,24,25] Other 'virgin soil' measles epidemics, such as the well documented one in the Faroe Islands in 1846, only resulted in a 2-3% mortality rate, so why was the Fijian epidemic so devastating?

The factors contributing to the high mortality were:

a) the sheer scale of the outbreak affecting almost 150,000 people within 6 months
b) the famine and dysentery accompanying the illness
c) the exceptionally wet weather of the hurricane season that year, and
d) the fact that whole communities were struck at the same time with no one left to care for the sick, procure food and water, or even to bury the dead.

Two further possible contributing factors were:

e) the apathy and despair among the native population due to the large number of deaths, and

f) the worsening of the illness by the traditional practice of lying naked in rivers or pools for hours to cool the fever, which may have contributed to secondary pneumonia, particularly in young children.

Later Outbreaks

Quarantine measures and herd immunity mostly kept measles out of Fiji after 1875 until 1903, when there was another outbreak with two thousand deaths, mostly in young children with no prior exposure. The use of steamships from 1884, which shortened voyage times by half, increased the risk of transmission because there might be time for only 2-3 generations of measles attacks on board before arrival in Fiji.[29] Between 1910 and 1947, there were five more waves of measles epidemics in Fiji, but with low mortality, except for the 'virgin soil' epidemic in Rotuma in 1911 in which 350 died.

In some of the later outbreaks, the virus was introduced from India, since about a third of the 87 voyages to Fiji with indentured labourers between 1879-1916 had measles outbreaks during the voyage. But only eleven of the ships had active cases on arrival requiring quarantine on the island of Nukulau near Suva (which is where George Speight was later imprisoned in 2000). By 1921, Fiji's CMO, Dr Montague, opposed continuing the quarantine for measles because by then measles mortality was low and he wanted to ensure some exposure of the population to measles to avoid a non-immune adult population, since this was still long before a vaccine which was not developed until 1963.

A later measles outbreak occurred in 1936-7, involving 3,500 notified cases, 225 hospitalisations but no deaths. This outbreak was witnessed by David Hoodless of the School who described it as mild in Fijian children, but more severe in adult Polynesian and Micronesian migrant labourers. It lasted for 6 months in Suva but continued for 18 months in other districts.[24,29] Urban cases had a higher rate of hospital admission, which may reflect either access bias or increased severity due to crowded living conditions. There were no measles outbreaks in Fiji during the Second World War despite the presence and transport of many military personnel. However, Papua New Guinea did experience several outbreaks during the war, including Australian soldiers based there. The most recent measles outbreak in Fiji in 2006 with 132 suspected cases was due to poor vaccine coverage, and was controlled by a vaccination campaign.[31]

Measles Epidemiology

When humans replaced hunting and gathering with agriculture, domestication of animals and urbanisation, they also allowed the introduction of new diseases or exacerbation of existing conditions, particularly parasitic and contagious diseases. Measles is unlikely to have affected humans living as nomadic hunter-gatherers, or at least could not have persisted in such small isolated populations. It probably emerged with agriculture and large urban populations after 3000 BC in the fertile crescent, transmitted from domesticated animals since the agents of canine distemper and bovine rinderpest have molecular similarities to the measles virus. Thucydides described an epidemic in 430 BC which killed a quarter of Athenian soldiers, which may well have been measles although another infection is also possible. However, by the third century both measles and smallpox were present in the Mediterranean region.[29] David Morens, a paediatric epidemiologist at the US National Institute of Health in Bethesda has researched the 1875 measles epidemic in Fiji, and eschews the eugenics-inspired view that the isolated and inbred indigenous Fijians had failed to resist measles due to racial degeneration.[32] On the contrary, Morens argues that:

> a plausible explanation for the high mortality in the Fiji measles epidemic was the combined effects of vitamin A deficiency, supervening bacterial pneumonia and diarrheal diseases, and exposure and lack of adequate care in a

population reduced to near starvation by hurricanes and by the explosive epidemic attack, which cut off food gathering.[27]

It has also been suggested that children who died of measles were feeble, so would have died of something else if not of measles. This hypothesis was studied with the introduction of measles vaccination in Guinea-Bissau and showed to be false, at least in that setting.[33]

The author experienced severe measles epidemics as a paediatrician in Masvingo, Zimbabwe and Port Moresby, Papua New Guinea in the early 1980s. In both hospital settings, measles accounted for 7.1% of all paediatric admissions and had hospital case-fatality rates of 39.1% (53 deaths) in Zimbabwe compared to only 11.5% (34 deaths) in PNG.

Fig. 13: Severe Measles (TALC)

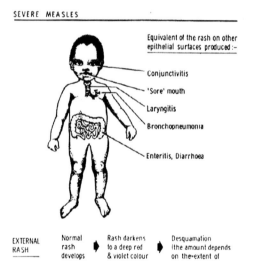

Severe measles was easily recognised by the darkening of the rash, and most early deaths were due to croup or pneumonia with some later deaths related to enteritis, new bacterial infections (due to the immune suppression) or malnutrition (Fig 13). All cases were routinely administered high dose vitamin A on admission, but many severe cases with conjunctivitis in Africa still developed xerophthalmia with blindness. At the local school for the blind in Zimbabwe, over half of the residents attributed their blindness to measles in childhood. Although malnutrition and immune suppression are important late consequences of severe measles in survivors, neither malnutrition nor lowered immunocompetence explains adequately why some children developed severe disease. Although the environmental factors mentioned by Morens were undoubtedly important in the Fiji epidemic, the host factors (e.g. malnutrition, vitamin A deficiency) are less convincing. We now recognise the importance of factors related to the infecting agent, the measles virus itself.

Working in Guinea-Bissau, the Danish epidemiologist, Peter Aaby, found "no association between nutritional status and subsequent risk of dying of measles. Instead, crowding and intensity of exposure were the main determinants of severe measles."[34,35] He differentiated index cases of measles contracted outside of home from secondary cases within the family, showing that the latter had a shorter incubation, more severe disease and a higher mortality. He attributed this to more intensive exposure to the virus from the index case, in other words a higher infecting dose. He also showed that severity was transmissible, so severe cases were more likely to transmit a fatal infection to a secondary case than a mild index case, and also curiously that severity increased when the virus was contracted from the opposite sex. It is also well known that primary measles infections in adults tends to be more severe than in children. Finally, it is now known from research on malaria, bubonic plague and the HIV epidemic that some genetic mutations are important in protecting some individuals from mortality, and so unknown host genetic factors may have also been a factor in survival or death in this measles epidemic. Thus, it seems likely that all of these host, virus and environmental factors combined in Fiji to explain the severity of the epidemic.

Although no higher later mortality in young children was documented after June 1875 in Fiji, the cell-mediated immunosuppression of measles has certainly resulted in increased late deaths from dysentery, malnutrition and other infections after measles epidemics in Africa.[36,37] The author also documented this in the 1984-85 Zimbabwe epidemic after retrospective analysis. Many of the acute deaths in this epidemic were related to severe croup (upper airways obstruction) with a haemorrhagic rash, although this was not documented in the Fiji epidemic.

Another dreadful complication of measles is persistence of the virus in the central nervous system, causing subacute sclerosing pan-encephalitis (SSPE) later in childhood. This has affected many children in Papua New Guinea after measles infection at a young age,[38] but appears to be less common following high mortality epidemics in Africa. In any case, this uniformly fatal chronic degenerative condition would not have been recognised as being measles-related after the 1875 epidemic in Fiji.

Measles and influenza were communicable diseases to which Europeans had already been exposed, recovered from and developed immunity, but natives of the Pacific islands were so-called 'virgin-soil populations'. Consequently, whole communities were affected simultaneously, leaving no one to look after the sick and get food from the subsistence gardens. For debilitating diseases such as measles, this resulted in high death rates, fatalism and social disruption. Evidence from epidemics in 'virgin-soil' populations show that social disruption may be as much a factor as the virulence of the disease on the high mortality.

Quarantine was obviously important for prevention of exposure, as it prevented the influenza epidemic of 1918 in American Samoa. In contrast, influenza resulted in the deaths of up to 20% of the Western Samoan population, where quarantine was not enforced effectively by the New Zealand administration.[39] A British colonial official commented that the general behaviour of the local populations was deplorable, as they not only showed no willingness to help themselves, but refused to help one another. However, this could be re-interpreted as an attempt by the colonial administration to blame native obscurantism and selfishness when the truth was that Western medicine failed to prevent or effectively treat an influenza epidemic in which many Samoans perished in a matter of a few weeks.[40] There are suggestions that this failure of Western medicine may have had adverse consequences for future European-Islander relations.

Thus, epidemics formed a crucial aspect of the history of this period of Pacific Island history, and led to serious reductions of the populations which took many years to recover.

Population Decline

As if the scourge of measles was not enough, the native population of Fiji and some other Pacific Islands continued to decline well after the effect of the epidemic. Demography has played a key role in the history of the region, particularly the decline of indigenous populations following European contact. For example, the official population estimates of the indigenous Fijian population were:

a) 200,000 in 1870;
b) 105,000 in 1891;
c) 87,000 in 1905; and a trough of 84,475 in 1921 (Fig 14).

Although the total population of Fiji did increase from 121,074 to 131,066 between 1903 and 1908, the proportion of indigenous Fijians decreased from 75 to 66% whereas Indians increased from 18 to 25% of the population.[41] By 1931 Fiji had a population of 185,573 of which 50.3% were indigenous Fijians and 41.3% of Indian descent. The birth and death rates were 35.3 and 22.2 per 1,000 for Fijians compared to 33.5 and 10.2 for Indians, demonstrating the impact of disease on the Fijian population. Thus, in contrast to the decline in the native Fijian population, the Indian population of Fiji increased rapidly until it had overtaken the indigenous Fijian population by 1946. These demographic trends were crucial in the subsequent events in Fiji which directly affected the School through political developments such as labour strikes, negotiations for independence and military coups.

The effect of epidemics on population growth is complex. With measles, for example, the effect upon population growth from recurrent epidemics is more marked because children are selectively affected. Although the initial 1975 epidemic affected all age groups, survivors were immune in subsequent epidemics, so only those born after the initial epidemic were susceptible, resulting in a heavy loss of young children before their reproductive age in later outbreaks. When this same pattern involves several diseases, the effect on population growth is obviously more marked. If venereal disease is also widespread, there may be an increase in infertile women, greater tolerance of promiscuity and higher marital breakdown, which affect fertility and further exacerbate the population decline.

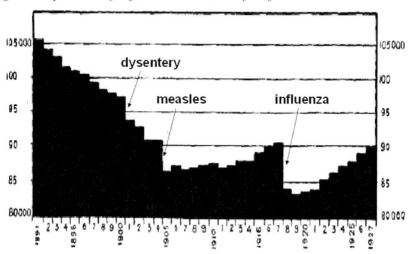

Fig. 14: Population of Fiji, 1891-1927, modified from SM Lambert.[42]

Another reason for the population decline—in addition to epidemic diseases—was the high burden of illness among native villagers. With respect to hospitalisations, for example, admissions to Suva Hospital were steadily increasing with 2,120 in 1911.[19] Provincial reports mentioned many cases of dysentery, typhoid, whooping cough, chickenpox, measles and German measles in 1910-12. There was also a mortality contribution from endemic yaws due to its high prevalence in children. Although hookworm was also highly prevalent, the worm densities were mostly low, so its contribution to mortality was modest among native Fijians.

Tuberculosis, on the other hand, was an important contributor to mortality in the urban setting, accounting for about 5% of admissions in Suva, 3% at provincial hospitals, but only 0.3% at plantation hospitals. In 1915, TB had an overall case-fatality rate in hospitals of 2.1%, although it was higher in Suva Hospital at 5.2%.[20] In addition,

Native Medical Practitioners from the School treated around 260 cases a year with 30 deaths (11.5%), which was a higher mortality because deaths in the community were recorded over a longer time period whereas many of the hospital cases died after discharge. There were, of course, no effective TB drugs at this time since Streptomycin only became available after 1947.

Other causes of illness at the time included an increase in dysentery cases in 1912, accounting for 24% of admissions to Suva Hospital (417 cases), but only 4.5% of provincial hospitals and 1.8% of NMPs' cases.[20] The mortality rate in both central and provincial hospitals was about 9% and for NMPs was 3.6% due to treating less severe cases. According to the annual CMO report of Dr AHB Pearce, the key health issues were leprosy, yaws, bacillary dysentery, typhoid fever, filariasis, tropical ulcer, epidemic dropsy, TB and trachoma. Mass treatment of hookworm had been administered to 28,551 people, so the prevalence of this disease had greatly decreased (see chapter 6).

Notably, there were almost no cases of rheumatic fever recorded at this time, despite it being a notifiable disease. This is striking contrast to recent times, where the highest prevalence in the world have been recorded in the Pacific islands, particularly in Samoa.[43,44] Annual reports also made frequent mention of cyclones destroying crops. Thus, in addition to epidemics, the burden of endemic diseases also contributed to the continuing population decline of indigenous Fijians.

Pre-Contact Populations

The actual pre-contact populations of Pacific islands has been a very controversial topic in the historical demography literature. The early explorers and missionaries often roughly estimated populations at the time of early colonisation as a reflection of pre-contact population of the islands, but these are usually considered inaccurate due to biases such as unknown populations in the interior of larger islands, counting only chiefs, influence of large gatherings and local conflicts keeping some groups invisible. In addition, views were influenced by European guilt at ruining a pristine environment and introducing diseases.[45]

The estimated population of Fiji before cession (and measles) has varied from 100,000 to 300,000, with many estimates based purely on guesswork, but the figure of 150,000 became the 'official estimate' of the population. An early estimate of 130,000 was made by Wilkes, the Commander of the US Exploring Expedition, who spent 3 months in Fiji in 1840. JB Thurston, who later became Governor in 1888, estimated the population in 1868 to be only 100,000-110,000. The missionary John Hunt's estimate of 300,000 in 1844 can be discounted as it was based upon the false assumption of an equally dense population in the interior as on the coast. The missionary Thomas Williams in 1856 modified an 1850 missionary estimate to 150,000, but pointed out that the Fiji population had decreased substantially over the 50 years before the measles epidemic due to both wars and other epidemics, so the actual pre-contact population may have been closer to 200,000. McArthur, a recent historical demographer, contends that the Fiji population before the measles epidemic was about 140,000 with a 20% mortality in the epidemic reducing it to 110,000-112,000.[21] (pp10-11)

McArthur argues that early Pacific explorers had overestimated the populations they encountered at first contact. She estimated, for example, that the pre-contact Tahitian population was only 30,000 on the basis of missionary accounts so concluded that the 'virgin soil' epidemics were not nearly as severe as previously thought.[21] At the other end of the spectrum is the historian of American colonisation, David Stannard, who maintains that historical demographers of the Pacific have seriously underestimated the pre-contact Pacific populations, arguing for a Hawaiian population of 800,000 to 1 million at the time of Cook in 1778 compared to the more orthodox estimates of about 200,000.[46] Some have sought to minimise the impact of European contact ('coloniser's complex') and others to exaggerate it ('white man's burden') for political motives. The true figure is likely to lie somewhere between.

In response to this controversy, the archaeologist Patrick Kirch and historical demographer Jean-Louis Rallu organised an international conference in French Polynesia to discuss Pacific paleo-demography, specifically the issue of the severity of the effects of depopulation in the first few decades following European contact with individual island societies.[47] The methods used by archaeologists include osteological demography, settlement demography, dating curves as proxy models and 'carrying capacity' approaches.[48] These techniques involve indirect and rather unreliable extrapolations of population numbers from:

a) analysis of skeletal remains in burial sites,
b) statistical methods such as use of life tables,
c) proxy measures of human settlements (e.g. 'house-count' method),
d) cumulative records of radiocarbon dates as a reflection of population growth rates,
e) estimation of the resource potential (e.g. food availability) as a measure of the theoretical maximum possible population or 'carrying capacity' of a region.

These are painstaking efforts (both time-consuming and expensive) and the authors readily acknowledge their uncertainty and underlying assumptions. Historical demographers have even developed complex models for Hawaii and French Polynesia starting with first settlement and postulating various population growth rates, from density-independent, exponential growth until stabilisation and thereafter density-dependent regulation of population.[45] There are many unknown factors which affect population growth rates in these models, such as date of settlement, number of initial settlers, onward migrations, natural disasters and wars. Nevertheless, the archaeological evidence appears to give an early indication of a higher pre-contact population than proposed by the classical historical demography of McArthur but less than Stannard's estimates.

The importance of establishing a reliable pre-contact population is, of course, a prerequisite to calculate the severity of depopulation after contact. The impact of certain diseases on mortality rates in a non-immune ('virgin soil') populations has been worked out as approximately: 300 for smallpox, 180 for influenza, 140 for whooping cough and 100 for measles per 1,000 cases, but these death rates will obviously vary according to factors such as ages of affected cases, nutritional status and population density (e.g. overcrowded housing).[45] This measles mortality rate was based upon the 1954 epidemic in Tahiti, but clearly the Fijian mortality rate was at least twice as high (280 per 1,000 or similar to smallpox) for the reasons discussed above. Of course, the long-term impact on a population is greater when child and young adult mortality rates are high than when mortality is mostly in older adults.

Other Pacific islands greatly affected by depopulation of the natives were Hawaii, New Zealand, French Polynesia and New Hebrides (Vanuatu), but it was not a universal phenomenon as Samoa and Tonga were much less affected. Samoa's population, for example, remained fairly stable at 29,300 from 1854 to 1884 despite inter-tribal wars, and then increased slowly despite approximately seven thousand deaths in the 1918-19 influenza epidemic.[49] The estimated Maori population at the time of Cook's visit was about 86,000 and life expectancy 32 years, but the population had fallen to 50,000 by the 1870s and male life expectancy to 25 years (compared to 39 in England and 52 for non-indigenous NZ) and its population continued to decline until before 1900 when it had fallen to only 42,000.[50]

The indigenous population of Fiji did not achieve its pre-measles 1875 population until 1956. In comparison with other Pacific islands, Tahiti's indigenous population was still less than a fifth of its 1774 population estimate of James Cook, whereas Samoa's population had doubled and Tonga's tripled since the 1870s.[21] This difference in Samoa and Tonga has been attributed to a smaller European settler population, fewer visits by European ships due to remoteness, maintenance of traditional customs and rejection of adverse European influences. The reasons for the depopulation of other Pacific islands with European contact and colonisation have been analysed extensively at the time, as well as by later social scientists and historians, as discussed below.

Perspectives on Depopulation at the Time

The colonial administration was genuinely concerned about the population decline in native Fijians, so appointed a Commission in 1896 to investigate the causes (Table 2). The most obvious factor had clearly been the measles epidemic in 1875 which killed around a quarter of the population. Dr Corney, who was one of the commissioners of the report, attributed the continuing population decline to outbreaks of disease: enteric fever (typhoid), influenza, dysentery and dengue fever.[51] There was substantial evidence to support the importance of the high burden of epidemic and endemic diseases contributing to the population decline in the native population, as discussed above. However, this was a rather biomedical model, which would be disputed by later commentators.

In an address to the chiefs at Kadavu in 1885, William McGregor is quoted as saying that "the people are dying from these causes:—First, bad houses; second, insufficient food; third, uncleanness of towns and bad water; fourth, neglect of women, children, and the sick."[52] In his 1900 Lancet paper, MacGregor stressed water quality and identified dysentery as the main culprit for depopulation, writing that

> the man who will work out an effective and practical means of dealing with contagious dysentery will be the greatest benefactor of the races that live in the tropics. He may claim to be the saviour of the Pacific Islander . . .[53]

However, the 1883 Commission on Depopulation in Fiji took a different view. The Commission believed that there had been a pre-European contact population decline in Fiji due to unremitting warfare, cannibalism, abortion, infanticide, superstition, taboos, unhygienic living conditions, epidemics and 'racial decline'. This latter term implied a degree of moral condemnation of heathen practices, perhaps to lessen the blame of destructive European contact. However, the Commission did not deny that there had been depopulation with European contact, but attributed it to:

a) changed ways of life and thought
b) psychological inertia and despair (fatalism), and
c) what they termed 'physical weakness'.

There was obviously an element of laying blame on the victims. As discussed below, implications of 'racial degeneracy' were strongly criticised by later writers. The Commission grouped the causes of depopulation into the following four groups:

Table 2: 1883 Commission on Depopulation Report. [54]

Predisposing causes tending to the degeneracy of the people as a race.

    i.   Polygamy.
    ii.   Consanguineous marriage.
    iii.   Epidemic diseases.
    v.   Communal system, with attendant customs of *lala* (tribute and service to chiefs and communities), *kerekere* (mutual appropriation of property), *bose* (councils) and *solevu* (festivals).
    viii.   Want of virility.

Causes more immediately affecting the Welfare and Stamina of the People individually.

    x.   Quality and supply of food and drinking water.
    xvi.   Abuse of *yaqona* [kava] and tobacco.
    xviii.   Treatment of sick persons. xix. Irregularity of living.

Causes more immediately affecting the unborn child.

xxiv. Work during pregnancy.

xxv. Fishing by child-bearing women.

Causes affecting the infant.

xxv.　Domestic dirt.

xxxvi. General insouciance of the native mind, heedlessness of mothers, and weakness of maternal instinct.

The Commission report even used the example of medical students at Suva Medical School to illustrate the psychological causes, since Corney had observed some of his students relapsing into apathy and inactivity, some of whom had to have their certificates withdrawn, which was attributed to 'flaws in the native character'. The missionary John F Goldie of the Solomon Islands Methodist church stated that:

> One of the saddest things in this sad land is the rapidly decreasing population. Men talk of the survival of the fittest, and the fate of the black man is to go down before the white man. But *is* this necessary? What is the cause of this racial decay? What can be done to arrest the decline? Of the many theories advanced, none seem to fit all of the facts . . . One thing is certain. The advent of the white man, though a contributing cause, is not the principal cause of the decline, which has been going on for years. Going into a heathen village for the first time, seeing the filthy condition of the people, the wonder is not that they decrease, but that they are not extinct.[55]

With the benefit of hindsight, what is striking about the Commission's report is its emphasis on tenuous links between mortality and factors of communal life, native customs and temperament. The report also downplayed the importance of introduced diseases. Perhaps since the document was intended as a charter for intervention, the Commissioners were paving the way for administrative intervention in the communal life of the indigenous population, as has been suggested by Thomas.[55]

Australian views on depopulation were no doubt influenced by the prevailing view of Aborigines, that they were 'a doomed race' which was destined to disappear.[56] This was not just the view of uneducated settlers, but of a noted anthropologist, Spencer Baldwin, in his 1913 report on the Aborigines of the Northern Territory as well as Darwinian evolutionists who claimed that the natural law of survival of the fittest destined Aborigines to extinction. However, rather than acknowledging the deleterious effect of European contact on Aborigines, Baldwin blamed 'Asiatic vices' (opium, whisky and prostitution) for the potent degenerate influence on them and downplayed European misdeeds. His response to prevent extinction of Aborigines was an authoritarian paternalism to protect them from contact with Chinese, stringently control their reproductive activity, remove children from their parents and make education compulsory. With respect to the native populations of the Pacific, Europeans at the time generally accepted the view of the inevitable decline of an inferior race with the advance of civilisation.

> A missionary's view of the situation in the Solomon Islands was probably typical of much opinion in the 1890s as well as the time of its writing: The author hesitates to single out any particular cause and is reluctant to accept the idea that a weaker race should or would necessarily die out, but is unable to categorically reject the sort of racial thinking upon which such a view is based.[55]

On the part of European settlers in Fiji, however, there was undoubtedly an element of vested interest and wishful thinking as they wanted native land.

Anthropology Perspectives

In his 1922 book on Melanesian depopulation, the anthropologist William Rivers adopted a more rigorous scientific approach to the issue.[52] He rejected as unproven the Commission's assertion that depopulation antedated European contact and was related to inherent faults in native culture and heathen practices such as inbreeding, polygamy and head-hunting. Since there was no evidence of deliberate attempts at extermination, as had occurred elsewhere, he considered that depopulation had not occurred by design.

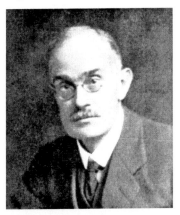

Fig. 15: WHR Rivers [57]

He also gave prominence to psychological factors as a cause of depopulation. Firstly, he examined the causes of increased mortality, of which the main culprit was introduced disease, particularly measles, influenza, dysentery and TB. He also recognised a second group of introduced causes of health risk in alcohol, tobacco and opium. A third direct cause of an increase in the death rate was the introduction of fire-arms, which transformed traditional warfare into a more lethal exercise. In terms of European influence on native customs, Rivers blamed the missionaries for the adoption of European clothing as a contributor to improper hygiene and skin infections, and enclosed housing for worsening TB propagation compared to the open traditional houses. But his main concern was the erosion of traditional cultural traditions, pointing out that:

> ... interest in life is the primary factor in the welfare of a people. The new diseases and poisons, the innovations in clothing, housing and feeding, are only immediate causes of mortality. It is the loss of interest in life underlying these

more obvious causes which give them their potency for evil and allows them to work such ravages upon life and health.[52]

Rivers argued that factors affecting the birth rate were as important as those affecting mortality, attributing the reduced fertility rate to a loss of interest in life or apathy. He used the example of the abolition of head-hunting in Solomon Islands, citing natives as questioning why they should bring children into the world if it was only to work for the white man. He suggests, somewhat implausibly, that instead of banning it outright, it might have been possible to substitute a pig's head and maintain the cultural significance. His proposed solution of the problem was for natives to renew old interests and create new interests. On one hand, natives need to be given a stake in the economic development of their country and, on the other hand, Europeans needed to better understand the indigenous perspective, according to Rivers. However, it is unclear just how much the mutual misunderstanding between Europeans and natives was contributing to native malaise and apathy.

Another key factor affecting fertility was the labour trade which took young men away from home instead of marrying and having children. Rivers stated that:

> It would be difficult to exaggerate the evil influence of the process by which the natives of Melanesia were taken to Australia and elsewhere to labour for the white man. It forms one of the blackest of civilisation's crimes. Not least among its evils was the manner of its ending, when large numbers of people who had learnt by many years' experience to adapt themselves to civilised ways were, in the process of so-called repatriation, thrust back into savagery without help of any kind. The misery thus caused and the resulting disaffection not only underlie most of the open troubles in the recent history of Melanesia, but by the production of a state of helplessness and hopelessness have contributed as much as any other factors to the decline of the population.[52] (p105)

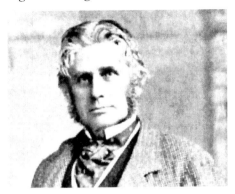

Fig. 16: George Pitt-Rivers [58]

The anthropologist and psychologist George Pitt-Rivers, published a book on depopulation in 1927 after five years of study.[59] He attacked many of the prevalent prejudices of the times, arguing that the aim of scientific inquiry was to trace the immutable laws of nature, however unpalatable they appear. He was adamant that missionaries were bound to destroy the traditional cultures of 'heathen and savage peoples' by imposing an incompatible culture, which was inevitably assisting the extermination of those they profess to protect. His demographic analysis led him to place great emphasis on gender distribution, with the following so-called 'laws of nature':

1. Disturbances in the sex ratio of reproductive adults greatly influence the population dynamics, with a progressive excess of males correlated with population decline.
2. Increasing populations tend to have a surplus of adult females of reproductive age over adult males.
3. With polygamy, polyandry inhibits reproduction, whereas polygyny (men with many wives) promotes population increase.
4. Miscegenation correlates with variations in the balance of the sexes.
5. The offspring of interbreeding possess greater adaptability to change, but are less adaptable to the traditional culture.[59] (p15)

Like Rivers before him, he attacked the view that the population decline was related to native culture, attributing this view somewhat unfairly to Sir Hubert Murray, Lieutenant Governor of Papua from 1907 to 1920, who had stated in a report that certain tribes with repugnant habits such as child marriage should be allowed to become extinct as their cultural practices were inconsistent with long-term survival. In Pitt-Rivers' view, the rapid change in the life of natives under European influence was the cause of depopulation, inducing general discontent and apathy. He stated that the colonisers had replaced wooden spears, native canoes and *tapa* cloth with muskets, Mother Hubbard dresses, boats and kerosene lamps, which had led to apathy and disorientation due to the destruction of native warfare, polygamy, the communal system, sorcery and the authority of chiefs.[59] Consequently, he called for more sympathetic studies of native customs and ideas, and to teach the native population to be proud of positive features of their culture.

In another book on the topic in 1927, Stephen Roberts of the University of Melbourne criticised the prevailing anthropological view that all natives were the same, based on the assumption that primitive societies had little inherent organisational structures.[49] He stated that:

> the problem is to deal with a mind very complex, reacting in a different manner from our own to any given set of conditions, always liable to relapse into uncontrolled barbarism, and limited even under ordinary conditions by an emotional waywardness so unbalanced as to defy discipline.[49] (p139)

From his demographic analysis, he concluded that overall for the total population of the Pacific Islands in 1927, 35% of the islands' populations were increasing, 39.3% were stationary, 25.5% were decreasing and only 0.16% faced extinction.[49]

In terms of remedies for depopulation, Roberts proposed that since depopulation was due primarily to psychological factors, the remedy should focus upon the effect of the transition from old to new traditions on the native mind.[49] He gave numerous examples of mysterious behaviour which was incomprehensible from a Western individualistic perspective because it involved concepts of collective responsibility and superstitious beliefs. For example, a district official in inland Fiji, recounted the story of an old woman who kissed the magistrate's feet, which by traditional custom obliged acceptance of her petition for her son, who was nevertheless found guilty, to the incredulity of both the woman and the provincial chief (*Roko*).[60] Another anecdote illustrates the peculiar attitude of the native towards medical treatment, when a native who was cured after many months of care by a practitioner, who—when refused the request of a musket for allowing himself to be cured—burned down the practitioner's drying-house. This was a cultural misunderstanding, as the surgeon's cutting creates a blood debt in traditional societies, including in Aboriginal culture.[61] (p103)

Consequently, one of Roberts' solutions was that:

> Education is rightly emphasised as perhaps the most important method of regenerating the native, for it will do much to dispel those mists of misinterpretation which arise from native ignorance. The drift of the native, and the consequent attitude of despair towards the problems of life, come largely from the fact that the native finds himself enmeshed in a net of change, the magnitude of which appals him, and the nature of which he cannot in the slightest understand ... Education is the force which transmutes the native life from darkness to understanding, and which makes him a consciously purposive force instead of a passive obstacle dragged along against his own volition.[49] (p189)

The key issue was the appropriate kind of education for the native peoples. The prevailing model of Western religious education had undermined their belief in their own culture, encouraged rote memory at the expense of wise judgement, and alienated them from their traditional way of life. Consequently, Roberts called for a new form of native education, linked to his traditions and what is useful in his life. This meant a change to vocational education, with agricultural subjects for boys and domestic science for girls in order to teach natives the value of work which benefits them and their society instead of the white man.

In order to reverse the personal and cultural apathy and despair of native populations, Roberts proposed a three-pronged approach involving governance, education and economics. For governance, he proposed modified indirect rule or government by the natives and in their interests, but still under close European supervision, not unlike what Gordon had tried to institute in Fiji. Secondly, for education, he sanctioned vocational training, and thirdly, for economics, he encouraged peasant-proprietorship on co-operative lines. With a better understanding of the native culture by Europeans and gradual accommodation by the natives to their changing conditions, Roberts felt that the outlook would change and these three groups of reforms, along with good colonial administration, would help solve the native population problem.[49]

A related issue discussed by Roberts was miscegenation, pointing out that the prevailing prejudices against it were unjustified from a scientific perspective. He asserted that race-mixture, whether for good or for evil, is 'one of the most important transforming agencies at work in the Pacific'.[49] New Zealand, Tahiti and Hawaii had been much more successful than Fiji in the integration of the races. In Hawaii, for example, in 1925 there were 21,145 pure race Hawaiians, 13,837 Caucasian-Hawaiians and 8,345 Asian-Hawaiians. But miscegenation had occurred there in rather different circumstances than Fiji in that the total European population in Hawaii was 65,396 compared to 128,068 Japanese, 49,335 Filipinos and 24,335 Chinese out of a total population of 323,645. Yet, for whatever reasons, the lack of intermarriage between Fijians and Indians in Fiji was an important aspect of Fiji's evolution.

Before finishing with anthropological perspectives, it is worth touching briefly on a more modern perspective on the Pacific, which relates to sexual behaviour rather than population. The true nature of traditional societies in the Pacific Islands has been a subject of considerable controversy in anthropology, as illustrated by the widely divergent views of Samoa by Margaret Mead and Derek Freeman.[62] In her classic 1928 book on *Coming of Age in Samoa,* Mead suggested that casual premarital sex was accepted and encouraged as natural pleasurable adolescent activity in contrast to the transitional difficulties of American teenagers.[63] Not only were these observations based upon inadequate and misleading fieldwork without any knowledge of the language, but they were also prejudiced by romanticised European views of Polynesia as a sexual and environmental paradise ('free love without guilt . . . under the swaying palms' as Albert Wendt put it).[64] The NZ anthropologist Derek Freeman published his critique of Mead in 1983 after forty years of meticulous research and a profound knowledge of the *fa'a samoa*, pointing out that Samoan society was not sexually permissive and most of Mead's other assertions about the Samoan way of life were also erroneous.[65] This myth of a paradise of sexual freedom amongst noble savages has been prominent in European views of the region in folklore, novels, cinema and even anthropology.

Public Health Perspectives

Dr (later Sir) Raphael Cilento, an Australian public health administrator, entered the depopulation debate in 1923 and again in 1928, mostly from data and experience in New Guinea.[66] He strongly disagreed with the view that miscegenation was needed to reinvigorate threatened native populations, contending that depopulation was a direct result of the high burden of disease, particularly malaria in Melanesia. This was meticulously documented in his studies of the Western Islands of the Bismarck Archipelago, where malaria had recently been introduced by travellers from the mainland, who infected the endemic anopheles mosquitoes which had not previously been infected in these remote islands. Due to the poor soil on atolls, he noted that they had resorted to growing 'swamp taro' (*fula*) as their staple crop in sunken gardens, which provided a breeding ground for the *Anopheles punctilatus* mosquito which is an efficient malaria vector in the Pacific. Not only did this reliance lead to nutritional deficiencies, but the breeding of mosquitoes also exacerbated filariasis (which can be transmitted in the Pacific by at least 22 species, including *Anopheles*, *Aides* and *Culex*,[67]) Additionally, the dense smoke of smudge fires to repel the mosquitoes would have exacerbated the high rate of respiratory diseases from passive smoking.

Cilento did not deny the responsibility of Europeans for depopulation through both introduced diseases and destruction of the native way of life. Although he acknowledged the psychological causes of depopulation, he attributed the native hopelessness and apathy to sickness rather than to disruption of native customs, since he alleged that healthier disrupted communities did not show apathy and reduced fertility. In his assessment, the main factors contributing to depopulation were:

a) introduced diseases
b) environmental factors
c) poor nutrition, and
d) abortion and infanticide.

On this basis, his recommendations for remedying population decline included:

1) improved medical services for natives by European Medical Assistants (since he opposed Native Medical Practitioners)
2) regular health checks
3) universal twice-weekly quinine prophylaxis
4) provision of bednets
5) mass hookworm treatment
6) improved water and sanitation
7) supply of implements for agriculture and fishing, and
8) assisting natives to market their produce fairly.

We encounter Cilento later in the story due to his refusal to send New Guinea students to the School in Suva (see chapter 8).

In 1949, Fiji's CMO McGusty, presented a paper at the Seventh Pacific Science Congress on the decline and recovery of the Fijian race, presenting it as a 'clash of civilisations' with the more primitive in danger of extinction.[68] He estimated the Fijian population to have been 250,000 before Western contact and its lowest point in 1919 was 83,000. In his view:

> the outstanding lessons from Fiji are centred in the endowment from the earliest Colonial days of its people with practical responsibility in the management of their own affairs and in the fact that, because the ancient form of their society was not entirely destroyed in the clash of civilisations, it is possible to form a mental reconstruction of its main features and from this to obtain a realistic picture of how ancient man existed.[68] (p61)

RF Scragg was the Director of Public Health in the Territory of Papua and New Guinea, and he carried out a study in 1957 on the causes of depopulation in New Ireland. He attributed the population decline to reduced fertility from venereal diseases, mainly gonorrhoea, and to increased mortality from malaria.[69] Finally, the epidemiologist Richard Taylor and colleagues found considerable uncertainty as well as variability in the pattern of mortality in Pacific Island states. Life expectancy, for example, ranged from 55 to 75 years between countries, with markedly higher rates of adult mortality in some countries, particularly for males, despite relatively low levels of child mortality.[70]

Contemporary Perspectives

Fig. 17: Thomas Nicholas [71]

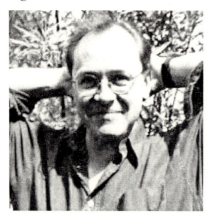

Professor Nicholas, Director of the Museum of Archaeology and Anthropology in Cambridge, has argued that the depopulation issue was a central concern of the colonial administration and facilitated the exercise of state power in colonial Fiji, particularly through regulations to improve hygiene, water supply and sanitation.[55] The fear of native assimilation, westernisation and moral degeneracy from imposing European culture (the worst features of white-native contact) was a factor in the emphasis upon preserving village life and chiefly authority in order to preserve the native race. But the lack of a specific cause of depopulation in the 1883 Commission report allowed the state to impose European bourgeois values on village life in the name of hygienic measures to reverse depopulation. Thus, many of the perceived shortcomings of Fijian hygiene were used to justify regulations which did little more than bring Fijian practice into a degree of conformity with European values. Thus, in spite of paying lip service to the preservation of the Fijian way of life, there was a good deal of cultural colonialism. In terms of the Indian population, Thomas points out that:

> Indentured labour and the paternalistic insulation of native society from the market were, in terms of the colony's socioeconomic structure, two sides of the same coin; hence the 'logic' of the shocking gulf between the violent punishment in plantations and coolie lines, and the indirect and paternalistic discipline in the villages over which Gordon's net of state power was just being cast.[55]

How successful was this repressive reordering of village social life in the name of hygiene? In spite of these native regulations having legal sanction, Fijian resistance took the form of evasion rather than confrontation, making enforcement difficult and frustrating the colonial administration. Nicholas argues that the underlying rationale of the regulations was to impose state control rather than change hygiene behaviour, but at least it gave the appearance of a tangible government in rural Fiji.

Recent opinion has also tended to view indigenous populations as far more resilient and adaptive than previously thought. The newer social science attempts to explain the demographic and epidemiologic patterns in terms of 'social organization, patterns of European contact, and social and economic change.'[39] It has tended to deny any biologic determinism about the impact of European contact on native populations, acknowledging the widespread population decline, but pointing out the differences in the responses of virgin-soil populations to newly introduced diseases due to social forces. On the other hand, recent social science has also tended to shy away from social determinism, such as the view that Western scientific medicine was largely irrelevant to mortality declines. Although controversy remains about the relative contributions of economic development versus health services in improving health, at the time of early colonisation it was improvements in living standards which were more important.

Stephen Kunitz of New York has made the bold statement that the major determinant of differences in contemporary health between colonised peoples in Africa, Asia, Oceania, and the Americas was the different ways in which governments have dealt with indigenous peoples.[39] He acknowledges that the colonial experience for Europeans in Africa was very different from Oceania due to the diseases in the former making it a so-called 'white man's grave', so their different disease ecologies had a profound impact on the Europeans and on the consequences of European colonization for the native peoples. That aside, however, he argues that the health consequences of differing colonial policies were particularly visible. The impact of disease on population is shaped by the context in which it occurs, as in Samoa compared to Fiji for epidemics.

Fig. 18: Prof Stephen Kunitz [72]

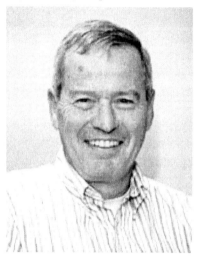

Two other key factors, in Kunitz's view, were the needs of labour and land. Where only land was needed, as in the Australian Aboriginal context, the native population was isolated on reservations and missions. Where only labour was needed, as in Samoa, a colonial system developed with a planter class and indigenous people continuing to live and work in their own villages. Finally, when both labour and land were necessary, as in Hawaii, the natives were integrated into the lowest social class of an emerging capitalist society. What about Fiji? Although he does not mention Fiji as an example, it was the benign attitudes of Gordon and the Colonial Office towards the native population at the time which led to the importation of indentured labour from India and a degree of protection of Fijian land from settler encroachment, which has had equally important ramifications, confirming once again the importance of labour and land, as discussed in chapter 5.

From his comparative study of colonised indigenous populations in Canada, Australia, NZ, America and Polynesia, Kunitz argues that neither biological, social, nor economic theories alone can adequately explain the evolution of population and mortality over the past 200 years. He concludes that:

1. diseases are shaped by the contexts in which they occur
2. in the 20th century, preventive and curative interventions *have* had a definite impact on the health status of populations, and

3. the health consequences of social change are mediated by economic factors, cultural values and social organisation.[39] (p177)

Indian Demographic Dominance

For the period of Indian migration to Fiji between 1879-1919, Ralph Shlomowitz of Flinders University has drawn the following conclusions about the infant mortality rates:

1) the age-specific mortality rates during the voyage and indenture showed high infant death rates, consistent with a life expectancy of 30 years at birth
2) infant mortality rates on the sea voyage were double the rates on land in Fiji (50 *vs* 21 per 1,000 per month from 1887-1916)
3) the stillbirth rate was also high at 99 per 1,000 live births
4) infant mortality rates of 241 per 1,000 showed no decline between 1880-1910
5) infant mortality rates had plummeted to 122 per 1,000 by 1918, mostly due to fewer post-neonatal deaths (between 28-364 days of age), and
6) unexpectedly, there was no excess male infant mortality compared to females, suggesting gender bias in the level of maternal care.[73]

Although the sea-borne infant mortality of Indian indentured labourers was almost twice that of European migrants of the same period, the land-based infant mortality once they were settled was initially similar between Fiji and India (280 per 1,000), both higher than in Australia (120 per 1,000), but by 1910 it had dropped below India. Thus, from the infant mortality perspective, Indo-Fijians were better off in Fiji than in India by 1910, although only for about a decade. The main reasons for this drop in mortality were improvements in domestic hygiene, water supply, sanitation and infant feeding which reduced the mortality from diarrhoeal disease and malnutrition. The contribution of medical care in this reduction was negligible. It was not until the 1930s or later, when the importance of dehydration was better understood and managed that curative services could have affected child mortality from diarrhoeal disease, other than by improved domestic hygiene.

Figure 19 is a graph of the annual population growth rates for Fijians and Indians in the decades prior to 1936, 1946 and 1956, illustrating the higher population growth rates for Indians. Registration of births and deaths was introduced in 1877 in Fiji. Population growth is a function of both fertility and mortality. Indian fertility rates were about 30% higher than indigenous Fijians due to younger age of marriage and greater frequency of births at all ages. By 1956, half of the Indian population was under 15 years of age compared to only 42% for indigenous Fijians, so the Indian population also had a higher reproductive capacity. The infant mortality rates (per 1,000 live births) in 1946 were 81.5 for Fijian males and 70.9 for females, compared to 50.5 for Indian males and 43.6 for females. But a decade later, the Fijian rates had dropped to 49.4 (males) and 44.9 (females), which had narrowed the gap with the Indian infant mortality rates of 47.1 for males and 39.0 for females.

Fig. 19: Annual Population Growth Rates (%) by Decade for Fijians and Indians in Fiji, 1927-56

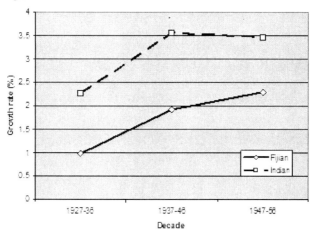

By the 1946 census, the rate of population growth of Fiji had increased to 2.6% per annum, which was up from the 1.56% increase per annum in the 1936 census. But the rate of increase was not uniform between the two main ethnic groups, since the native Fijian population rose by 20.9% compared to 41.7% for the Indians in Fiji. Consequently, Indians had become the dominant ethnic group at 46.5% of the total population compared to 45.5% for indigenous Fijians. In addition, 84% of the Indian population had been born in Fiji and considered it their home. An Australian demographer who analysed the 1946 census in detail at the time, pointed out that if existing trends continued, the numerical ascendancy of the immigrant Indians would be ensured, which was already causing a current of deep anxiety for the future running throughout the Colony.[74] Native Fijians were losing the population race due to later marriages, smaller families and higher mortality rates.

In addition to numerical dominance, the Indians were also gaining economic ascendency, displacing Europeans in the control of agriculture, trade and commerce. By 1946, there were only 4,593 Europeans and 6,142 part-Europeans in Fiji. The number of native Fijians in paid employment was 4,442 which was only about 4% of the total indigenous population. The estimated average income of independent Fijian market-gardeners was about £6 per annum and for copra-growers was £14 per annum, which compared unfavourably to £94 per annum for Indian contractors growing sugar cane on leased land.[74] Two other features brought out by the census were the increased mobility and urbanisation of indigenous Fijians. For example, on census night in 1946 nearly 22% of Fijians were enumerated as being away from their villages, compared to only 5.25% in 1921. Between 1936 and 1946, the population density of Suva suburbs had increased some 1.7-fold.[74]

In conclusion, the aetiology and consequences of epidemics and depopulation on the native population of Fiji have generated great controversy over the last 130 years. With the benefit of hindsight, there is little doubt that it was European contact and the resulting epidemics of disease which were the major contributors to depopulation. Measles, influenza and dysentery were the key epidemic diseases, for which there were no effective treatments. Although of secondary importance, there is little doubt that both the high mortality of epidemics and the cultural dislocation of colonisation also had psychological effects on the native population, which may have contributed to lower fertility.

Quarantine was a potentially effective preventive measure against epidemics, but there were notable failures of its application which allowed some of the worst outbreaks (e.g. measles in 1875 and influenza in 1918). In addition, endemic diseases such as yaws, typhoid, diarrhoea and pneumonia were also important contributors to mortality. Although Native Medical Practitioners did play an important role during the influenza pandemic of 1918, it was really only with the emergence of effective treatments for yaws and hookworm that the NMPs reputation was enhanced over traditional medicine and sorcery.

In terms of fertility, Indian women had a higher rate than Fijians due to the younger age of marriages. The higher population growth rate of the Indian population causing them to overtake the Fijian population by 1946 was a harbinger of future problems for Fiji and the School.

Chapter 3

Colonialism with a Human Face

Sir Arthur Gordon

Fig. 20: Sir Arthur Gordon

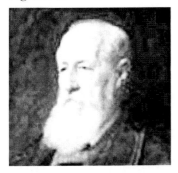

Britain had annexed the Fiji Islands on October 10, 1874 at the request of King Cakobau, so it is referred to as 'the cession of Fiji'. Cakobau's motives for requesting to become a British colony were largely related to paying off an American debt—which, incidentally, was clearly unfair[75]—and rivalry with Ma'afu, the Tongan chief in Lau. Britain's traditional reluctance for further colonial expansion at the time was overcome by humanitarian and missionary pressures. British public opinion was incensed by descriptions of 'blackbirding' in Oceania, so humanitarian, anti-slavery and Christian mission organisations joined forces in urging British acquisition of Fiji as a means of ending these labour practices.

In order to understand the background to the establishment of the School, we need to understand the change in British colonial policy towards the native population and the character of one of its chief architects. Fiji's first Colonial Governor, Sir Arthur Gordon, sought to avoid the consequences of conflict, landlessness and poverty associated with colonisation elsewhere, so he instituted policies intended to preserve Fijian land, labour and traditional lifestyle from exploitation by white settlers. When Gordon arrived in Fiji as its first governor in 1875, shortly after the measles epidemic, he had to face the problems of labour shortage, land and revenue, as the Colonial Office expected the colony to be cost neutral. This meant that revenue generation to pay for his administration was dependent upon labour supply.

These were not unfamiliar issues to Gordon, as in his previous posts as Governor of Trinidad and of Mauritius, indentured labourers, called 'coolies', had been recruited from the British Colony of India. His previous experience made him acutely aware of the danger of exploitation of labourers by European settlers. In 1870, for example, there had been a Royal Commission into the poor treatment of Indians in British Guiana, largely due to concerns of Gordon's friend William Des Voeux, who was a magistrate there when Gordon was Governor of Trinidad and who replaced him in 1880 as Governor of Fiji. Later, shocked by planter callousness and police brutality as Governor of Mauritius, Gordon himself ordered a Royal Commission into labour conditions which resulted in legislation to protect Indian labourers.

Gordon was responsible for recruiting Dr William MacGregor to Fiji as his Chief Medical Officer (CMO). Although both were Scots, Gordon was the converse of MacGregor. He was born into privilege as the youngest son of the Earl of Aberdeen, educated at Trinity College, Cambridge, and he had entered Parliament in 1854 as a Liberal. When his father had been Prime Minister, he had been his private secretary and then became private secretary to Gladstone in 1858, so he was extremely well connected in Britain and could have had a distinguished career there if he had not chosen to serve in the Colonial Service. He was greatly interested in history, including primitive societies and social institutions, so he viewed native Fijian society, somewhat condescendingly as 'guinea pigs' for experimentation. Thus, Gordon is often described as a very capable administrator, aristocratic, lacking in humour but not lacking in vanity.

Here is how he was described by his private secretary in Fiji:

> A short man, dark, not good-looking, careless of appearance, short-sighted... Nowhere has he been popular since he has a very bad manner with strangers, and he is perfectly aware of it and regrets it much. He is very determined, and puts aside all opposition when his mind is made up, but with people with whom he is in sympathy, though agreeing, he is perfectly open to discussion... He is a high Churchman with strong religious opinions which he does not air. He professes to be a thorough liberal, but his aristocratic leanings come out insensibly. He is very proud of his family and descent. He is very large-minded, and in some things almost an enthusiast. Well-read, particularly in history in some curiously odd subjects. Very fond of nature and scenery... Active, a good walker, utterly careless of what he eats and drinks—or rather, I don't believe he knows what he eats or drinks.[76,77]

Due to his contacts in the Colonial Office, Gordon was able to stipulate most of his subordinate officers, many of whom later also became colonial governors. In addition to MacGregor, there was Captain Arthur Havelock, Charles Mitchell, George Ruthven Le Hunte and John Thurston, who was already in Fiji as acting Colonial Secretary. Gordon's most urgent initial challenge was finance, so he designed a native taxation scheme with the help of Thurston, which required Fijians to work in their village plantations as a communal 'in kind' contribution as opposed to working for wages on European plantations for revenue to pay their taxes. This encouraged them to produce and sell excess agricultural produce, for which they needed to be ensured sufficient land, so Gordon also developed a land policy to curtail excessive land claims by European settlers. Needless to say, this was very unpopular with traders and planters, but was popular with the chiefs and highly successful in raising revenue for Gordon's administration, collecting almost £20,000 in 1879 which was as much as customs revenue.[78]

After revenue and labour issues, Gordon's other major task was to develop a native policy. He firmly believed that he possessed an instinctive understanding of natives, but the true nature of this understanding has been questioned.[79,80] The historian, Ian Heath, has acknowledged Gordon's key contribution to the concepts of indirect rule, but has argued for a re-interpretation of his role in Fiji:

> In many ways the main failing of Gordon's administration was his success at preventing rapid change . . . He believed that 'the more the native polity is retained, native agency employed, and changes avoided until naturally and spontaneously called for', the less likely was the Fijian to 'perish from off the face of the earth'. He undoubtedly felt that the integration of native society would be upset by imposed change and sought to avoid this consequence. What he failed to understand was that his system was too easily institutionalized, and **change therefore became impossible or at least difficult to achieve**.[79] (p87, my emphasis—also my experience, see chapter 15)

Under pressure from humanitarian and missionary groups in Britain, the Colonial Office had made some concessions to prevent exploitation of native labour by settlers in their colonies. It is clear from his correspondence that Gordon had a genuine desire to protect native Fijians and their culture from destruction. With the support of MacGregor and Thurston, Gordon paid great attention to the views of Fijian chiefs, despite strong opposition from both settlers and missionaries. Perhaps his most important innovation was the establishment of a Great Council of Chiefs as a kind of 'native parliament'. The Colonial Office wished at all costs to avoid a repeat of the Maori wars in the New Zealand colony, so they supported Gordon's native policy of self-government by chiefs, as it promised less conflict with the native population.[78]

Gordon's experience as governor of New Zealand and Fiji convinced him that a self-governing colony would not treat the indigenous population fairly, which is why he opposed Queensland's ambitions to govern New Guinea. He felt that settlers in Fiji, Australia and NZ had showed a crass and inhumane attitude to the native populations, and so was intolerant of their opposition to his native policies. He expressed his views on Queensland's proposed annexation of New Guinea in 1883 to the Colonial Office in the following terms:

> I have heard men of culture and refinement, of the greatest kindness and humanity to their fellow whites ... talk, not only of wholesale butchery, ... but of the individual murder of natives, exactly as they would of a day's sport, or of having to kill some troublesome animal. This is not the spirit in which to undertake the government of native races. ... I should still more earnestly protest against its [New Guinea] being placed under the control of the government of Queensland, than which I can hardly conceive any government more unfit for such a task.[78] (p295)

Another important component of the native policy, with the support of the chiefs, was 'industrial schools' to educate the native population while maintaining acceptable native customs, which of course did not include cannibalism, infanticide or the sale of wives.

Throughout his time as Governor of Fiji, Gordon carried out a regular correspondence with the British Prime Minister Gladstone. His letters demonstrate very well his sincere humanitarian instincts and his competence as a colonial administrator.[76] But he was also given a very free reign by the Colonial Office due to his high connections, operating as a benevolent dictator—the proverbial philosopher-king of Plato. He saw his role as protecting the natives' interests against those of rapacious white settlers and traders, introducing the system of indirect rule in which the tribal chiefs were involved in governing, so as to preserve the traditional village structure and native institutions.

The key planks of Gordon's native policy were a separate code of laws and a system of communal taxation in produce, rather than money.

Shortly after arriving in Fiji, he wrote to Gladstone about his initial impressions:

> The white planters are not as a body by any means such *mauvais sujets* as they have been represented to be, though there are among them, heaven knows, as foul and abominable scoundrels as defile this earth, and their general tone on all subjects connected with the natives is one which to you at home would be unintelligible. The natives themselves I like very much. I was by no means prepared to find them either so intelligent or so civilized. They nearly all read and write and are very great scribes, always writing letters to one another. Two things have struck me especially as shewing that they are a good way from barbarism, the high position of women, and their respect for agricultural labour. [. . .] I have the very greatest objection to the not unindustrious native population of these islands being forced from their own homes & cultivation to cultivate for others. But this is in fact what the planters demand.[76] (p67)

With the hope of extending this protection to a wider region, he persuaded the British government to appoint a high commissioner for the Western Pacific, a position to which he was then appointed as High Commissioner under the Colonial Office and Consul-General under the Foreign Office in order to enhance his position in Fiji. The Western Pacific High Commission was eventually established in 1878, and was designed to give Britain control of British subjects in those islands not already governed by a civilised power, and to enforce the Pacific Islanders Protection Act of 1872 which was designed to stop Britons from kidnapping islanders to work on plantations in Fiji and Queensland. But without any naval backup for the position, Gordon was unable to protect other Pacific islands from European adventurers.

Indirect Rule

There were two unsuccessful models of native administration in the Pacific which Britain wanted to avoid in Fiji. The first was the traditional British *laissez-faire* model which had allowed unscrupulous European settlers to exploit natives, capitalising on their lack of administrative experience for the new ways of governance once their traditional cultural structures had been abrogated, and leading to gunboat diplomacy when European interests were threatened. The other unsuccessful model was direct rule, adopted by France until about 1910, which was also highly destructive of native customs. These failures of the British theory of native independence and the French system of direct rule led to a new British policy of indirect rule, which was applied to Fiji by Gordon. It aimed to build upon native traditions through education and using native institutions to allow them to control their own destiny as much as possible. It meant that colonial administrations should act in the interest of native populations so both natives and colonials would benefit, rather than exploiting natives for their labour and imposing European models of administration.

The key proponents of this new idea were Sir Arthur Gordon in Fiji, Sir William MacGregor, when he moved on to New Guinea, and Sir William Lugard in Nigeria. MacGregor, for example, argued for looking at issues from a native perspective by putting 'natives first' and helping them to develop for themselves. This went as far as using jailed murderers as native constables on their release, since natives who could carry out a successful murder and escape the wrath of the injured kinsmen had the qualities needed to make them a respected member of society, and jail gave them unparalleled exposure to European civilisation. MacGregor attempted to maintain the desirable features of traditional native society, including the authority of the chiefs. In Gordon's case, his aristocratic background fitted in well with the principle of indirect rule in Fiji, since governing a subject people in their own interests meant through the chiefs (aristocracy). He protected Fijians from exploitation by the plantation system, labour market, and loss of their land to European settlers. Needless to say, this made his administration very unpopular with settlers who were struggling with low commodity prices, labour shortages and renewed competition from America in cotton production.

His administration was equally unpopular with missionaries, who objected to the retention of the traditional chiefly system, which destroyed individual freedom and incentive. Missionaries also opposed the so-called 'Polynesian' labour traffic or blackbirding, which they saw as akin to slavery, with humanitarian organisations such as the Anti-Slavery Society, the Aborigines' Protection Society and Christian missions raising public awareness about exploitation of natives. Although Gordon was not unsympathetic to these views, he needed labour for the colony to prosper so never actually abolished 'blackbirding' which only ended once the sugar industry stopped employing islanders because they were less productive than indentured Indian labour. So economics dominated ideology.

Thus, the essence of Gordon's native policy was: indirect rule through Fijian chiefs, entrenchment of native rights to the land, protection of the indigenous population from exploitation by labour recruiters, and promotion of native cash cropping through tax payments in kind. His policy also had to provide political stability so as to attract foreign investment and promote economic prosperity.[81]

At the heart of this new British colonial policy of indirect rule was a paradox. Gordon had to reconcile the preservation of the Fijian communal system with absolute state control by the colonial power. During his first address to the Council of Chiefs, for example, he explained his wish to retain good native customs, while also making clear his administration's power over them. His successor, Governor Thurston (1888-1897) continued his policies, but his benevolent administration was more intrusive, even at times repressive, perhaps revealing something about the nature of colonial power.[82] For twenty-three years after cession, Thurston exerted enormous influence in Fiji as Colonial Secretary, Administrator, Lieutenant-Governor; and then full Governor.[83] During those years, he followed a consistent policy of governing according to Fijian aspirations as expressed in regular councils of chiefs. This participation of natives in the administration was also a means of stimulating new interests to allay their apathy, which was seen as a contributing factor to depopulation.

Indirect rule was generally received favourably by Fijians because it recognised Fijian interests as paramount and precluded transformation of Fijian village society, and it has also been reviewed favourably by expatriate historians because of their politically conservative views, according to Thomas.[55]

Perspectives on Colonialism

The colonial history of Fiji and the Pacific Islands was very different from the nationalist struggles of African nations, so much of the academic literature on colonialism is not directly relevant. Frantz Fanon's *Les Damnés de la Terre* (The Wretched of the Earth),[84] for example, examined the relationship between violence and nationalism largely from the war of liberation in Algeria, but his decolonizing paradigm does not take into account the considerable variations in cultural and political circumstances in colonial experiences. Fiji was ceded to a reluctant British Empire and was handed back to the indigenous Fijians without any violence or even much political activism. Perhaps this was why Fanon's third phase of decolonisation—a new unified national identity—never evolved in Fiji as part of independence, because the ethnic issues between the two main racial groups were never resolved.

Michelle Keown argues in her book on *Postcolonial Pacific Writing*[62] that Fanon's three decolonising phases still occurred in the Pacific in the development of national cultures through writers such as Albert Wendt in Samoa, Alistair Campbell in Tonga and Keri Hulme in New Zealand. The first phase was the passive assimilation of the culture of the coloniser, which was followed by an artistic phase when the writers are finding their own voice, followed by the third 'fighting phase' which awakened the people to a new post-colonial order. She illustrates these phases by allegories from these NZ-Polynesian authors, who are all of mixed race. However, none of her examples includes Fijian writers because there is no such revolutionary literature in Fiji. Indeed, Fiji's public intellectuals have largely been Indo-Fijian, like Brij Lal and Satendra Nandam, with the possible exception of Ratu Joni Madraiwiwi, the former Vice-President.

However, other contemporary commentators have not been so generous to Gordon's 'indirect rule' policy in Fiji. Here is what Robertson says about it:

> Despite the laudable humanitarian principles used by the British to justify the incorporation of Fiji within their extensive Empire, these counted for little in the final analysis. First and foremost, Britain wanted the colony to pay its own way. Its decision not to employ Fijians in the canefields had less to do with missionary concerns at the exploitation of indigenous labour than with the pressing need to establish a stable environment for the operation of colonial capital. After all Fijians vastly outnumbered Europeans. And the recruitment of Fijian labour could have only one effect: the destabilization of Fijian society and attendant political, possibly military, repercussions.[85] (p7)

Many are sceptical of the view that this strategy was one of benevolence, a strategy which 'saved' the Fijians and ensured the survival of the Fijian 'way of life'.

'Atu Bain, a USP sociologist, has also questioned the official ideology of benevolent protectionism instituted by Gordon and Thurston, particularly "the sweeping generalisations about the privileged condition of indigenous Fijians under British colonialism."[86] He contends that the colonial policies in apparent conflict with settler interests were only intended to ensure the viability of subsistence agriculture in the villages and prevent the "growth of a class of Fijians divorced from tribal associations and dependent for their livelihood on the economic conditions of the labour market." He continues that "in many respects, indentured Fijians were subjected to a scale of oppression comparable with that of their Melanesian and Indian counterparts."[86] Thus, the ideology of state protectionism masked an array of legislative measures which ably defended the interests of plantation capital. Fijian labour laws were progressively liberalised through the late 19th and early 20th centuries in order to meet the expanding needs of European planters.

The Pacific historian, Annie Stuart, also describes this favourable attitude of British colonialism as profoundly paternalistic:

> Colonial views of the time believed in an Anglo-Saxon mission to civilise the dark races, which was tied with views of racial and cultural superiority. Thus, the factors at play were the new advances in western medicine, the commercial advantages and the new sense of moral responsibility for indigenous populations which had become the 'white man's burden', an expression first used by Rudyard Kipling, these gave impetus to renewed efforts in public health and medicine in the British tropical colonies, including in the Pacific.[12]

These conflicting perspectives make it difficult to understand the true implications of colonial rule on the story of the School, which is our present task. Stuart has proposed the postcolonial cultural concept of 'hybridity' to understand relationship of colonised and colonisers. This refers to the 'cultural collisions' of colonisation leading to formations of new identities as cultural categories converge.[87] The Western scientific medicine taught at the School, which was originally assumed to have purely humanitarian motives, has been reinterpreted by cultural theory as a technique for extending control over subject populations to ensure their labour productivity, which also implied a need for reversing depopulation.

One analytical approach, political economy, suggested that the colonial state was largely responsible for indigenous ill-health by entrenching unequal access to power and resources in the interests of expatriate investors and settlers, whose demand for labour also determined subsequent uneven treatment policies designed to return populations to a functioning level. In addition, cultural imperialism analysts discerned the steady imposition of western biomedical knowledge, diffusing from imperial centres and replacing local understandings of health, disease, and indigenous practice, as 'modern' medical services contributed to the purposeful restructuring of colonised societies. However, whatever their utility in re-examining triumphalist narratives of scientific medicine, both analytical models have their shortcomings, with their tendency to represent western culture as homogenising and western medicine as monolithic.[87]

Speaking of 'triumphalist narratives of scientific medicine', it is worth pointing out that such 'grand narratives' by medically-qualified historians and others have gone out of fashion in the contemporary climate of postmodernist relativism. Our narrative in this book avoids heroic bombast, and is only one version of many historical perspectives.

Of course, the early NMPs were a good example of cultural 'hybrids' as intermediaries in the 'programme for civilised modernity'. Later, with the role of the Rockefeller Foundation in the Central Medical School, we see a complex interaction between American philanthropy, British imperialism, settler interests and also an emerging Australian nationalism, manifested both as a desire to promote its own interests in its backyard without meddling American business interests, and as the 'white Australia' immigration policy (see chapter 8).

Gordon's labour policy was necessary for his experiment in protecting the native Fijians from exploitation of their labour.

Gordon's biographer argues that he could not have foreseen either the consequences of Indians remaining in Fiji and becoming the majority despite Fijians owning the land, nor the persistence of Fijian semi-feudal society much longer than anticipated. Nevertheless, he contends that Gordon's native policy was still "eminently more successful than the alternatives would have been." [78] (p219) There can be little doubt that without men of the calibre of Gordon and MacGregor in the Fiji colonial administration and without their sympathy and interest in the native population, it is doubtful whether the medical school in Suva would ever have been established. So we should acknowledge that both indirect rule and native practitioners were innovative concepts emanating from a new form of colonialism with a human face, but which also held indigenous Fijians back educationally and commercially by delaying their liberation from an archaic feudal social system.

Chapter 4

The Empirical Tradition

In order to better understand the story of the medical school for natives in Suva which commenced in 1885, we need to appreciate the differences in medical education, practice and knowledge from the present day. In this chapter, we give the background of medical education in 19th century Britain so as to understand the kind of medicine which was taught at the Suva Medical School in Fiji by colonial doctors who had trained in Scotland and England.

British philosophy at the time was dominated by the empiricism of David Hume and John Locke, which also had a strong influence upon scientific and medical thinking—which we have called the empirical tradition in this chapter, meaning that medicine was based upon experience and observation.

Physicians, Surgeons and Apothecaries

By the beginning of the 19th century in Britain, there were three distinct kinds of medical practitioners; physicians, surgeons, and apothecaries. Physicians had the longest tradition and were the most respected and privileged group. They were university educated in the classics, and their medical activities were confined to offering advice, for which they did not charge a fee as such, but expected reimbursement of expenses and gifts in gratitude for their advice. Incidentally, in contemporary usage, a physician means a specialist in internal medicine or paediatrics in the UK and Australia (e.g. Royal College of Physicians), whereas in north America it is a generic term for doctors. We use it in the former sense only in this book.

Surgery, on the other hand, was seen as work beneath the dignity of gentlemen and was forbidden to clerics due to the mediaeval rule against them shedding blood. It was an apprenticed craft which treated patients by the operation of the surgeon's hands. Surgery had only ended its association with barbers in 1745 and the Royal College of Surgeons in London was created by charter in 1800.

The third group was the apothecaries, who were originally retail druggists who sold their concoctions in shops, so were considered of lower social status then either physicians or surgeons. By this time, apothecaries had become the equivalent of general practitioners, particularly in combination with surgeons. In order to function in this role, theoretically they should have had diplomas from both the Society of Apothecaries and the College of Surgeons, but most had no formal qualifications at all. They depended for a living on the sale of drugs, so were seen as tradesmen, but extended their practice to prescribing and dispensing their own medications, which tended to lead to over-prescribing.[88]

In terms of their educational pathways, a physician's education in the 19th century was very different from today, aiming primarily to produce a cultured and highly educated gentleman. Culture and education in those days meant scholarship in the classics in Latin and Greek. The degree of Bachelor of Medicine at Cambridge, for example, required residence for nine terms or about five years, but students only had to witness two dissections and keep one 'Act and Opponency'. This refers to the mediaeval disputation, which was an archaic form of examination by disputation and opposition from medieval times, which had more to do with debating skills than an assessment of the medical knowledge of the candidate.

Thus, an adequate knowledge of medicine was entirely secondary to a physicians training, with no clear medical curriculum and many physicians having only one year of medical training after completing their long general university education. Of course, the amount of medical knowledge needed to work at that time was small, mostly involving the writing of complicated prescriptions of largely ineffective herbal remedies. The examination for the Licence of the Royal College was not demanding in medical knowledge and students usually prepared themselves for the exam by attending a London hospital to listen to lectures and 'walk the wards'.

Surgical education, on the other hand, was highly practical with little pretention about being a learned profession, so there was no need for a university education. Although surgeons, like physicians, tended to be the sons of clergyman, doctors, and other professions, they also included the less privileged who were seeking higher social status through medical practice. Since there were almost no anaesthetics, speed and manual dexterity were essential skills for the successful surgeon at this time. However, surgery was largely relegated to conditions visible externally, since the internal parts of the body were inaccessible to the knife due to the risk of fatal infection in the peritoneal, thoracic or cranial cavities. Although surgeons had detailed knowledge about the anatomy of hernias, for example, they could still not repair them, although they could drain hydrocoeles using a cannula. Another difference from physicians was that their training and membership of the Royal College of Surgeons were much less expensive.[89]

Apothecaries tended to come from the lower class of shopkeepers and other lower middle-class groups, but might also include the youngest or wayward sons of curators or village schoolteachers. Like surgeons, their education was entirely practical, but required a detailed knowledge of botany and chemistry. Apothecaries were expected to avoid infringing on the domain of the more learned physicians. Since he was basically a shopkeeper, his method of training was also mainly by apprenticeship. Although by the 1850s apprenticeships for apothecaries were disappearing, medical students still continued to be licensed to practice without the need for a university degree, although by the 1890s, they had to pass examinations in Greek, Latin, English and mathematics before commencing their non-university medical studies.

Medical Education in England

The main reasons why medical students in England did not attend university to study medicine at this time were the constraints of religion, time and cost of attending Oxford or Cambridge. University education was denied to Roman Catholics and Jews since only members of the Church in England could graduate, and religious tests were not abolished until 1871. Other constraints were the cost and length of courses, since Oxford, Cambridge and Dublin required medical students to spend up to seven years for a Bachelor's degree, and an additional four years before obtaining a medical degree. Although students did not have to spend all this time in residence, it still took eleven years before students could practice as physicians. Moreover, Oxford and Cambridge only graduated a small number of doctors a year and Latin remained the language of final examinations at universities until the 1830s in Britain.[90]

By the 1840s, there was a surplus of medical practitioners in England, with a rate of about 107 per 100,000 population, which was twice the density of France at the time, so there was fierce competition between doctors, apothecaries and non-professional medical practitioners. Although the number of medical practitioners per 100,000 population had dropped to 66 by the 1880s, many medical practitioners still struggled to make a living.[91] These figures compare to about 50 for Fiji and 250 for Australia at present (Fig 2). But incomes varied enormously, from the successful London physician earning up to £10,000 a year, those in provincial towns on £1,000 a year, and surgeon-apothecaries on £400 per year. Overseas options for medical practitioners included the North American colonies, the East India Company and the army or navy, but there was still a significant risk of illness in tropical settings. The rank of physicians in the army was higher than surgeons with twice the rate of pay, with even a novice physician was given seniority over an experienced surgeon despite treating similar patients and conditions.[92]

Apprenticeships in medicine often started at a young age, sometimes at 13-14 years of age. Many medical students (excluding university-trained physicians) had completed their training by 21-22 years of age. Perhaps related to their youth was the reputation of medical students for rowdiness, indecency and callousness.[90] They were often described as lowly-bred, with drinking, smoking and brawling very common in the dissecting room. In those days, of course, there were no women medical students to moderate their behaviour. But to be fair, their vulgarity reflected the coarseness of the society at the time, including the teachers themselves. Another factor contributing to their poor public image was the practice of 'body-snatching' from graves and mortuaries due to the great shortage of cadavers for anatomy dissection.[89,90]

The training of medical practitioners for rural settings required a different training programme, as it was recognised that rural practice paid too little to attract men who had undergone an expensive university education. Rural medical practitioners were generally considered to be second-class doctors, similar to the Native Medical Practitioners of Fiji. In England, it was often the unqualified surgeon-apothecaries who tended to practise in a rural setting, although not exclusively.

Medical Education in Europe

Human dissections were a key component of training. They had originated in Bologna in the 14th century, although the first medical school in Europe at Salerno in Italy (1096-1270) had used pigs for dissection and anatomical teaching since the previous century.[93] The medical course at Salerno lasted five years with an additional apprenticeship year, and was the first time medical graduates were called 'doctors'.[94] Montpellier was the second European medical school, established in 1181, and attached to the cathedral. Its scholastic medicine was based upon Greek and Roman theoretical teachings, modified by Christian theology and supplemented by apprenticeship and practical experience. As all university-trained physicians were clerics, who were forbidden to shed blood, surgery was relegated to craftsmen or barbers.

The French medical profession had been reorganised after the Revolution, and the best medical education was provided by the *coles de Santé* of Paris, Montpellier, and Strasbourg. In order to attract rural doctors, the positions of *officiers de santé* and *médecins de deuxieme classe* were created requiring a 3-5 year apprenticeship of practical training. Germany also developed an equivalent *Landarzt* or *Routiniers* for rural practice, and Russia trained *feldshers* to treat the peasants.[95] But by the 1850s, there was a strong campaign to eliminate these second-class medical practitioners, who were seen as socially inferior to university graduates, although they still constituted a significant proportion of medical practitioners in rural settings. By 1893 in France, for example, the position of *officiers de santé* had been abolished.[91]

The London Hospitals

Medical education was still very unstructured in Britain in the early 19th century. Other than the tiny minority of elite university-educated doctors with the MB degree, most medical practitioners served an apprenticeship with an apothecary or a surgeon for a variable period of time followed by collegiate licensing. Most sought a dual license (MRCS/LSA or MRCS/LRCP) after hospital apprenticeship training. Glanville Corney, who ran the Suva Medical School and was CMO in Fiji until 1907, had followed such an apprenticeship and licensing programme.

The London St Thomas's Hospital started some sort of teaching in 1695 and St Bartholomew's (Barts) started an anatomical and surgical museum in 1726, and lectures and dissections for anatomy commenced in 1734. By 1893, Barts taught 53 subjects to 498 students with a staff of 41.[96] At the London Hospital, students were enrolled from 1782 and the physicians and surgeons were allowed by the hospital Governors to build a suitable classroom for teaching purposes at the east end of the hospital, so by 1785 the London hospital was the first complete school of medicine and surgery in London.

In 1828, the University College Hospital in London was opened as the first non-sectarian university in England which could give degrees to those debarred by the religious tests at Oxford and Cambridge. By 1858, there were medical schools at a dozen London hospitals, and students went about attending lectures and 'walking the wards' at the various London hospitals. Besides the London hospital medical schools, by 1858 there were another dozen or so provincial schools in England which did not grant degrees, but prepared medical students for licenses from the College of Surgeons, Society of Apothecaries, and for medical practice with the armed services.[89]

Conditions at public hospitals were often appalling in the early 19th century with overcrowding, poor hygiene and inadequate facilities resulting in a mortality rate of 25% at the 1,200 bed *Hotel Dieu* in Paris and a 10% mortality rate in most English hospitals. Infant mortality rates were even higher at foundling hospitals for orphans, as safe alternatives to breastfeeding did not exist. It was George Newman, a public health doctor in London before the First World War who first documented the importance of good mothering and breastfeeding on child mortality from diarrhoeal disease.[97]

But it was not just overcrowding at hospitals which increased mortality, as overcrowded urban housing was also a major contributing factor to high mortality. For example, in Glasgow in 1901, families with four rooms had mean mortality rates of 11.2 per thousand compared to 32.7 for those living in a single room.[97] Such data is of course confounded by socio-economic status, as underlying poverty was a major contributor to high mortality rates. But the rapid growth of towns and cities had resulted in very high population densities in urban slums.

It was the development of the technique of eliciting and interpreting physical signs which attracted students to the London hospital schools (as well as to Paris) where there were many patients with good physical signs. Between 1805 and 1820, there were about a thousand new students a year in London studying anatomy and requiring bodies for dissection. The only legal sources of bodies were executed criminals and purchased bodies from relatives. The resulting shortage of bodies for anatomy dissection was the origin of body-snatching. This even resulted in criminals murdering individuals in order to sell their bodies to medical schools. Consequently, the Warburton Act regulated supply of bodies to the medical schools in London, increasing the supply from legitimate sources, which finally put an end to the practice of body-snatching.[89]

Scottish Medical Education

Compared to England where medical education was largely based at hospitals, in Scotland it was in the hands of the universities, which established an excellent reputation for medical education. As mentioned, William MacGregor, who founded the Suva Medical School, was a Scottish university graduate. His medical course took four years and he attended classes in anatomy, surgery, *materia medica*, pharmacy, the theory and practice of medicine, clinical medicine, midwifery, chemistry, and botany courses consisting predominantly of lectures (Table 3).

Table 3: Scottish Curriculum for a Medical Degree. Report of the Commissioners of the Universities and Colleges of Scotland, 1830. (Adapted from Rosner,[92] p175)

1st Year	2nd Year	3rd Year	4th Year
Anatomy	Anatomy	Surgery	Practice of Medicine
Chemistry	Practice of Medicine	Midwifery	Infirmary
Materia Medica	Theory of Medicine	Clinical Surgery or Medicine	Clinical Medicine
Practical Chemistry	Clinical Medicine	Hospital Attendance	Clinical Surgery or Medicine
Practical Pharmacy	Hospital Attendance	Practical Anatomy	Botany

In 1858, the Universities (Scotland) Act instituted the four year Bachelor of Medicine / Master of Surgery degree, which was increased to five years in 1889.[98] This move towards university education for the majority of doctors was led by the Scottish universities in Edinburgh, Glasgow, Aberdeen and St Andrews.

Edinburgh dominated medical education in Scotland from its establishment as a medical school in 1726 until the mid-Victorian period, with 2,200 students attending medical classes by the 1820s, but the pass rate was only around 10-15%. Its distinction as a centre of medical education was attributed to its openness to outside influences, particularly from continental Europe. Glasgow became more prominent around the time that William MacGregor attended medical school, when the city's population had increased to over 200,000 and there were 1,500 students enrolled in medical classes. Aberdeen was considered a second-rate medical school, but improved just before MacGregor was a student there (and later in Glasgow, graduating in 1872). Scotland also had a strong scientific surgical tradition, possibly due to the influence of John Hunter (after whom the new hospital was named in Newcastle, Australia) and Joseph Lister in Glasgow.[98]

Regulation of Medical Practitioners

The state in Britain played little role in regulating medical practice in the early 19th century, adopting a *laissez-faire* attitude to non-professional healers and charlatans. This was in marked contrast to France, where the French Revolution had led to much more state regulation of medical practice.[91] This created in Britain a competitive medical market-place where patients could seek advice from professionals, folk healers, itinerant cure-all peddlers, magicians and other 'quacks'. It is undoubtedly this competition in the marketplace which forced the fusion of surgeons and apothecaries into general practitioners.[99] By the early 19th century, it was the surgeon-apothecaries who formed the majority of medical practitioners in Britain. Although these divisions between physicians, surgeons and apothecaries ultimately broke down, the class distinctions between them persisted.

It was the threat of quackery and exploitation which finally led to government regulation of medical practice in Britain. An initial bill in 1806 had specified minimal ages and periods of study for physicians, surgeons and apothecaries, making it possible for the public to know who was properly qualified. The 1834 select committee on medical education acknowledged the need for some form of 'inferior doctor' to provide medical services in rural districts as well as in the colonies, particularly for preventive medicine. But it was not until 1858 that the British Parliament passed the Medical Act to regulate the qualifications of practitioners in medicine and surgery, establishing a general council of medical education and registration (GMC) which consisted of members chosen by each of the licensing bodies, including colleges and universities. This Act established the principle of the profession's self-regulation and established an official register of practitioners. However, it did not abolish unlicensed practice. A separate role for pharmacists (apothecaries) was established by the formation of the Pharmaceutical Society of Great Britain and the Pharmacy Act of 1868.[89]

The new General Medical Council's (GMC) priorities were to improve the general educational level of students entering medicine, encourage university training and ensure that graduates were of good moral character. The GMC recommended that examinations for entry into the profession should include the compulsory subjects of English language, arithmetic, geometry, and Latin, but gave a lower priority to scientific subjects such as chemistry, physics and biology initially. However by 1867 the GMC included the following subjects as essential to the curriculum: anatomy, general anatomy, physiology, chemistry, *materia medica*, practical pharmacy, medicine, surgery, midwifery and forensic medicine. These were also the subjects taught to native practitioners in Fiji, albeit it at a much more rudimentary level. Two years later, the GMC added physics, chemistry, practical chemistry, medical chemistry and botany to the list of essential subjects.[89] Later, the GMC and Royal College of Physicians insisted on registration of students to ensure attendance at lectures and student discipline.[96]

It was not until 1859 that a woman was allowed to practice medicine in Britain. She and the later pioneers encountered enormous resistance to allowing women into medicine, since nursing was seen as the most appropriate role for women. The medical profession was genuinely concerned about exposing women to the horrors and immodesty of medical practice due to the strong Victorian view that the study of anatomy and dissection of the body would destroy the special sensitivities of women. At a more prosaic level, there was also concern about the indecent and vulgar behaviour of both students and teachers during lectures and anatomy dissection. It was America which led the way in integrating women into medicine, establishing four medical colleges for women between 1850-70. By 1876, all restrictions on the registration of women as medical practitioners had been removed in Britain. This finally opened the medical profession to applicants of both sexes, although it would take another hundred years for them to be more equally represented at medical schools.[89,90]

British Empiricism

The approach to medicine in Britain until about 1880 was empirical, from the philosophical tradition of British thinkers such as John Locke and David Hume who argued that knowledge should be based upon observations and experience rather than reason or intuition. In medical education, the new empirical tradition implied an emphasis on anatomical and clinical observations, including evidence from post-mortems and surgery. William Cullen (1710-90) at Edinburgh, for example, had divided medicine into three pillars; namely, physiology, pathology and therapeutics. His nosological classification was based on the patient's symptoms and pathology from post-mortem examinations. It was holistic rather than based upon organ systems or aetiology, since causes of disease were largely unknown at the time.

Therapeutics was also very limited, with reliance on the Hippocratic armamentarium of cathartics, emetics, sudorifics (to induce sweating), antipyretics and bloodletting. More recent medications included digitalis (foxglove), quinine (Peruvian bark), guaiacum for syphilis, ipecac to induce vomiting, various other herbal remedies and the metals arsenic, mercury and antimony. Dietary advice was also important for correcting perceived imbalances, including citrus fruits for treating scurvy.[88]

Other than treatment, there were two important differences in medical practice in the early 19th century; namely, the lack of physical examination of the patient and a complete absence of any clinical investigations, either laboratory or radiological. It is surprising how physical examination was ignored in the early 19th century. Of course, in Victorian culture it would have not been deemed appropriate, in most circumstances, for a male doctor to infringe upon the modesty of women of higher social status, but this barrier also seemed to apply to the lower classes.

The principal method of teaching was by lecture and the art of lecturing had been perfected in the middle ages. In addition to attending lectures, students 'walked the wards'. This expression amounted to little more than looking at the cases from the end of the bed and listening to the remarks of the medical attendant. The clinical teacher informed the students of the daily progress of each patient at the bedside, but without any teaching of physical signs. Physical signs were hardly mentioned in medical textbooks of the period with the exception of the face, tongue, and pulse and possibly comments on the appearance of blood, urine and faeces. Doctors did not generally perform a thorough physical examination of patients, although they might take careful histories and look at the facies and the tongue, feel the pulse, observed the appearance of excretions. Thus, medicine at this time was essentially based upon the consideration of symptoms and the application of a complex pharmacopoeia, mostly of dubious efficacy.

There were also remnants of 'humoralism', which was the medical tradition which considered illness to be the result of a disturbance in the natural balance of the humours within the body.[100] Humoralism had a long tradition in Greek philosophy and Western medicine commencing with Hippocrates of Cos (*c*.450-370 BC) and Galen of Pergamum (c.129-200 AD) who consolidated the theory of the four humours of blood, phlegm, yellow and black bile in the heart, head, liver and spleen, respectively. These humours varied with the four seasons, but illness reflected imbalances between them, such as 'plethora' from too much blood, which was treated by blood-letting.[95]

The four humours were also analogous to the four environments (hot, cold, dry, wet) and four elements in Greek philosophy (earth, air, fire and water). But Galen and Hippocrates believed that illness was the result of imbalances within the body, so treatment involved restoring the balance by eliminating poisons through sweating, urinating, defecating, vomiting, bleeding and other practices which punished the body. Ancient medicine had depended heavily upon mystical explanations of disease, linked to magic, divinations, dietary protocols and codes of behaviour. Hippocratic medicine taught that disease was a natural event, not caused by supernatural forces. Such views had dominated medicine for almost two thousand years.

Persian philosophers and physicians, including Rhazes (865-925) and Avicenna (980-1037) also contributed to medical theory, with Rhazes the first to differentiate measles from smallpox.[97] There was also a theory of how the environment caused epidemics and disease through miasma or polluting agents in the air, often with foul odours such as stagnant marshes, decaying materials, excreta, etc. This was further developed by Thomas Sydenham (1624-1689) into the effects of environmental factors, such as the atmosphere, humoral imbalances and the seasons on disease.

Clinical Examination

The introduction of the stethoscope, microscope and medical laboratory as medical tools was met with considerable resistance by traditionalists, who defended the empirical art of bedside clinical medicine against threatening scientific advances. The Scottish medical schools were more open to continental innovations than in England, where there was much greater resistance at the London hospitals which remained more traditional.[96,98]

There was a similar resistance to specialisation in medicine, with 'generalism' seen as a gentlemanly ideal. Nevertheless, specialist hospitals did emerge in the larger cities, including hospitals for children and ophthalmology departments within hospitals, and specialist services were introduced into teaching hospitals in the competition for students. This in turn led to a more academic model of medical education and scientific practice of medicine with greater use of the laboratory under German (Virchow, Koch) and American (Osler) influence.[96] Sir William Osler (1849-1919), a Canadian physician who was Professor of Medicine at Johns Hopkins and later the Regius Professor of Medicine at Oxford, laid the foundation for modern clinical diagnosis through analysis of the patient's symptoms, signs and laboratory investigations.[101,102]

In the early 19th century, the French had led the way in medical education with the Paris School of clinical medicine by inventing the new science of physical signs which developed into clinical medicine. This occurred in France because of scientific advances and the excellent clinical experience of students in the Paris hospitals. Yet medical teaching in France still involved lectures in the hospital amphitheatre with little actual bedside teaching due to the large number of students who flocked to Paris from all over Europe and America. This was also true of Britain, but the lack of clinical contact by medical students was more related to resistance by hospitals and protection of patient privacy. Student feedback was consistently that there was too much lecturing and not enough bedside teaching and experience.[90]

The hallmark of hospital medicine in France was the integration of medicine and surgery with an emphasis on pathology, physical diagnosis and clinico-pathological correlation, leading to advances in clinical diagnosis through careful observation, classification and analysis despite a lack of knowledge about the aetiology of diseases.[88] This led to the use of inspection, palpation, percussion and auscultation on hospital patients, although there was still a certain reluctance to undress private patients.

According to the renown medical historian, Bynum, the four key features of French hospital medicine were:

1) bedside diagnosis from the patient's background history
2) signs and symptoms with lesions confirmed by pathological anatomy
3) clinical judgement from observation and interpretation of clinical signs (inspection, palpation, percussion, auscultation), and
4) symptoms, and expression of medical information quantitatively.[88]

The most important innovation in physical examination was the stethoscope developed by René Laënnec (1781-1826) whose book on auscultation was published in 1819. It took some time before the stethoscope was adopted in England and still longer before auscultation sounds were correlated with morbid anatomy findings in patients, but it did mark a revolutionary change in medical education from symptoms to physical signs, which only came into use after auscultation. In addition to the stethoscope, the diagnosis by physical examination also included the ophthalmoscope, laryngoscope, and measurements of pulse, temperature and blood pressure.

The teaching of physical examination as a technique and its application to the description of diseases transformed medical education, just as laboratory diagnosis revolutionised medicine in the first half of the 20th century. Although there were impressive advances in the understanding of physiology, pathology and bacteriology, they did not yet translate into reductions in mortality from diseases. So the experimental physiology of Claude Bernard (1813-78), cellular pathology of Rudolf Virchow (1821-1902), and germ theory of Louis Pasteur (1822-95) and Robert Koch (1843-1910) did not immediately transform medicine's ability to cure.[91]

Pierre Louis (1787-1872) used mathematics to demonstrate the inefficacy of commonplace remedies such as bloodletting.[88] Soon, conventional forms of therapy such as bleeding, purging and many other remedies were discarded by sceptical practitioners as ineffective, leaving a treatment void (therapeutic nihilism) exploited by unorthodox therapies such as homeopathy, osteopathy and chiropractic, herbalism, hydropathy and vegetarianism.[99] Another important use of mathematics was for vital statistics in public health to describe quantitatively the health profile of populations (e.g. prevalence of diseases, mortality rates, life-tables).

In conclusion, medicine at the time of the establishment of the medical school in Fiji involved clinical diagnoses based on history taking with almost no physical examination, a system of pathology based on pure theory, and treatments which attempted to relieve symptoms with little concern about causation of disease. The medical profession in Britain had consisted of three different kinds of medical practitioners (physicians, surgeons and apothecaries), each of different social status and with different educational paths. However, by late 19th century these distinctions were becoming blurred with a more homogeneous and scientific profession due to the start of government regulation of medical practice. Incidentally, governments had also instituted compulsory vaccination against smallpox and quarantine, which resulted in a libertarian backlash in Britain against both measures, so the politics of anti-vaccination campaigns has a very long history.

The major revolution in medical education and practice beginning at the time was the development of the physical signs of disease as a means of diagnosis, by correlation of physical findings and post-mortem pathology to establish an anatomical pathology. Later, bacteriology added the causes of disease. Sir Kenneth Calman outlines five themes of medical education which emerged in the 19th century, namely:

a) the importance of the clinical examination
b) the new paradigms of disease
c) regulation of the profession
d) sanitary reform,
e) and the student life.[94] (p175)

As the medical historian Newman put it:

> By 1900, medicine had settled on a system of diagnosis based mainly on the elucidation of physical signs, a system of pathology based on the sciences of morbid anatomy, bacteriology, the beginnings of chemistry, and a system of treatment which attempted to counteract the physical causes of disease.[89]

So the state of medicine and medical education at the time of the start of the Suva Medical School was still empirical. These recent innovations in physical examination and laboratory medicine would have to await the next phase of the School's remarkable story as the Central Medical School (Part II).

Chapter 5

Labour and Land

The 'Polynesian' Labour Trade ('Blackbirding')

There had been numerous attempts at employing local and regional natives as labour sources on plantations, with limited success. Fijian villagers had little incentive to work on plantations as the benefit went to the chiefs with whom the labour contract was negotiated. So-called 'Polynesian' labourers from other Pacific islands had been recruited as part of the notorious 'blackbirding' venture, but Fiji paid lower wages than Queensland. These labourers learned a simplified form of English, which they took back to PNG as *'Tok pisin' (Pidjin)*, to Solomon Islands as *'Pijin'* and to Vanuatu as *'Bislama'*, as a *lingua franca* where there were many indigenous languages, but Fiji, Samoa and Tonga did not participate in this labour trade and had single languages, so 'pigeon' English was never introduced.

But the quality of Islander labour was considered poor, because they would only work hard for short periods, and were poorly motivated for the drudgery of the long hours demanded by European settlers. Gordon initially promoted an increase in Islander labourers in Fiji as a substitute for indigenous Fijian labour which he sought to protect from European exploitation, but at the same time he negotiated the importation of indentured labourers from India as had occurred in other British colonies such as Mauritius.

Between 1878 to 1881, over seven thousand Islander labourers were imported to Fijian plantations, with an alleged annual mortality rate of 17.8% and up to a 9.3% mortality rate on the voyage.[103] This compared to mortality rates of around 5% in Queensland between 1863-1907, although Kay Saunders of the University of Queensland has documented appalling health condition among islander labourers in Queensland with mortality rates of 11-16% in 1883-4 in Ingham, Townsville and Mackay, compared to only 1.6% for whites.[104]

More recent documentation of Pacific Islander labourers to Fiji between 1865-1911 has documented a total of 488 voyages, with 81% occurring between 1870-84. Excluding deaths at sea, out of a total 17,381 labourers there were 255 deaths after arrival in Fiji, 144 rejects and 18 deserters, so the official recorded mortality rate was only around 1.5%, which is considered an underestimate. Only about 8% of the labourers were women. More recently, Seigel has provided evidence of a higher total number of Pacific island labourers of over 27,000 from 1865-1911, mostly to Queensland and Fiji.[105]

The origin of these so-called "Polynesian" labourers was in fact Melanesia, with most from New Hebrides (Vanuatu, 14,198) and Solomon Islands (8,228) and smaller numbers from Kiribati (2,398) and New Guinea (1,618). By 1883, the CSR company was relying exclusively on Indian labour, no longer employing Islanders who had 'inferior stamina' for work. Governor Des Voeux, who succeeded Thurston, confessed in his memoirs that he would have ended the labour trade earlier if his career in Fiji had not been cut short by illness. He doubted whether the benefit of 'Polynesian' migrant labour was sufficient to compensate for the evils which accompanied it.[106]

Pacific Islanders had been first introduced into Australia as labourers in 1842 but did not thrive in the cold climate of southern NSW. In 1863, sixty-seven Melanesians, who were referred to as 'Kanakas', were imported to grow cotton in Queensland and by 1886 the Melanesian population of Queensland peaked at 10,036 (90.8% male) who were mostly employed in the sugar industry. The Pacific Island Labourers' Bill of 1901 ended the system of Kanaka labour in the Queensland sugar industry, and the Sugar Bounties Act of 1903 provided for rebates on sugar produced by white labour as part of the

'White Australia' policy which restricted immigration by a dictation test as a means of excluding unwanted immigrants until the 1960s.

Hence, importation of Melanesians ceased with nearly all repatriated such that by 1921 there were only 1,869 Melanesians left in Queensland.[14] The historian Clive Moore of the University of Queensland has documented the devastating effects of binge drinking after pay periods on the Melanesian labourers in Queensland, which affected their health and contributed to violent behaviour. This remains a huge problem today in Papua New Guinea, but is less of a problem in Fiji and Polynesian countries where kava is a more popular and cheaper drink. Alcohol-induced violence and crime in Oceania has been seen as a substitute for traditional warfare with drunkenness viewed by Pacific Islanders as culturally-sanctioned spirit possession. The contributors to alcohol abuse in Queensland were the anxiety, aggression, alienation and powerlessness which they felt in response to their racist treatment and cultural dislocation.[107] The prohibition of the sale of alcohol to the native populations was in force in Queensland and most Pacific colonies from the 1860s, with the exception of French colonies including New Hebrides (Vanuatu). Binge drinking and chronic alcoholism were also problems for some European medical officers, and NMPs were also affected when posted away from home such as in New Hebrides where alcohol was readily available.

Indian Indentured Labour

The British colonial experience in New Zealand had an important influence on colonial labour policy in Fiji, since the experience of a prolonged guerrilla war against a smaller Maori population precluded taking land by a war of conquest against a much larger Fijian population. Thus, Robie suggests that Fijians have the Maori people to thank for the fact that they still own 83 percent of their land.[108] The need for Fiji to exploit the land to gain revenue to fund the colonial administration virtually obliged Gordon to bring Indian immigrants, as had happened in other British colonies. In the words of the historian IM Cumpston, who published a book on *Indians Overseas in British Territories:*[109]

> by introducing laborers from India, Sir A. Gordon redeemed the Fijian from the possible fate of the *deraciné* migratory laborer, coerced into labor on a distant island, leaving desolate and declining villages in his own. The Fijian became instead a wealthy landlord, and his £20,000 rent roll appeared to him ample compensation for parting under lease with portions of uncultivated land.[110]

By 1878, Gordon had gained approval from both British and Indian governments to supplement Islander labour with indentured labourers from India. The labour contracts were for a fixed period of five years, after which the labourer was entitled to repatriation. Abuses by employers were penalised, and plantations with a high mortality rate were denied any allotments of immigrants in the succeeding year. The agreement specified that planters had to provide two-thirds of the cost of transport of almost £20 per person, making it more expensive than islander labour.[110] In addition to sugar, the possibility of coffee plantations was also explored using labourers from Ceylon, but there were concerns about: a) ethnic conflict with Indians, b) the leaf rust disease which broke out in 1879 and c) the drop in world commodity price for coffee in 1881 compared to sugar.[81]

The first shipload of 480 labourers arrived from Calcutta in 1879 aboard the *Leonidas*. But 32 passengers on board had died of cholera, dysentery or smallpox during the voyage, so MacGregor put the ship under strict quarantine for 90 days. He had not forgotten the lesson from the recent measles epidemic. He also trained three young Fijians as 'vaccinators' against smallpox and sent them out to vaccinate at risk communities. Due to these quarantine measures being applied to subsequent ships, there were no cholera or smallpox outbreaks in Fiji.

With the shift of the Fijian capital to Suva, the quarantine station was moved to Nukulau island. Compared to Europe at the time, Fiji was very fortunate to have avoided endemic or epidemic cholera, smallpox, diphtheria and typhus, as well as being malaria-free. Dorothy Porter has detailed the enormous historical impact of these epidemic and infectious diseases on Europe and America at this time.[97] Nevertheless, measles, influenza and dysentery did affect Fiji, and played an important role in health, demography, politics and of course the founding of the School.

Contrary to popular belief, indentured labourers did not come only from the lower castes of Indian society but were representative of rural society. Although called "coolies", they called themselves *girmitiyas*, from a mispronunciation of the English word "agreement" (*girmit*), which referred to the indenture contract. They provided agricultural labour instead of using indigenous Fijians, who were insulated from the capitalist market for their own protection by colonial policy.

At the time, there seemed to be little foresight of the potential for future ethnic strife by introducing another race with different religions. Indeed, the British policy was specifically to recruit Indians of different ethnicities, languages and religions from the colony. The gender ratio was regulated by India at five men to two women, and 15% of migrants were Moslems. Once in Fiji, the administration ensured that they were dispersed and their mobility restricted by an 1886 ordinance, lest they form ethnic groups and agitate politically.[111]

The conditions under which Indian labourers worked were appalling, described as 'a new system of slavery'. However, it was still a better situation for most of them than in India at the time due to the risks of unemployment, famine and even lower wages.[81] Here is a labourer describing conditions at the time:

> *Kulumbars* [overseers with whips] were bad—the Australians were especially bad, while the New Zealanders were good as they took pity . . . We woke up at four when the mill whistle blew. At six we started to work, cutting grass in the larger cane field and dug drains. Some—those who knew the work,—finished their tasks early. But most of the others

would carry on and, depending on their relative skill and strength, complete their tasks [by sunset].[108] (p204)

These conditions undoubtedly contributed to a high suicide rate among Indian men.

Thus, Fiji's national economy was built on what Robie calls 'the unholy trinity of European capital, Fijian land and Indian labour', which he summarises as follows:

> As Indo-Fijian labourers ended their *girmit* contracts, the sugar plantations were eventually carved up into plots leased by Indo-Fijian small planters. But they remained dependent as they were forced to sell their cane to the Colonial Sugar Refining Company on company terms. Strikes to improve their existence were suppressed by the company and the colonial government. Their claims, however, gradually led to slow improvements, while the indigenous Fijians clung to their communal pattern of life.[108]

In addition to labour, the sugar industry, settlers and foreign investors all needed land. Under the Deed of Cession, European settlers who had acquired land before 1874 had to prove their claims, and they had laid claim to 850,000 acres of the best land in Fiji, although only about 15,000 acres was actually being cultivated.[78] Land was essential for economic development and foreign investment, but it was also sensitive issue for chiefs whose views could not be ignored. The Council of Chiefs had declared in 1879 that by tradition, native land was inalienable. Fijians did not appreciate that if a settler or company purchased land from a chief, it meant that they had acquired exclusive rights over the land.

Gordon appointed a commission to examine land claims, which resolved the delicate issue by granting only 517 of the 1,683 claims as *bona fide,* most of which was lying idle at the time. In addition, Gordon had negotiated with the Australian Colonial Sugar Refining

(CSR) Company to build sugar mills in exchange for permission to buy land, and by 1903 they owned 15 sugar mills and sugar exports constituted half of Fiji's export earnings, valued at over £400,000.[81] From 1908, land sales ceased due in part to pressure from Gordon—or Lord Stanmore, as he was then known as. Although he had left Fiji for NZ in 1880, he continued a keen interest in Fiji's affairs. By the time indentured labour migration ceased in 1916, over 60,000 Indians had been imported to Fiji, with only about 24,000 returning to India at the end of one or two contracts.[111]

In 1910 and 1914 India appointed two Commissions (Sanderson and McNeill-Lal) to look into conditions of Indian immigration to Fiji, which concluded favourably that the advantages far outweighed the disadvantages. They were impressed by the health and living conditions of the Indians in Fiji, with relatively few having returned to India, although they retained strong links to the mother country.[111] Economically, Fiji had trebled its foreign trade in the last decade, and Indians had sent considerable sums of money back to India as remittances or savings.[110]

Despite these economic advantages of Fijian labour to India, it was India which stopped the flow of indentured labourers in 1916 with the last contracts terminated in 1920. This decision was based upon humanitarian grounds. The anti-indenture protest was one of the first protest movements of Indian nationalism with mass public appeal in India, which began over the treatment of Indians in South Africa. But soon Fiji became a focus of attention, when Gandhi's friend CF Andrews visited Fiji, and the stories told by Indians returning home after working as indentured labourers caused anger in India. Fijian Indians read Indian nationalist newspapers and pamphlets and enrolled nationalist leaders in their cause, such as Manilal, who came to Fiji in 1912 and led strikes that shut down the Fiji sugar industry and a nonviolent boycott of European employers until he was deported in 1920.[111] The assertion of Indian rights meant the sugar industry was plagued by strikes, with the first major Indian trade union formed in 1937, and a strike lasting six months in 1943 while Britain was at war.

The American anthropologists John Kelly and Martha Kaplan argue that:

> many of the problems faced by the *ex-girmitiyas* and their descendants in Fiji followed from the fact that the tools they imported for community representation, as means to deal with "the Indian problem," the means to initiative, were tooled in fact for different political purposes, even when they were already colonial-era hybrids. What nation, exactly, was a Fiji Indian National Congress working to forge? How, exactly, was an Arya Samaj to address the reality of South Indian descended people in Fiji (Dravidians?), let alone Muslims of more than one form of commitment? As events moved fast in India, what was in the interests of the so-called "Indians" of Fiji?[112]

Indian Permanent Settlement

The permanent settlement of Indians in Fiji took place without apparent Fijian resentment or opposition. In 1910, Governor Im Thurn spoke of 'indifference' between the two races: there was very little contact, no intermarriage or co-habitation, and apparently no ill-feeling, although some sources suggested that Fijians treated Indians with contempt. Brij Lal attributes the apparent indifference to specific policies of the colonial administration to prevent Indians and Fijians joining forces against the colonial power.[111]

The CSR company reacted to the ending of indentured labourers by leasing them 4-hectare plots out of their almost 54,000 hectares of company land. The main problem with the leases was the small size of land plots which kept Indian cane growers poor. However, Indians also acquired larger leases of 10-20 acres of native Fijian land through the Native Land Department. According to Robie, many of the later problems arose from the disproportionate level of land rents which went to the chiefs rather than to villagers, in spite of most chiefs rarely having enough resources to meet their customary obligations to their people.[108] Europeans were threatened by the entrepreneurial skills of the Indians as traders and agriculturists, so most opposed further Indian immigration to Fiji. In 1973, the embattled CSR company sold its sugar interests to the newly independent government of Fiji.

The labour unrest was followed by conflicts over voting and land-owning rights. The protection of indigenous Fijians resulted in the permanent reservation of 83 percent of Fiji's land for indigenous Fijians, leaving Fijian Indians virtually landless. Gordon's legacy of official colonial empathy for Fijians was never extended to Indians, as reflected in one official's statement:

> The Indian is disliked and feared by Europeans principally because he is politically conscious and is aiming at placing himself on a level with Europeans. The Fijians are superficially a much more attractive people ... and the position of Europeans towards them is roughly that of the guardians of attractive, promising, but not yet quite fully developed children.[108]

Such British views were reinforced during the Second World War, when Fijian males responded by becoming soldiers, whereas Indo-Fijians demanded equal pay with British soldiers. Brij Lal points to evidence that Indians were strongly discouraged from enrolling in the military, quite aside from the pay dispute.[111] Similarly, the bitter sugar strike by Indian growers and labourers, which allowed the sugar cane to rot in the fields while Britain was fighting a desperate war, was seen as disloyalty. Consequently, the European-Fijian alliance was strengthened with chiefs gaining a more important role within the colonial administration.[108]

Two north American geographers carried out a survey of Fijian and Indian attitudes to land in 1978.[113] Fijian attitudes to the land had been formed from the security of land, forest, and sea; whereas Indian consciousness had sprung from insecurity, and from an immediate need to survive. They documented widely divergent views between the two ethnic groups and envisaged two possible scenarios for resolution. Firstly, views could become increasingly polarised until the growing population forced the two races into open strife, Alternatively, Fijians and Indians could see the need to compromise and expand their awareness of each other's views. Although this might be seen by some as a loss of ethnic integrity, the achievement of better understanding between the two races was seen as the major problem Fiji must face for the future. But they also point out the importance of the European influence:

> For a century and a half, Westerners in Fiji, in introducing advanced technologies and alien cultural values, must have caused the Fijians to feel that the very essence of their life was being eroded. To assuage some of the guilt felt toward Fijians, the linear Westerners sought to preserve the Fijian way of life through defined, stable, and uniform land tenure, systematic government, and the introduction of outsiders to prevent social dislocation and to support the Dominion's economy.[113](p12)

The anthropologist John Kelly contrasts indigenous Fijians with Indo-Fijians, contended that the former were loyal colonial subjects, devout Christians, and non-capitalistic; whereas Fijian Indians resisted colonial authority and Christian missions, and were actively capitalistic.[114] Thus, there were a total of 557 Indian business registrations in Fiji between 1924-1945, including 298 by Gujaratis who represented less than 10% of the Indian population. The colonial government failed to diversify the single-crop economy, and neglected education.[115] Despite a literacy rate in their own languages of 84 per cent in 1936, indigenous Fijians had limited secondary school access and almost none to tertiary education.[116]

Over the period 1920-40, the Indo-Fijians experienced population growth, increased prosperity and better educational levels. In order to control this new Indo-Fijian assertiveness, Europeans aligned themselves politically with the indigenous Fijians. A minority even suggested repatriation or re-settlement of Indo-Fijians in New Guinea. With Indo-Fijians having attained majority status during the war, they favoured an electoral system with a non-racial common roll with independence. These issues really needed to be resolved by negotiation and compromise before the granting of independence. As they were not really resolved, they were to emerge later to cause problems for Fiji and the School, as we shall see in Part III.

Chapter 6

Rockefeller Philanthropy

The partnership between an American capitalist philanthropic foundation and the British colonial administration is an important part of the story of the medical school in Fiji. JD Rockefeller's philanthropy commenced in 1901 with the Rockefeller Institute for Medical Research. By 1909, it had embarked upon a successful hookworm campaign in the southern states of America, since the disease was affecting the productivity of workers.

In 1913, the Rockefeller Foundation was established with a US$50 million grant, and it formed an International Health Commission, which became a Board in 1916 and then a Division in 1927.[117] President George Vincent of the Foundation launched a mammoth international public health programme, which encompassed medical education. Since the Standard Oil Company, which was the source of Rockefeller's wealth, was a multinational corporation with a reputation for ruthless capitalism, the Foundation and its international health programmes had to be seen to distance themselves from the company. However, despite its nominal political neutrality, the Foundation was not averse to wielding its influence in order to implement the kind of programmes it wanted.[118]

Since Standard Oil had earned its profits in many countries, the Foundation sought to expand its successful US hookworm campaign into a global initiative of disease control, at least partly as a show-case of American laboratory-based medicine. Dr Victor

Heiser, who was Director of the Rockefeller International Health Board for the East, made his first visit to Fiji in 1915 as part of a world tour to assess its suitability for a hookworm campaign. Perhaps because of its malaria-free status without the confounding effect of malarial anaemia, Fiji was chosen as one of the sites for hookworm eradication.

The Foundation approved funding for a medical officer, microscopists, equipment and medicines for the campaign, on condition that Fiji provided staff quarters, space and transport costs. The Ministry of Health was also expected to improve sanitation so that the anticipated success in reducing the prevalence of hookworm would be sustained by prevention of reinfection.

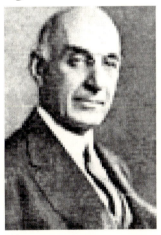

Fig. 21: Victor Heiser

The primary focus of the campaign was the Indian population due to its economic importance for the sugar industry but it was hoped it might also contribute to halting the population decline among Fijians, which was a major concern at the time of the colonial administration (chapter 2). Not surprisingly, it was found difficult to translate the American experience to the Pacific Islands context, but the main constraint was the campaign's focus on treatment alone, which placed too heavy a responsibility on the health department for expensive preventive activities such as health education and sanitation (e.g. building latrines).

Hookworm Campaigns

Fig. 22: The Hookworm

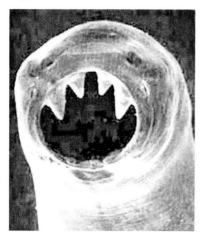

The initial hookworm survey in 1917 showed a mean prevalence of 94% among Indians and 79% among Fijians, which was higher than expected for Fijians. But the survey was flawed by not measuring worm loads, so could not differentiate light infections of little significance from heavy infestations with anaemia, which were largely confined to high rainfall regions. There was also a hookworm species difference between the two groups, with *Ankylostoma duodenale* affecting Indians and *Necator americanus* affecting Fijians and other Pacific Islanders. Incidentally, this difference showed that Indian migrants had not infected Fijians with hookworm, as had been assumed. There was also a high prevalence of ascariasis (roundworms), which tended to migrate within the gastrointestinal system when 'irritated' by the oil of chenopodium (American wormseed) treatment for hookworm. Chenopodium with purgatives was already a very unpleasant form of treatment, but migrating roundworms could add significant morbidity by obstructing bile or pancreatic orifices.

The Queensland campaign

After this initial survey in Fiji, Dr Sylvester Lambert was recruited by the International Health Board of Rockefeller to continue the hookworm campaign in the Pacific. Lambert had been rejected by the American army because of poor eyesight, and Heiser only reluctantly appointed him temporarily, while looking for a better candidate. Lambert arrived in Australia in October 1918 during the pandemic of influenza and actually contracted influenza on the voyage. The ship was quarantined, and Lambert was publically scathing about Australian health officials, which was not a good start in international diplomacy.[12] However, Lambert partly redeemed himself with the Queensland hookworm campaign through his directness and joviality, which contributed to the campaign's success and his future career with the Foundation.[87]

It was the Queensland's premier, DF Denham, who had pushed for a hookworm program for Queensland while on a visit to London because it was a cause of debility among white settler communities in north Queensland, threatening the productivity of white labour in the tropics and the racially-based immigration policy of keeping Asians out. Although Queensland's concern was white colonisation of the Australian tropics, Fiji's was the health of indentured Indian labourers for the sugar plantations.

Lambert worked in collaboration with the Australian Institute of Tropical Medicine, which had been established in Townsville in 1909 under the Austrian researcher, Dr Anton Breinl, in an effort to research how to ensure good health and work productivity of white Australians in a tropical setting. The 1919 stool survey found a hookworm prevalence of only 21% for whites, but 81% of the Aboriginal population of tropical Queensland were infected. With Lambert's departure for Papua in 1920, Dr Raphael Cilento took over the hookworm campaign in north Queensland, although it was ultimately controlled by Cumpston at the new Commonwealth Department of Health in Canberra.[12] Hookworm was greatly reduced in the white population due mostly to improved sanitation, but high rates persisted in the Aboriginal population into the 1990s when the routine use of the single dose antihelminthic drug, albendazole, finally reduced its prevalence dramatically.[119]

Melanesian Campaigns

It was not until after Lambert's successful Papuan campaign that his reputation was established as well as his good relationship with Heiser.

The first administrator of British New Guinea from 1888 to 1898 had been none other than Sir William MacGregor, who had started the native medical school in Suva while CMO in Fiji. The Papuan protectorate had been transferred to Australia in 1905, and Hubert Murray was appointed as Lieutenant-Governor from 1908 until 1940. Murray shared MacGregor's concern for native welfare, but his main health efforts were towards improving labour productivity.

By the time of Lambert's arrival in Papua in 1921, there were only four doctors (three of whom were described as 'elderly hacks' by Lambert), and the CMO, Dr William Strong, who was unconvinced of the importance of hookworm disease as a public health priority. There were no native medical assistants in Papua at the time (unlike New Guinea), although a simple travelling medical service was established in 1922.[12] Rather than a constraint to health prevention, native beliefs in magic and sorcery were used by Lambert in his hookworm campaign, explaining the need to kill the invisible snakes in the body causing illness. He also became sceptical of the prevailing European view that the native races in Australia and Melanesia were doomed to extinction. He employed Papuans to assist with the bothersome chenopodium and purgative treatments, and even suggested training native assistants to treat common medical conditions such as hookworm, malaria, yaws and other skin diseases, under supervision from visiting medical officers.[12]

Lambert's next campaign was in the Australian mandate of New Guinea, on the island of New Britain, since the highland population was yet to be 'discovered' by Europeans. This territory had been training native medical assistants, known as *tultuls,* since 1903 under German rule, who had been given simple first aid training to deliver basic medical care at village level. This confirmed Lambert's belief in the possibility of medical training of natives. He also learned *tok pisin* (pigeon English) in which he gave idiosyncratic talks about hookworm control to the local population.[12,120,121]

Although the main focus of the hookworm campaign was therapeutic, Lambert also embarked upon a research project using prisoners to compare various regimes of chenopodium. His methods would be considered highly unethical by today's standards, and were even considered unpublishable by the Rockefeller Foundation using the standards of the day. In his hookworm campaign, Lambert gained the support of the new Director of Health for New Guinea, Dr Raphael Cilento. However, this did not prevent Cilento from opposing Lambert's later proposal of sending students from Papua and New Guinea to the new regional Central Medical School in Suva (chapter 8).

Lambert's next survey was in the British protectorate of the Solomon Islands, where there had been no government health services until 1910 so missions and plantations had provided health services. Indeed, it was the company Levers Plantations' concern about native labour which led to the survey. But Lambert's experiences in three areas of Melanesia had already convinced him that training native assistants was better than relying on poor quality European doctors.

In 1922, the International Health Board of the Foundation posted him to Fiji for the next phase of the hookworm campaign, where he found that 57% of Indians and 46% of Fijians were positive for hookworm ova on stool surveys.[12]

Carbon Tetrachloride Treatment

Meantime, Lambert had changed the treatment of hookworm from chenopodium to carbon tetrachloride, which allowed for quicker and more effective treatment. Its use had been reported by Maurice Hall, a Washington zoologist in 1926.[122] Lambert describes seeing Hall's report as a kind of 'eureka' experience in his book, but the timing of these events fails to corroborate his version of events.[121] He did, however, carry out human studies, reporting his extensive experience with the new drug in three articles which included a total of 286,486 treatments.[123-125] However, other Rockefeller researchers in Sao Paulo had carried out experiments on the toxicity of the drug in dogs in 1923, and found toxic effects on liver and kidney.[126] Lambert reported seven deaths and acknowledged the danger of roundworm migration due to irritation without killing them.

Lambert's behaviour as an investigator leaves one with an impression of an 'impresario' instead of a cautious scientist.

Recent studies have examined the toxic effects of carbon tetrachloride on the liver.[127] Metabolism of the drug in the liver generates free radicals which initiate lipid peroxidation, and the by-products result in liver toxicity and a risk of cancer. Chenopodium fares even worse in recent studies as it has been found ineffective against intestinal worms and to have serious toxicity.[128] However, it is possible that Lambert's combination of chenopodium with purgatives may have transiently paralysed worms long enough for them to be expelled by the laxative, hence explaining his belief in its efficacy. Ironically, Heiser described how the hookworm campaign in Fiji miraculously transformed the inhabitants from 'a dejected, downcast, docile, uninterested people' into one which was healthy, alert, and mentally progressive.[120] The truth may have been more prosaic.

Other Pacific Campaigns

Lambert's next campaign in 1924 was in the Gilbert and Ellice Islands (Kiribati and Tuvalu) which included Ocean Island and the Union Group (Nauru and Tokelau). The Colony's medical department was largely staffed by NMPs with only one doctor since 1921. Lambert was accompanied by his favoured NMP as assistant, Malikai Veisamasama. They documented a high prevalence of yaws and tuberculosis, with some leprosy, dysentery and influenza. Although the Polynesians on the Ellice Islands had high rates of filariasis and hookworm, these were uncommon among the Micronesians of the Gilbert Islands.[12] Lambert attributed the lower hookworm prevalence to defecating into the sea rather than on soil around villages. An innovation for this campaign was to include yaws treatment with NAB injections, which were curative with less need for a preventive programme. It was the first real example of a highly effective Western treatment for a local disease with high morbidity.

In May 1924, Lambert went to Tonga where hookworm disease was uncommon. A major advantage of the work in Tonga was his developing a close relationship with Queen Salote and her husband, whose support for his Central Medical School proposal was crucial. However, he came to loathe the CMO, Dr Dawson, who no doubt felt threatened by his friendship with the Queen.

From Tonga, he moved on to Western Samoa, where he gained support for his plans for the medical school as they had serious shortages in medical staffing. The Samoans had already developed a scheme for training local medical assistants or cadets at Apia hospital, which they were happy to transfer to Suva. Rather than hookworm, Lambert concentrated on a yaws campaign in Samoa since yaws was considered an important contributor to the high infant mortality rates. Samoa's infant mortality rate was 149 per 1,000 live births in 1924, in comparison to 43 for New Zealand at that time.[12] By 1933, the infant mortality rate had dropped to 114 per thousand, although the contribution of yaws treatment to this fall was unclear. High-ranking Samoan women were recruited to lead the Women's Committees in the villages which focussed on child welfare and improved village hygiene, which did contribute to the reduced infant mortality. In 1927 the *Mau* rebellion encouraged Samoans to refuse to participate in medical treatments, so health standards declined as a consequence.

The Foundation approved a further hookworm campaign in April 1932, and Lambert was assisted in the campaign by two NMPs, including Ielu Kuresa. This survey found that 60% had yaws, and 74,080 injections were given. Unfortunately, this corresponded with the time of a polio epidemic, thus contributing to at least 150 children developing paralysis. This was a devastating iatrogenic complication, since injections during a polio outbreak make limb paralyses more likely.

The Cook Islands was the last hookworm campaign in the Pacific by Lambert, from November 1925 to January 1926. He was accompanied by NMP Malakai Veisamasama, and they screened most of the population, finding a high hookworm prevalence of 70% in the Polynesian population, but low parasite density rates. Lambert recommended a mass treatment campaign combined with hygiene education and latrine installation.[12] As on other islands, Cook Islands also had great difficulty recruiting expatriate medical staff.

In conclusion, the hookworm campaign in the Pacific region treated a large number of individuals, but ultimately failed to significantly control hookworm due to the poorly implemented hygiene and sanitation measures to prevent relapse. But a new bore-hole latrine represented a more affordable and acceptable solution to the longstanding problem of re-infection from soil contamination with hookworm ova. Lambert's persistence eventually obtained Foundation funding for constructing 35,000 of these latrines in Fiji.

In spite of the hookworm campaign failing to achieve prevalence targets, the population was educated about sanitation issues and many households acquired latrines. On the other hand, the yaws treatment program with arsenicals by injection proved more sustainable and helped convince the native population of the value of Western medicine and also of NMPs. Fiji's Council of Chiefs passed a resolution to record its gratitude to the Rockefeller and to Dr Lambert.[12] But our main interest in these Pacific island hookworm campaigns was the role of Rockefeller philanthropy and Lambert in founding the Central Medical School, which is the subject of Part II.

PART II

CENTRAL MEDICAL SCHOOL
1928-1961

Chapter 7

A Regional Medical School

Sylvester Lambert

In this chapter, we explore in more detail the role of Dr Lambert in establishing Central Medical School. He appears as a rather flamboyant American, who was sent to the South Pacific by the Rockefeller Foundation from 1919 to 1939.[121] As discussed in the last chapter, his primary responsibility was with the International Health Board, attached to the hookworm project. Lambert was a colourful character, who became greatly attached to the peoples of the South Pacific, especially indigenous Fijians. In spite of being overweight, a heavy smoker and myopic, he endured considerable physical discomfort on his tours of many Pacific islands. He demonstrated profound concern for the health and welfare of islanders, and acquired from experience the skills in negotiating with a large philanthropic organisation like the Rockefeller Foundation as well as the British colonial administration, eventually establishing for himself a solid reputation. Although he had carried out many community health surveys of hookworm, yaws, and tuberculosis prevalence, his orientation was more to public health programmes than to research.

Lambert was born in New York State and attended Syracuse Medical School. During his third year of medical school, he made a trip to Mexico where he met his future wife Eloisa, the daughter of an American mining engineer and a Mexican mother. Following graduation, Lambert was admitted to the Costa Rican Medical Faculty and then spent four years in Mexico, including during the Mexican civil war in 1914 during which he had many adventures. These included excising a large tumour from the groin of a rebel Colonel, who absconded from hospital and subsequently died of peritonitis. Consequently, Lambert was thrown in jail and sentenced to execution. It was apparently only last minute American gunboat diplomacy by the Secretary of State, William Jennings Bryan which obtained his release. Bryan was of course more famous as an unsuccessful three-time presidential campaigner and anti-Darwinian in the Scopes trial in which he was an eloquent opponent of evolution.[129]

Lambert arrived in Fiji in 1924, when there were about 22-24 British medical officers, with whom, incidentally, he was mostly very unimpressed. Indeed, he was very critical of the average white colonial doctor in his 1926 Memorandum to the Rockefeller.[130] Annie Stuart is a Pacific historian who has examined in detail the primary sources of the exploits of Lambert and the Rockefeller Foundation in the Pacific in a PhD thesis for Canterbury University,[12] on which I have relied greatly for this chapter, along with library archives at the School.[131] From Lambert's correspondence, Stuart cites the following statement of his views about expatriate medical officers in the Pacific:

> He comes out to the islands, often with no knowledge of tropical medicine, frequently an alcoholic, usually a medical cripple of some sort . . . He does what he chooses. Often at the start he wants to learn his work and do his best for the native but he is handicapped by lack of knowledge of the languages and customs and his best efforts for something better are apt to be opposed by his lay superior, who is sure from his experience (and lack of knowledge) that such efforts are useless. The result is that good men get out and the others resign themselves, each year more easily, to letting things take their course.[87] (p130)

Thus, European doctors cost too much, were unfamiliar with the culture and found working conditions too hard, often resorting to drink. The obvious solution was to train native doctors, but native educational standards were too low for a Western-style medical school, and it was believed that trying to make them into Western doctors would also make them unwilling to work in the remote settings where they were needed.

Even before arriving in Fiji in 1922, Lambert had formed a favourable opinion of Native Medical Practitioners (NMPs) during his hookworm projects on other islands. In his initial projects in Queensland and Papua, he had relied on European assistants, but in Fiji he was given two NMPs as assistants and found that they could not only carry out his medical instructions accurately, but could also communicate with the Fijian patients to explain exactly what was required of them. When Lambert continued his project in Tonga and Samoa, he requested permission for a NMP to accompany him. He was particularly impressed by the recent graduate, Malakai Veisamasama.[13]

Lambert formed a close friendship with Dr Aubrey Montague, who was the Chief Medical Officer (CMO) of Fiji at the time, describing him as one of the three best men he had known in the Pacific.[121] It was an unusual friendship in that their character traits were very different: Lambert was fat, jolly and ostentatious whereas Montague was frugal with sensible British reserve. In collaboration with Montague, Lambert planned the enlarged regional medical school for NMPs in Suva, a model leprosarium at Makogai Island, and a unified medical service for the Pacific Islands. But Lambert had to win a number of battles before the Central Medical School could be established.

Right from the beginning, Heiser had reservations about Lambert. His initial appointment was only temporary, and he certainly started on the wrong foot initially by openly criticising Australia's quarantine practices on his first posting, which was not exactly the kind of diplomacy the Foundation was looking for in its employees. A similar incident occurred in Papua when Lambert criticised the spendthrift health policies of Governor Murray using rather tactless language. But Lambert's reputation within the Foundation was starting to change due to his 'boisterous energy and romantic tales of cannibals in the South Seas'.[12] Since the difficult early days, Lambert had implemented highly successful hookworm campaigns under difficult field conditions, he had learned to speak a sort of idiosyncratic 'pidjin' English, and—as we will see—he had a major diplomatic success in establishing the new School despite opposition from within the Foundation. Above all, he had gained the unequivocal support of the local Fijian administration, so his tactlessness was overlooked by Foundation officials and Heiser began to view him in a more favourable light.[120] However, Heiser retired from the Rockefeller Foundation in December 1934 after being rejected for promotion to head the Department of Medical Education.

There were also changes in the Foundation which affected Lambert's role in the organisation. In 1928, the International Health Board had changed its focus from disease control, such as Lambert's hookworm projects, to scientific research in public health. Lambert attempted to adjust to the change by publishing his hookworm and yaws treatment results[125,132,133] and surveying TB prevalence by means of tuberculin skin reactions. Realising the poor laboratory support for research in Fiji, he pushed the Foundation to provide new laboratory facilities and a better qualified pathologist in order to upgrade research and improve NMP training, in keeping with the new Foundation focus.

Origins of the New School

Even before Lambert arrived in the region, Dr VG Heiser of the International Health Board of the Rockefeller Foundation had carried out a survey of the training school for NMPs in 1916, when he had felt that improvements were required to give them more status in the region. It was Heiser who first proposed that the High Commissioner of the Western Pacific establish a Central Medical School in Fiji for the training of natives from Fiji and regional colonies such as the

Solomon Islands. By then, the School in Suva was already accepting students from outside of Fiji, with two students from Tokelau (known then as Union Island) graduating in 1916. But the next regional student to complete his studies was not until 1927 with the graduation of Ielu Kuresa of Western Samoa.[23]

Heiser also called for the inclusion of Fijian Indian students in the Fiji quota. The first Indian graduate was not until 1926. But it was really only with the establishment of the Central Medical School in 1928 that the school became a truly regional medical school. While working on the hookworm campaign in Papua in 1922, Lambert had proposed training native assistants to treat common conditions like hookworm, yaws and malaria, under the supervision of travelling medical officers. This was at a time when Papua had no native medical assistants, but his idea was not taken up at the time.

There were great expectations for this new Central Medical School and it was assumed that the best NMPs would progress to full training as doctors at a university overseas. A major incentive for the new enlarged medical school was the opening of the Colonial War Memorial Hospital in Suva in 1923 with 106 beds, which had been named in memory of soldiers killed in the First World War. The original scheme provided for 20 students from Fiji, four each from Tonga, Gilbert and Ellice Islands, British Solomon Islands and Western Samoa, and two each from the Cook Islands and the New Hebrides, for a total of 40 students who would live in two new dormitories. The staff was to consist of one full-time tutor along with at least eight honorary lecturers. The regional nature of the new school meant that teaching in Fijian, as had occurred at the old school, would now have to be changed to English for regional students.[13] Although this made it easier for the teachers, the English requirement remained an important barrier for many students.

At the old Fiji Medical School, NMPs had proved to be a highly successful model as a cost-saving measure both to provide health care to the indigenous population and to convince them of the merits of Western medicine as part of the civilising mission of the British Empire. Indigenous medical practitioners were not unique to Fiji as they had also been trained as native assistants in Goa by the Portuguese, in Calcutta by the East India Company and in Bengal at the Medical College.[12] In spite of the success of native practitioners, it was not smooth sailing for Lambert to get approval for an expanded regional school. Although the new Governor of Fiji supported the proposal, the Colonial Office procrastinated.

Rockefeller Opposition

There was strong opposition to Lambert's proposal from within the Department of Medical Sciences of the Rockefeller Foundation, particularly from the Director of the Division of Medical Education, Dr Richard Pearce, who had a large budget to fund medical education projects anywhere in the world. Pearce was only interested in first class medical schools, following the academic model of Johns Hopkins in the USA, which promoted the need for appointments of full-time clinical professors. He was strongly opposed to the idea of funding what he saw as a third-rate medical school for medical assistants in Fiji. Lambert's proposal apparently made Pearce and the New York office feel physically ill, insisting that Rockefeller must stick to the policy of aiding only first class schools.[117]

Pearce was not ill-informed about the School as he had sent a questionnaire to Montague on student education levels, facilities, faculty and the curriculum, and on the basis of this information had rejected the school as unacceptably sub-standard and ineligible for Rockefeller funding.[12] He had even questioned the need for a Pacific medical school given the small population and difficulties of inter-island travel, suggesting that doctors for the region should be trained at proper medical schools in Australia or NZ. Even an official request by the Governor of Fiji for Rockefeller support to train NMPs in Fiji to meet the shortage of medical practitioners in other Pacific Islands was to no avail.

Pearce's views were supported by the Director of the International Health Board of Rockefeller, Dr Frederick Russell, who agreed that the Foundation should have nothing to do with a low quality medical school for natives. Since Lambert's hookworm project came under the International Health Board, he tried to convince his immediate bosses of the merit of his proposal face-to-face while on leave in New York in 1926. He did manage to gain the support of his immediate superior, Dr Heiser and also of Dr Wilbur Sawyer, with whom he had worked on the hookworm project in Australia. Sawyer was an important ally as he was Head of the Division of Laboratory Services at the time and became Director of the International Health Program from 1935-1944.

Although the Department of Medical Sciences remained opposed to the proposal, Lambert eventually obtained funding through the International Health Board, which was a separate division of the Rockefeller Foundation. This was the first time the Board had given financial support to a medical school, since up to then it had always been from the medical education division of the Department of Medical Sciences. This department did not support the project until after Peirce's death when his successor, Dr Alan Gregg, finally acknowledged the importance of Lambert's project as a medical education initiative.

Critiques of Rockefeller Philanthropy

Rockefeller philanthropy has come in for considerable criticism as a manifestation of American imperialism. Peirce's Division of Medical Education is probably a case in point, particularly in its attitude to Fiji's medical school. Christopher Lawrence, for example, has described the Foundation in the following terms:

> The scale of Rockefeller international intervention is staggering. Practically every country in the world received some form of assistance although those with strong colonial

governments were touched least . . . The Rockefeller public health programme largely targeted diseases . . . susceptible to laboratory investigation and were eradicable by some combination of vaccines, straightforward public health measures, and education. Hookworm, yellow fever, and malaria roughly fulfilled these criteria. Leprosy and TB, in which there was clearly some extremely complicated relation to the socio-economic causes of poverty, did not . . . Public health schools were supported by the Foundation when they conformed to the model of the School of Hygiene and Public Health at the Johns Hopkins University. . . . On the one hand Rockefeller intervention was seen as part of sinister American imperialism, on the other it simply did not work because it ignored (frequently deliberately) local practices.[117] (pp 29-30)

In a similar vein, Gillespie re-assessed the contribution of the Rockefeller Foundation in the following way:

A more radical view has emerged since the Rockefeller Archives were opened in the 1970s . . . Abraham Flexner's report on American medical education and the subsequent campaign by the Rockefeller Foundation . . . [used] the lure of endowments to impose a particular model of medical education . . . [The] Foundation required its beneficiaries to establish a closer relationship between clinical and theoretical instruction, with full-time teaching staff, modelled on the Johns Hopkins Medical School. The public health work sponsored by the Rockefeller Foundation was a more directly political extension of these concerns, involving both labour market considerations . . . In short, it was the application to public health of the same mixture of high-minded altruism and the ruthless pursuit of commercial and cultural domination which animated the "open door" and other aspects of early twentieth century American imperialism.[134] (p65)

Final Preparations

Following the initial Rockefeller refusal to fund the School, Lambert looked for other sources of support. An early enthusiastic supporter of the medical school was Queen Salote of Tonga, from when Lambert first discussed the proposal with her in 1924. With her support, he proposed that the island governments share the expense of new buildings and equipment for the medical school, which he reduced to only about £1500 per island group by reducing the building proposal and living costs. Fiji would have had to pay for most of the teaching and capital expenditure costs, as well as donating a suitable site for the school. Nevertheless, he was concerned that the scaled down model would compromise the quality of training, since his highest priority was to train competent NMPs to meet the health needs in the region.[12]

Another key supporter was Sir Maui Pomare, an American-trained Maori medical officer. It was at Pomare's request that Lambert first visited the Cook Islands towards the end of 1925 for a hookworm survey. However, Pomare withdrew Cook Island support for the medical school in 1927 due to a personal racialist insult by a young British medical officer when accompanying leprosy patients from the Cook Islands to Fiji. On his arrival at the Makogai leprosarium, Pomare was told by the medical officer that coloured people should go this way, not realising that Pomare was a proud Maori chief and the New Zealand Minister of Health. However, the situation was resolved when Lambert visited Pomare in Wellington to apologise, by agreeing with him that *pakeha* could not insult a Maori chief with impunity.[12]

Lambert returned to Fiji in January 1927, anticipating that the Central Medical School would commence that year. Largely due to Heiser's suggestions, the first year course was now comprised of 78 lectures in physics, chemistry, anatomy and physiology, including dissection and practical demonstrations. Pathology and bacteriology were added to lectures in medicine, surgery, *materia medica* and therapeutics in the second year, with practical work in the hospital in the latter half of the second year. The third year covered eye diseases, obstetrics and childhood diseases. Infant welfare was covered in 12 lectures, but hygiene, medicine and surgery had 39 lectures each. There were also classes in store-keeping and accounting.[12] Although not up to the Johns Hopkins model, the new syllabus was certainly an improvement in the scientific quality of professional education over the old School. The changes accommodated the scientific advances in medicine, including in clinical examination, and basic and laboratory sciences.

It was also a new venture in education by the colonial administration as this had generally been relegated to missions. But it was the Fijian Chiefs who put pressure on the colonial administration for better educational resources, such as the Queen Victoria School at Nasinu, and a scholarship fund to send Fijian boys to Wanganui Technical School in New Zealand. Thus, it was the Council of Chiefs which established a scholarship which was granted to Ratu Jone Dovi Madraiwiwi to study medicine at the Otago Medical School in NZ in 1928.[12]

The changes proposed by Heiser had to be approved by the High Commissioner for the Western Pacific and the other participating Pacific administrations. The Western Pacific High Commission included Fiji, Solomon Islands, Gilbert and Ellice Islands, but Tonga, Western Samoa and Cook Islands were not yet included. One difficulty with the proposal was that Fiji's CMO was to have control over the other island health departments, but a compromise was reached requiring name changes to Central Medical Authority and Medical Adviser to the High Commissioner, which resolved this issue. The New Hebrides Condominium Government (now Vanuatu) was a particularly delicate political problem due to reluctance from the French side.

Initially, the Rockefeller Foundation agreed to contribute a proportion of the total expenditure for the first four years, provided that the High Commissioner for the Western Pacific guaranteed continued funding. The cost of the buildings and equipment was estimated at £8,000 with additional costs of £1,200 for a student dormitory and the land to be donated by Fiji. The annual cost per student, excluding capital expenditure, was estimated to be £90 plus travel costs. Until then, the School had only had part-time teachers but Rockefeller insisted on the appointment of a full-time medical tutor, who would be responsible to the Governor for the administration of the school. There was also provision for an Advisory Board, consisting of the CMO, the Secretary of the Western High Commission, the Resident Medical Officer of the War Memorial Hospital, a representative of the Rockefeller Foundation, and representatives of other participating regional governments when in Suva.[12]

It took until March 1927 before Governor Hutson finally obtained approval from the Colonial Office and May before Rockefeller approved the sum of £15,247 for the maintenance of the school for the initial 4 years. Lambert's proposal for the Central Medical School was not approved by the Rockefeller Foundation until 1926, when it granted US$10,000 that year for public health education in the South Pacific. This was out of a total budget for public health education projects worldwide for the Foundation that year of US$1.5 million.

The funding approval arrived just in time to reverse a Fijian decision against a regional school in which only students from Fiji would have been accepted. The Rockefeller funding for half of the expenses of the new school was conditional on it including students from other Pacific islands. Annie Stuart concludes that:

> the final success of the Central Medical School initiative was a remarkable achievement by Lambert and had taken seven years of planning with difficult negotiation through complex bureaucratic and diplomatic channels.[12]

Central Medical School Opening, 1928

The official opening of the Central Medical School in the Western Pacific was on the 29th of December 1928. Official guests included Sir Maynard Hedstrom, the US Consul, the Secretary of Native Affairs, the Colonial Secretary and his Excellency Sir Eyre Hutson, Governor General of the High Commission. In his opening speech, Hutson acknowledged the key roles of Lambert, the Rockefeller Foundation and Montague in the project, acknowledging Lambert's strong faith and persistent advocacy for the School. In a press interview, Lambert also acknowledged his partnership with Montague and the important financial assistance and support of Queen Salote of Tonga. At the Rockefeller Foundation, Lambert was now seen with some admiration as a 'memorable character' who had successfully challenged Pearce's powerful Division of Medical Education.[12]

The Fiji Council of Chiefs also expressed their gratitude to the Rockefeller Foundation. However, it was not the Rockefeller but the colonial government that was responsible for the ongoing funding of the School. Critics of the choice of the new name for the School pointed out that it did not locate the School geographically (e.g. Pacific Islands) and it was unclear what it was the centre of, as there were no peripheral medical schools.

Fig. 23: CWM Hospital [13]

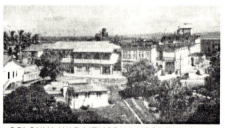

COLONIAL WAR MEMORIAL HOSPITAL, SUVA

The new school opened for the 1929 academic year with 40 students. The new one-storey concrete main building would still mean quite cramped quarters for the 40 students since space was needed to teach pathology, bacteriology, biochemistry and dissection. There was also a new two-storey dormitory for 28 students, a dining room and a house for the full-time tutor.

Construction of the dormitory and classrooms, which had begun in August 1927, was completed before the official opening in late 1928. Unfortunately, this was also the time of the Great Depression, which threatened the region's relative prosperity and reduced Fiji's revenue by around 20%. The resulting financial constraints of health administrations in the region put the viability of the school under threat. Thus, over this period, Cook Islands only sent one student, Solomons halved its quota and Western Samoa decided not to send any students. Lambert used his influence in the region to ensure that the School survived the economic crisis, but it was not until 1935 that Western Samoan students returned, and American Samoa, Nauru and New Hebrides also started sending students for the first time.[12]

Although the tuition fees had been calculated as £90 per student, the mean expenditure was only about £75 per student for the first 5 years of the new school. This was largely due to the cautious budget control of Montague, since Lambert was more extravagant and visionary by nature. The resulting savings were used for improving the dining room and laundry.

Fig. 24: Central Medical School Buildings [13]

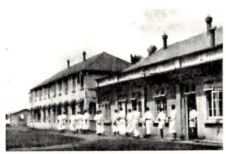
STUDENTS LEAVING LECTURE ROOMS FOR THE SCHOOL HOSTEL

The new school retained the term 'Native Medical Practitioner' (NMPs) for its graduates, with 'Indian Medical Practitioner' used for Fijian Indians. Students were expected to wear a standard traditional *lavalava* and a shirt, and were discouraged from wearing European dress, including shoes and trousers. The school tried to maintain a delicate balance between training medical practitioners in the Western model and retaining native culture so NMPs would return to their communities and still be accepted by the native population. In this regard, the main challenge was Cook Island students who had attended NZ high schools, which had made some of them rather disdainful of native practices.[12] Upon graduation, NMPs were assigned to a district by the government and were not allowed private practice. Their responsibilities included general medical treatment, minor surgery and preventive activities. After six years, NMPs could apply for speciality training in Suva, but there were always accommodation shortages limiting opportunities for further training. Nevertheless, many developed specific expertise in surgery, carrying out surgical procedures when referral was impractical, often assisted by another NMP to administer the anaesthetic.

Lambert was aware of the importance of adequate supervision of NMPs in the field by competent medical officers. This was also the basis of Fiji's agreement with the Foundation to provide a travelling medical officer, although was never implemented due to the financial constraints during the economic depression. Although some medical officers did carry out regular district visits, most spent their time in private practice in relatively wealthy areas such as Nausori where the sugar mill was based. However, Dr Victor McGusty did manage to visit most NMPs in Fiji at least once a year and reported that they were providing a good service to the population and maintaining high standards of professional conduct. When McGusty was promoted to CMO, supervision dropped off again and the travelling medical officer position was only filled in 1936 when the first fully qualified Fijian doctor, Dr Doviverata, returned from New Zealand. So most NMPs did not have regular supervision by a medical officer.[12]

It was taken for granted at the time that only men would become NMPs, with women relegated to nursing. Of course, these sexist attitudes reflected the prevailing views in Europe at that time. Lambert managed to get Rockefeller funding for a European nurse in Fiji to be trained in the modern theory and practice of nursing education in the United States. She returned to Fiji in 1940 and opened a school for native nurses. These nurses were often posted with NMPs to the district, with nurses focusing on maternal and child health. Predictably, this led to many marriages between nurses and NMPs.

The English language was a major difficulty for medical students from Pacific islands, so most were required to take a preliminary course in English before starting the medical course. Melanesian students from New Hebrides and Solomon Islands, in particular, had lower educational standards, so they had difficulty recruiting enough suitable students for the School. Lambert suggested that the best students from Melanesia could do a preparatory year at Queen

Victoria School in Fiji, but this never happened as QVS was seen as a uniquely Fijian institution. Polynesians were generally considered to be superior intellectually to Melanesians at the time, although this was largely related to better educational opportunities. There was considerable rivalry between these Pacific 'ethnic groups' at the school, but Melanesians gradually caught up with the Polynesian students. Sir Maynard Hedstrom offered a gold medal for excellence in public health studies in the senior year, for which there was strong competition. Lambert was acutely aware of the difficulties for students in making the transition from traditional-native to Western-scientific learning, and realised that too demanding a course, such as recommended by Heiser, would result in many students failing.[12]

The old Fiji Medical School had relied exclusively on teaching of NMPs by Suva-based medical officers, the Matron and the CMO on a part-time basis, but the Central Medical School was to have a full-time Principal. The part-time teaching staff were considered a well-qualified and capable group of practitioners and teachers. They included:

1. Dr AHB Pearce, Chief Medical Officer (Obstetrics)
2. Dr Aubrey Montague (Internal Medicine)
3. Dr Thomas Clunie, Medical Superintendent (Surgery)
4. Dr W Foskett, DMO Rewa (Diseases of Children)
5. Dr Regina Roberts (Infant Welfare)
6. Charles Bula, NMP Hospital Dispenser (*Materia Medica*)
7. Dr CHB Thomson, MoH (Ophthalmology)
8. Matron Pankhurst (Demonstrator)
9. various other practitioners and scientists, and
10. Dr Lambert of the Rockefeller (Public Health).

Apparently, Lambert sought the position of Principal, but Fiji appointed David Hoodless in spite of initial resistance from Heiser, who wanted a fully-qualified and more experienced medical officer as Principal. Although there is evidence that Lambert and Hoodless got on well initially, it is notable that Hoodless does not even rate a mention in Lambert's book, despite his key role at the new school.[121] In contrast, Hoodless is very gracious in his mention of Lambert's role in the origin of the School.[13]

David Hoodless

Fig. 25: Hoodless and Lambert (right) [13]

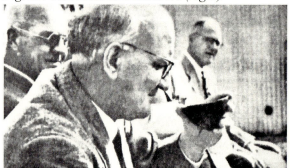 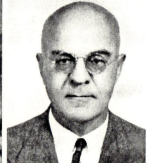

Hoodless was from Sheffield, UK, but had also spent time on his grandfather's farm in Nottinghamshire and with his uncle who ran a dockside inn in Hull, which catered for rugged sailors. So Hoodless was greatly influenced as a child by both farming and tales of the sea. He retained a Yorkshire accent all his life, and his daughter described him as having the Yorkshire quick temper with mood changes from being dour and disagreeable to *bonhomie* and the art of the *raconteur*. He won a scholarship to King's College, London where he obtained a BSc in mathematics in 1909.

In December 1911, he was appointed as Assistant Master at Queen Victoria School in Nasinu (near Suva), Fiji, with an annual salary of £200. This school had been established in 1907, following a request in 1902 by the Council of Chiefs to the Governor to educate Fijian boys who would be future leaders of Fiji in the tradition of English Public Schools. This Queen Victoria School and its 'old boys' played an important role in the history of the medical school in Fiji, both as students and staff members. When Hoodless was appointed, there were

32 students who studied subjects such as English, Pacific History, Typing, Surveying and Tropical Agriculture, so it was oriented to local educational needs.[135]

Hoodless travelled from Liverpool to Vancouver on the *SS Baltic* in the company of Dr Victor McGusty, who was taking up a position in the Colonial Medical Service in Fiji. In 1912, Suva was still a backward town with muddy streets and no electricity, but telephones and inter-island wireless were just being established. With the outbreak of the First World War, Hoodless repeatedly requested home leave to volunteer as a soldier. This was a source of irritation for his colonial superiors, who consequently banished him to the provinces as Acting Headmaster of the Lau Provincial School, where he commenced in July 1915.

He clearly started off on the wrong foot with the local chief, Ratu Finau, who wrote a devastating letter to the Native Commissioner in Suva in September accusing Hoodless of frequenting prostitutes and drinking whisky with natives. The real cause of his concern is probably revealed in the last sentence about Hoodless not having consulted him over school matters as his predecessors had done. This was eventually sorted out and Hoodless settled well into life on Lakemba Island, befriending Gustavus Hennings, a wealthy copra plantation owner on a neighbouring island, whose German ancestry was an issue in this British colony.

After the First World War, Hoodless decided to study medicine in the UK using his accumulated home leave. So in August 1918, he commenced medical studies at Kings College, returning to Fiji in 1921 as Superintendent of Schools. In this role, he arranged for two chiefs' sons, Jone Doviverata and Edward Cakobau, to be sent to Wanganui Technical College in NZ. The former, whose father was the paramount chief Ratu Jone Madraiwiwi, trained in medicine at Otago, later returning to Fiji as a medical officer, and the latter had a distinguished military and political career. In 1923, Hoodless married the newly appointed headmistress of the Suva Girl's Grammar School, who was from NZ. Although she resigned from the school, she did later run a benevolent correspondence school for European children on outlying islands.[135]

By 1928, Hoodless had accumulated enough leave to continue his medical studies at Charing Cross Hospital, London. However, he was unable to graduate as expected due to an episode of serious haemorrhage from a peptic ulcer, which troubled him for much of his life. Despite his failure to complete his medical degree, Hoodless returned to Fiji in 1929 as the first full-time Tutor of the Central Medical School. So the first full-time staff member of the School was himself a medical student, and a second full-time member of staff was not appointed until 1952.[136]

By August 1934, Hoodless had accumulated enough leave to return to Charing Cross Hospital in London to complete his medical degree in 12 months. He successfully completed his training, despite his peptic ulcer flaring up yet again. During Hoodless's absences for study and illness, Lambert tried to help out by doing extra teaching and taking on additional responsibilities in the short term. At this time, the School tried unsuccessfully—the first of a number of attempts—to recruit a medical educationalist from overseas.[12]

Upon his return to Fiji in August 1935 as a fully qualified medical officer, Hoodless was finally appointed as Principal of Central Medical School, since prior to that his title had only been Tutor. His clinical work was at both the Suva Gaol (Jail) and the Public Lunatic Asylum, which he changed the name to Suva Mental Hospital. He visited the jail three times a week, and assigned an Indian Medical Practitioner to be based there. He discovered many cases of scurvy and beriberi among Indian prisoners, so introduced fresh fruit and vegetables into the prison diet. The mental hospital had 80-120 patients, of whom about 60 were hopeless long-stay patients. In addition to two European assistants, the remainder of the staff were all Samoans whom Hoodless found had a special aptitude for caring for the mentally ill.

In 1936, Hoodless was offered the position of Dean of the medical school in Singapore, but turned it down because of concern about the lack of availability of fresh milk for his peptic ulcer. In 1939, the Colonial Office arranged for Hoodless to go on a tour of medical schools, including Singapore, Ceylon, Egypt, Uganda, Senegal and ending up in London on leave. The Second World War broke out while he was at Makarere Medical School in Kampala, so he taught mathematics at the local high school until he could arrange a return passage to NZ and Fiji. However, his duodenal ulcer flared up again in 1943, so he returned to NZ where his wife had been living, since the war in the Pacific had made it unsafe for her and their daughter to stay in Fiji. Hoodless was not coping well without her in Fiji, but had to return to the school in 1944, where he continued to suffer from depression.

In June 1946, his duodenal ulcer bled again and he became seriously ill. His wife managed to catch the 'flying boat' from Auckland to Laucala Bay in Suva, which was an eventful flight when lightning struck the plane and removed the cabin door, exposing her to freezing cold. She contracted pneumonia and joined her husband as an inpatient at CWM Hospital. Hoodless had been due for retirement in 1942, but a replacement for him was found in the person of Dr AS Frater. He retired in Fiji in February 1947, but still helped out with locums at Nadi airport and the Gilbert and Ellice Islands in 1948. His chronic duodenal ulcer eventually perforated causing his death after his retirement to England in 1955.

With the benefit of hindsight, it is likely that Hoodless had *Helicobacter pylori* infection as the underlying cause of his peptic ulcer, which flared up during times of stress. This bacteria causing peptic ulcers was only discovered in 1984 by Warren and Marshall of Perth,[137] so with hindsight a course of combined antibiotics could have cured his ulcers had it been available at the time.

The Curriculum

The 1929 curriculum for the new school continued the 3-year course of the old Fiji Medical School, with the first 6 month subjects including English, chemistry, physics and biology. At the June examinations, any student failing more than one subject was terminated. The next 12 months involved anatomy and physiology, followed by a second set of examinations. The final 18 months was the traditional apprenticeship, with practical work at the hospital in the mornings, and lectures in the afternoon on materia medica (pharmacology), bacteriology, medicine, forensic medicine, surgery, anaesthetics, paediatrics, obstetrics, dietetics and book-keeping.[13] There was also practical instruction from senior European nursing sisters on surgery, midwifery and infant welfare. Public health and post-mortem knowledge and skills were also taught by the Chief Medical Officer and Pathologist, with some students rotating to Makogai for leprosy training. The final examinations included both written and oral assessments at the end of each rotation.

Central Medical School had provision for an Advisory Board to supervise the new curriculum of the school, which included Montague, Lambert, the Medical Superintendent of Colonial War Memorial Hospital, and the acting Colonial Secretary as members. In view of the need for more NMPs, the Board kept the course as 3-years of study. However, on Heiser's visit to Suva in 1928, he recommended more basic science and a review of the curriculum by experienced medical educators. Medical academics from Uganda and Singapore were chosen for the review, as it was felt that British or American reviewers might not understand developing world circumstances and the requirements for training natives in the Pacific.

The key recommendation of the 1929 review was that the course should be increased to 4 years. Although the reviewers felt that there should be more biology in the initial year, they acknowledged that the basic science year was unsuitable for local conditions and too difficult for the students. In response, Dr Clunie, who was the surgical tutor and hospital superintendent at the time, defended the ability of the students, but agreed with the need for an additional year as the new role for NMPs was different from the old 'dresser-dispenser' role which required direct supervision by a medical officer. The aim of the new four year course was to train natives to practice medicine under the distant guidance of a medical officer, but without the need for direct supervision. The recommendations of the review were accepted and the

Advisory Board agreed to establish the 4-year course with a modified curriculum commencing in 1931.[12]

The implications of the new 4 year course placed restrictions on the number of students able to be admitted each year, and this caused serious staffing problems at the War Memorial Hospital, which relied heavily on the students for routine clinical duties and dressings. In 1932, for example, there were only eight senior students instead of the expected 22 students. New accommodation had to be built for additional students, and the original dilapidated dormitories still had to remain in use for students.[12] The old school had accommodated 16 students, but the new Central Medical School increased enrolment to 40 students, of whom half were from Fiji and the other half from other Pacific Islands. The inaugural enrolment included two Fijian Indians, and provided for four students from each of Tonga, Western Samoa, Solomon Islands, and Gilbert & Ellice Islands, and two each from Cook Islands and New Hebrides, with Nauru and American Samoa joining the School from 1935. Once new additional accommodation was built, the number of students increased to 50.

As there were more applicants than places, an entrance examination was instituted in Fiji to prevent favouritism. But the regional differences in educational levels mitigated against a uniform selection procedure, so each administration set its own requirements. Tonga, for example, sent the best student to Australia, while the next best students went to Fiji. Western Samoan medical students tended to come from the medical cadets at Apia hospital. Gilbert and Ellice Islands medical students were selected from government schools without an entrance examination. Medical students from Cook Islands had usually attended high school at Te Aute College in New Zealand, so had good English language skills. According to Hoodless, the educational standards were highest for Fijian, Indian, Tongan, Samoan and Cook Island students, whereas Melanesian and Micronesian students had more difficulty with English and the academic requirements of the course.[13]

The most popular extra-curricular activities for the students at the school were rugby, cricket and the school band. Rugby provoked great rivalry, especially between Fijians and Polynesians. Indeed, ethnic stereotypes are invoked in school reports of the time, contrasting sanguine Polynesians to phlegmatic Melanesians and choleric Micronesians. However, Hoodless claimed that during his years at the School, "there has never been any racial friction or lack of co-operation among the students themselves."[13] The school rugby team competed against other organisations such as the police, winning the shield one year with some players chosen for the all-Fiji team.

The third year of the new school in 1931 saw the first 11 graduates and also inaugurated the new 4 year course, including biology and clinical obstetrics. The graduating class included the first Solomon Islander, 2 Tongans and Cook Islanders and a Gilbert and Ellice Islander and 2 Fijian graduates who were posted to Solomon Islands and New Hebrides, including Mesulame Taveta (see below). The Fijian graduates joined an established NMP service, which consisted of 54 Fijians and 5 Indians. Reports reviewing the performance of NMPs in Fiji documented considerable accomplishments, despite little supervision from European doctors in many cases. Only 15 worked under direct medical officer supervision, with the remainder in charge of dispensaries and smaller provincial hospitals.

In November 1930, Clunie introduced a medical journal for continuing professional education which was called *The Native Medical Practitioner,* which continued until September 1941.[131] It published many practical and interesting review articles on local health issues, including many by NMPs.

Pathology Laboratory

Despite the new buildings for Central Medical School, there was still too little space for the expanded number of students. Lambert described how the full-time Tutor had to use his office as both a classroom and a laboratory. Lectures and dissections in pathology were particularly overcrowded. Consequently, Lambert drew up an ambitious building project which included a new pathological laboratory, and took every opportunity to seek support from wealthy Americans, including his friend Templeton Crocker with whom he had travelled to Rennel and Bellona islands in the Solomons. In 1935, an Australian mining executive donated £5000 for a new children's ward in the hospital which was to be built close to the School. However, Lambert managed to change the site as he felt that the noise would disrupt lectures. According to Stuart, he was rather paranoid about the hospital wanting the School to be moved out of the hospital grounds.[12]

With the economic depression ending, Lambert raised the issue of a new laboratory for the School directly with the Rockefeller Foundation when on leave in New York in 1931. He stressed the importance of a properly equipped bacteriology laboratory, as the current one was grossly inadequate with a non-medically trained bacteriologist who had only limited specialised training. It was particularly inadequate for research into disease aetiology and prevention, which was needed to improve the quality of medical practice and to attract overseas research projects in Fiji.

Such projects had begun quite early in Fiji with research on dysentery and filariasis by the famous Dr Manson-Bahr in 1910,[138] after which a small laboratory was built for the Medical Officer of Health, which was now inadequate for the needs of the new School. Lambert even got his influential American millionaire friend, Templeton Crocker, to write directly to the Foundation in support of the project. Although it was strictly outside of the Foundation's brief (as indeed was the School itself), the new laboratory was approved by the Foundation in October 1934 with a capital grant of US$11,000 once the Fijian government had agreed to maintain it.

On his visit to Fiji in 1935, Heiser reviewed the plans for the new buildings, including a post-mortem theatre which seated the entire student body. He saw the importance of a new laboratory for teaching NMPs bacteriology, pathology and hygiene, but made the appointment of a full-time medically-qualified pathologist and the provision of equipment as conditions for the grant. He also recommended establishing a health centre where NMPs could gain experience in practical hygiene and preventive medicine. This visit ended with Heiser and Lambert travelling to Tonga and Western Samoa to inspect the work of the NMPs there.[12]

Unfortunately for Lambert, the Foundation requirement for a medically-trained pathologist revived awkward issues of professional jealousy in Fiji. Since 1924 the government bacteriologist in Fiji was Mr Campbell, who spent his time doing tasks such as testing water supplies and doing cultures for suspected typhoid cases in the hospital. Despite his lack of medical qualification, he performed his job well, so was sent in 1930 to do the Diploma of Bacteriology at the London School of Hygiene and Tropical Medicine. During his absence, Dr Margaret Kidston of NZ was recruited as his replacement. It was rather progressive at the time for Fiji to employ an expatriate woman, as Queensland and Samoa had refused. Incidentally, Stuart quotes her as describing Lambert as 'a very short-sighted, overweight and jolly man with a great stock of awful stories.'

Upon the return of Campbell, his annual salary had increased to £900, which was higher than most colonial medical officers, provoking resentment among his colleagues. But he built up the bacteriology laboratory for public health investigations and involved himself in some teaching and research, including the training of an NMP in bacteriology. But without a medical degree, he did not satisfy the Foundation's requirements for the new laboratory, so Dr Duncan MacPherson was appointed to head the new laboratory. He had been a medical officer in the Gilbert and Ellice Islands, and had studied public health at Johns Hopkins in Baltimore on a Rockefeller Foundation fellowship, returning to the Pacific in January 1935.[12]

With the arrival of MacPherson, Campbell was informed that his position had been abolished. Predictably, Campbell protested with an appeal to the Secretary of State and Colonial Office insisting on his adequate qualifications and outlining his ideas for bacteriology in Fiji, arguing that the laboratory should remain in the hospital and independent of the medical school, invoking the traditional 'town-gown' conflict. MacPherson was also unhappy with the position, due to his lower salary at the District Medical Officer level of £650 plus £100 allowance, which was less than Campbell and did not recognise his recent American qualification.[12] Undoubtedly, his discontent was also related to his unwitting role in Campbell's dismissal and the ensuing enmity.

There was also confusion about the new laboratory's status as a regional or Fiji donation and its role in hospital pathology, training of NMPs and research. This story is one of the earliest documented episodes of unpleasant medical politics and professional jealousy at the School, which notably only involved expatriates in this instance. The laboratory was opened in April 1930, and in addition to the main laboratory, it included rooms for biochemistry, parasitology, post mortem theatre, offices, library, vaccines, darkroom, sterilisation, storage and an animal house. There was also equipment to assess the chemical composition of native foods.

The Foundation granted £4200 and Fiji another £2000 for the laboratory and the Foundation contributed another £1750 towards equipment. Its running costs were also an issue, so the budget had to be increased for it by both Fiji and the Foundation in 1936.[12] The new laboratory did not live up to expectations as a regional resource or for research into Pacific health problems, such as nutrition and dietetics. Lambert proposed using some of the space in the new building for a nursing school, but this proposal encountered strong political opposition.

Conclusions

In her thesis entitled *Parasites Lost? The Rockefeller Foundation and the Expansion of Health Services in the Colonial South Pacific, 1916 to 1939*,[12] Stuart shows how Lambert played a significant role as the Rockefeller Foundation representative in the region by negotiating with philanthropic organisations, governments, medical departments, the local population and the wider scientific community in his attempt to improve health services, community health and medical training of indigenous peoples. Rockefeller philanthropy towards improving Pacific Islander health allowed colonial governments to extend their administrative control over indigenous populations by providing them with health services. It also allowed Central Medical School to build infrastructure, adopt the biomedical model and become a regional School. The new laboratory was an important new asset for the School allowing it to modernise its curriculum in keeping with new trends in medical education (chapters 4 and 10), but it had also aroused professional rivalries and failed to achieve its regional research mission by the outbreak of the Second World War.

With Lambert's departure from Fiji in 1939, the Foundation direct representation in the Pacific ended. From his retirement, Heiser wrote him a very positive letter about his important contribution to Pacific health. Clunie also praised Lambert in his annual report of the School, even getting photographs of Lambert and JD Rockefeller to hang in the school library. Although some personal animosities had marred his relationships in Fiji in the later years, the success of Central Medical School was a lasting legacy. Lambert and the School were also written up in Harper's magazine in 1937 in a melodramatic article full of inaccuracies, which described the school as "unique in the world's educational institutions".[139] (p377)

Chapter 8

New Guinea and Micronesia

In this chapter we explore other models of medical education in the Pacific Islands region, specifically the experience in Papua New Guinea and the Pacific Basin or Micronesia. This allows us to examine Australia's role in providing medical education for the natives of the Territories of Papua and New Guinea, and the reasons for its refusal to send students to the Central Medical School. Later, we examine how the School failed the Micronesian countries by imposing educational standards which were unsuitable for them, and how they responded to the crisis in human resources for health. So the story is directly relevant to the history of the School in Fiji.

Papua New Guinea

Papua New Guinea (PNG) refers to the eastern part of the island of New Guinea, which was divided in colonial times into 'New Guinea', which was claimed as a colony by Germany in 1884 and handed over to Australia after the First World War, and 'Papua', which was claimed by Britain from 1884 and then handed over to Australia in 1906. Australia progressively brought it under a single colonial administration until PNG gained its independence in 1975. The western part of New Guinea was a Dutch colony which became part of Indonesia in 1963, so is not considered part of the Pacific Islands.

In pre-colonial times, natives were affected by endemic diseases such as yaws, malaria, filariasis and skin diseases such as the fungal infection, *tinea imbricata* (Figs 11-12). But deaths were related less to endemic diseases than to acute infections such as pneumococcal pneumonia and bacillary dysentery. The relative isolation of communities, especially in the highland regions, protected them from epidemic diseases and the altitude limited malaria transmission. Although sorcery was widespread, traditional herbal remedies were not. Curiously, the role of traditional birth attendants hardly developed at all, so women gave birth on their own or with the assistance of a female relative. This contributed to the very high maternal mortality rates, with no experienced elder women to assist in labour and delivery.[140] Although the adult population was generally healthy, it was at the cost of a high infant mortality, short life expectancy and chronic nutritional stunting.

PNG has an extremely rich medical history which has been written and reviewed elsewhere.[141-152] Our aim in this chapter is to tell only the portion of the story which relates to regional medical education, since PNG followed a different path in the training of indigenous health workers from Fiji. However, there is no doubt that the quality of health care services has deteriorated over recent decades.[153-155]

Papua and New Guinea Medical Students

The main issue for our discussion is the failure to send medical students from the Australian Territories of Papua and New Guinea to the new regional Central Medical School. This was a source of great disappointment for Lambert, although the Australian Board of Missions did send two privately-funded Papuan students to the School. The issue was raised several times in the Pacific Island Monthly (PIM) magazine at the time, deriding Australia for its refusal to send students.[156] After the first year of the new course, there was praise from a number of highly respected sources, including the Pacific Health Report for the League of Nations in 1929 by Hermant and Cilento, and also from the renowned Australian medical specialists Sir James Barnett.[12,42] As Cilento, himself, was a key player in the opposition to sending Papua and New Guinea students to the School, this paradox needs to be further explored.

From his experience in both Queensland and New Guinea between 1918-24 with the Rockefeller hookworm project, Lambert was very critical of Australia, linking the decision not to send students to Fiji with the racist 'white Australia' immigration policy. Despite an obvious need for native practitioners, the Australian administration decided that Papuan and New Guinea natives were not yet ready for higher education and were only suited to a more subordinate role as medical orderlies. In New Guinea, the German administration had already trained 'medical *tultuls*' who were continued by the Australian administration, with training in dressing wounds, recognising illnesses requiring hospitalisation, administering treatments under supervision, assisting at operations, and instituting sanitation and quarantine measures.

Although this may sound superficially like NMPs in Fiji, in fact it was a very different role and only involved about 6-12 weeks training of uneducated villagers as *tultuls*, who then returned to their villages with a supply of drugs which was replenished 3-monthly by patrol visits by medical assistants. However, in practice supervisory visits were erratic, with only about 38% of the proposed 4,000 visits taking place in 1938-9, when it was found that 17% of *tultuls* were performing poorly.[140] So they were village health workers, who functioned at a very much more rudimentary level than NMPs.

Lambert contacted Dr Tom Brennan, the Director of Public Health in Rabaul, to propose the NMP model as suitable for New Guinea as a medical school in Rabaul. Even this proposal for a local school on the Fiji model was opposed by the triad of Cumpston, Cilento and Strong who favoured the *tultul* or hospital orderly model of the army rather than 'quasi-medical men'. In 1932-3, the acting Administrator of Papua and Dr Brennan proposed setting up a school for training native medical practitioners locally or even sending students to Fiji, pointing out the success of Solomon Island students from the British Melanesian colony. There was strong opposition to the proposal from Canberra's Department of Territories on the basis of being unworkable due to New Guineans 'low stage of civilisation', so natives should remain at home and train as orderlies. It was a rather patronising perspective.

Nevertheless, Dr Strong devised his own scheme for training primary school leavers as Papuan medical assistants, and trained 12 boys from the village of Hanuabada near Port Moresby. Three batches of them were eventually allowed to go to the School of Public Health and Tropical Medicine in Sydney in 1933-35, but the programme was closed down after that, apparently due to pressure from Australian settlers and missionaries in PNG about their potential exposure to the 'fleshpots of Sydney', despite them having been placed in a highly protective setting.[157] Again, this was an even more patronising viewpoint, leaving suspicions about the real motives.

League of Nations Report, 1929

Between October 1928 and April 1929, the League of Nations Mission conducted a survey of the health conditions of the Melanesian region, including the Territories of Papua and New Guinea under Australian mandate, the British Solomon Islands Protectorate, the Condominium of New Hebrides, the French islands of New Caledonia, and the British Colony of Fiji.[42] Among the issues raised in the report was the medical training of the indigenous populations of these islands, comparing the three year medical practitioner (NMP) model in Fiji to the three months *tultul* scheme in New Guinea. Despite the obvious success of the Suva Medical School over the last 45 years, the Report clearly favoured the Australian *tultul* programme due to the strong views of Cilento. Some of the purported reasons for Australia's refusal to send students from Papua and New Guinea at the time can be surmised from this Hermant and Cilento Report of 1929.

Although superficially the Report appeared to praise the School in Fiji, a closer reading shows it was more a case of 'damning with faint praise'. Regarding the Fiji model, the Report expresses doubts about the acceptance of native practitioners by communities other than their own, where they would be seen as an interloper with no common ground of interest or attachment. Almost certainly, "the repressive activities of the older men and the ignorance and suspicion of the village would stultify his work." The Report continues that "the closest supervision by European supervisors is also necessary to prevent abuse, as yet, even in localities where there is no resistance, as in Fiji itself; while, where the people are opposed to the scheme, native hostility is impervious even to European persuasion, and the problem can only be met by prior native education."[42]

The Report then turned to the native 'medical orderly' model in New Guinea at the time. In 1929, the government budget for medical services of the Territory of New Guinea was high at £52,000 or 18% of total government expenditure for the year. The health services were under the control of the Director of Public Health in Rabaul, with nine other medical officers, ten senior medical assistants and twenty medical assistants with no right of private practice. The Report describes the experience of indigenous medical training in the following terms:

> From every village, a native medical orderly is selected as a medical *tultul* for three months instruction at the native hospital in first aid, the treatment of ulcers, common diseases, sanitation and hygiene. He is then supplied with dressings and simple drugs and sent back to act as *doctor-boy* in his village, but with refresher courses of one to two months periodically ... The chief value of these natives is that they accustom the native mind to the use of European remedies; that they act as an intelligence force for the Department of Public Health; and as a reservoir of partially trained individuals from which it is hoped the most capable may be drawn from time to time for further instruction in the matter of medicine, until ultimately native medical practitioners may be evolved.[42]

The Report expressed no need to upgrade the 2,098 *tultuls* employed in the Australian Territories to medical practitioners for at least another twenty years. It clearly favoured to the model of medical training in New Guinea which relegated natives to the role of 'doctor boys' (medical *tultuls*) with only a few months training. Reading between the lines of the Report, one is left with the feeling that Cilento had a rather condescending view towards Melanesians and did not believe they had the intellectual capacity to study medicine for three years in Fiji. For example, referring to 'doctor-boy', the Report states that "every year he returns for a recapitulatory course, the memory of the native being proverbially short."[42]

Further support in the Report for the view that PNG natives were not yet ready for training as medical practitioners is contained in an Annex written by Dr WM Strong, who was the well respected Chief Medical Officer of Papua. He writes:

> The Papuan native has not yet reached the stage of being a medical practitioner. He can often do, and has often been trained to do, simple dressings, to hand out quinine, etc. In the Chief Medical Officer's office, a native does much of the work of packing and the despatching of drugs to the magisterial stations, etc., and keeps a card index of the issue and receipt of such drugs. A bottle of medicine used to be a panacea for every kind of illness. The universality of yaws in the community and the dramatic action of "914" [salvarsan] and bismuth in many instances has led the natives to have a great faith in injections for anything and everything or for nothing. Consequently, the native readily takes to the use of the needle and is capable of giving both intravenous and intramuscular injections. In one case, a native, who could neither read nor write, gave several hundred injections. Some few native medical assistants have learned to work alone, and to keep the records in quite a satisfactory manner

in the book provided for the purpose. There are now 2,098 trained "*tultuls*" in the territory. This will be for many years the full extent to which natives can be used for medical work—simply as dressers.[42] (Annex 1)

Dr Strong arrived in Papua on an ethnographic expedition in 1904 and stayed on. He was a Cambridge graduate, and was initially appointed as a magistrate but took on a medical role in 1910, eventually becoming Chief Medical Officer and government anthropologist under Governor Hubert Murray. During the 1930s, he organised the training of Papuan medical assistants and by 1936 there were 50 graduates. Their training involved 12 months instruction after primary schooling, and their role was in rural extension work or making up prescribed medications under supervision. The health department also prepared a *Handbook on the treatment and prevention of disease in Papua when medical advice is unobtainable* in 1917, a kind of predecessor of the popular *Where there is no Doctor* by David Werner.[158] By 1930, the *Handbook* contained 29 drugs and 18 dressings with a strong emphasis on purgatives, especially Epsom salts, but the main medical strategies remained quarantine and segregation.

So in spite of general praise for the Fiji School in the Report, it also contains clear evidence of reservations about the NMP model. It reflected Australia's attitude towards native education at the time, with the focus on basic primary education, which would lead to later criticism that it was holding back the Papua and New Guinea indigenous population from early independence by not promoting university education to produce future political leaders.[157] If Cilento had examined the evidence more objectively, he would have seen, firstly, that some Melanesian students from Solomon Islands and New Hebrides had already become successful NMPs through training at the medical school in Fiji and, secondly, that NMPs were readily accepted by indigenous communities, both in Fiji and in other territories of the Western Pacific. Indeed, rather than rejection by communities, it was the non-acceptance by European medical officers which caused most problems for NMPs.

Montague, the Chief Medical Officer of Fiji, also wrote an Annex to the Report in which he pointed out that:

> There has been in existence for forty-five years a system of training native medical students [in Suva] and there are at present forty-seven native medical practitioners in Government employment in Fiji, two in Samoa, two in the Gilbert and Ellice Islands, and one attached to a Methodist Mission in New Guinea. There are also two Indian medical practitioners, trained at the school, in Government employment. An enlarged native medical school [Central Medical School] taking students from Samoa, Tonga, the Cook Islands and the Solomon Islands, as well as Fijian and Indian students, was opened on November 1st, 1928.[42] (Annex 4)

There were political reasons, not discussed in the Report, which emerge in other correspondence to help explain why both Cumpston and Cilento (the Australian Director-General of Health and his Deputy at the time) opposed sending Papuan and New Guinea students to the Central Medical School in Fiji. Australian government officials were concerned about American influence in what was increasingly seen as their sphere of influence, and there was particular suspicion of the motives of Rockefeller Foundation due its links to an American corporation. The Central Medical School was seen by Australian officials as a joint British colonial and American commercial project, and Australia in 1928 was seeking to go its own way in its new Territories. Both Cilento and Cumpston were wary of American influence in Australia's backyard. However, this did not appear to extend to any personal animosity towards Lambert, who had also spoken highly of Cilento when they had met during his hookworm campaign in New Guinea.

The PNG 'Medical Orderly' Model

A later innovation in medical training in New Guinea, as a replacement of the *tultuls,* was the training of native medical assistants or more commonly called aid-post orderlies. They were uneducated villagers who were given a relatively short period of training at one of six schools. They had highly specific responsibilities to treat common conditions such as pneumonia, malaria, dysentery, meningitis, skin conditions and TB, following standard treatment protocols with pictures and under the supervision of visiting medical assistants or doctors. Dr Gunther, the Director of Public Health, established the Aid-Post Orderly Training School to provide basic medical services in the rural areas. By the 1960s, there were 1,400 aid-post orderlies in small rural communities. Thereafter, their role was marginalised and their supplies erratic, so their training was gradually phased out.

Nursing training of locals was entirely in the hands of missions at this time. Yet another group of health workers in New Guinea were the health extension officers (HEOs). In 1972, the House of Assembly called upon the Health Department to integrate government and mission health services. Although missions tended to provide better health services, it was becoming increasingly expensive for them without government assistance and the salaries which they could afford to pay local staff were much lower than for government. Integration occurred as part of the decentralisation of health services to provincial health authorities.

There is also a memo attributed to Cilento which is scathing of the Fiji model, accusing its graduates of being "poor, lacking in initiative . . . and temperamental disabilities that necessitate constant supervision."[140] (p55). The memo also makes condescending remarks about the 'low stage of civilisation' and presumed low intellectual capacity of natives in New Guinea. There were also concerns about the four year separation of medical students from their culture and village if they were sent to Fiji. The opposition of such influential Australian doctors as Cumpston and Cilento put an end to any proposals for native practitioners in the Australian Territories until after their departure from the scene.

An influential contemporary commentator, Daniel Denoon, is scathing of Australia's approach to native medical education at this time:

> In both dependencies [Papua and New Guinea], then, the provision of medical education reflected the fantasies of a small expatriate population surrounded by villagers whose lives were but dimly perceived through a miasma of racist and sexist stereotypes, and whose capacities were neither tested nor significantly stretched. The fact that those few Melanesians who were offered any opportunity whatever . . . responded eagerly and successfully to their new careers, should make us recognise the scale of the opportunity lost.[140](p57)

Although Cilento's condescending views of the natives warrant criticism, it was nevertheless true that Melanesians in the Australian Territories at the time were not nearly as ready for tertiary education as Polynesians and Fijians. However, there is still some significance to the contrast between condescending Australian attitudes to the indigenous population over this time in contrast to the 'enlightened' British colonial leadership of MacGregor and Gordon several decades earlier.

John Gunther

After the Second World War, public health concerns were the top medical priority in Papua and New Guinea when Dr John Gunther was appointed as Director of Public Health. Gunther managed to get a marked increase in the public health budget from £173,191 in 1946-7 to £605,735 in 1948-9.[140] Although only 35 years old at the time of his appointment,

Gunther had a forceful personality with a reputation for blunt speech, but good administrative skills and pragmatic efficiency.[159]

There was a serious shortage of medical staff after the war, with only about five doctors with a clinical role, five Australian nurses and 23 European medical assistants. Gunther recruited more male nurses, dressers and orderlies from Australia and medical assistants from Europe, so that by 1949 there were 93 European Medical Assistants and 32 doctors, although only 18 worked in government service and the rest with missions or other organisations.[159] Gunther also recruited 50 eastern European doctors (e.g. Hungarian, Polish, Ukrainian) whose qualifications were not recognised in Australia, and 40 white female nurses who were only expected to care for white patients.

Gunther expressed frustration at the sexist and racist attitudes of Australian colonial recruitment practices at the time. Denoon is much more positive about the Department of Health's contribution under Gunther as "the centrepiece of welfare colonialism . . . which was thoroughly empirical in seeking the best available methods, judged only by professional criteria . . . unusual only in its élan and its effectiveness."[140] (p75-6)

In 1947 an agreement was finally reached with the Australian government for Papuan students to attend the Central Medical School in Fiji. This was largely driven by the continuing shortage of doctors, difficulties of recruitment of even refugee doctors, and limited educational facilities locally. Gunther was keen to train local doctors, but was restricted by low educational levels and too few high schools. The only feasible course available was the one for Assistant Medical Practitioners (AMPs)—the new name for NMPs—at Central Medical School in Fiji. Seven students were sent to Suva in 1947, but the idiosyncratic selection process meant that one was found to have active TB and some of the others did not have a strong enough educational background to cope with the medical course.

Another group was sent in 1952, and by 1955 there were 26 students in training in various disciplines in Suva, with the last medical graduate in 1966.[23,159] Two notable Fiji medical graduates of this period were Gabriel Gris, who played an important role in the university administration, and Frank Aisi, whose son became PNG's Ambassador to the UN. After this, PNG students attended the new local university medical school in Port Moresby.

Sir Raphael Cilento

Cilento was the son of humble Italian immigrants who arrived in Adelaide in 1856, but apparently he invented illustrious ancestors to counter the disdain of his peers, and had managed to win a place in the Adelaide Medical School in 1914. He was posted with the Australian Army Medical Corps to New Guinea towards the end of the war, which was also the end of the German colonial period. It was from this experience that he became convinced of the importance of diet and nutrition in tropical health. After a year in the Federated Malay States, he returned to New Guinea as Director of Health, completing his MD on the nutritional status of native populations. During this time in the Malay States, he befriended Dr JSC Elkington, who was the Director of Quarantine in the Commonwealth Department of Health.

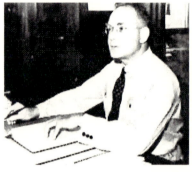

Fig. 26: Sir Raphael Cilento

He completed the Diploma in Tropical Medicine at the London School of Tropical Medicine and Hygiene. Upon winning the medal at his London graduation, Cilento's response to the question of what he would dedicate his life to, was "populating tropical Australia" to which the celebrated Dr Manson-Bahr of the London school replied "not alone, I hope".[160] (p51)

In 1921, he was appointed as a medical officer for tropical health to the Australian Institute of Tropical Health in Townsville. It had been established in 1910 by the Australian Commonwealth government with a threefold aim:

a) to gain knowledge of diseases peculiar to the Australian tropics,
b) to carry out research and teaching, and
c) to investigate whether the tropics is safe for 'the working white race' in Australia.

As discussed above, a distinguished Austrian scientist named Anton Breinl was appointed as inaugural Director of the Institute, recruited from the Liverpool School of Tropical Medicine. But Breinl's career was held back by his move to Australia, mainly because of limited resources, the inability to extend his research activities to New Guinea—since the Institute's aims were restricted at the time to the health of white settlement in the tropics—and because of a combination of professional jealousy and hostility towards a German-speaker after the outbreak of the First World War.

Breinl presented his research findings at a medical congress in 1920, in which he showed that by applying the science of public health, the tropics could be made safe for whites to live and work productively, contrarily to the experience of regions such as West Africa which were still seen as a 'white-man's grave'. Breinl had wished to pursue further the causes of tropical fevers in north Queensland but this work had floundered due to a lack of resources. He resigned the next year, possibly after a conflict with Dr John Cumpston, the Director-General of the Commonwealth Department of Health, under which the Institute had been placed.

Unlike Breinl, Cilento's responsibilities as Director of the Institute did include New Guinea. In the 1920s under Cilento, the Institute continued the tradition of researching tropical medicine from the perspective of making it safe for white settlement of the tropics. This was a serious economic issue for northern Australia at the time as there were doubts about whether whites could adapt to working in this environment. But such views were often conflated with frankly racist views about white superiority, extinction of Aborigines and eugenics. These formed the basis of the controversial 'white Australia' policy in immigration, a policy which Cilento strongly supported.

Modern readers may not appreciate the influence and popularity of the science of eugenics between the wars. The investigation of heredity and Darwin evolutionism were linked to ideas of racial improvement and the prevention of evolutionary degeneration. Francis Galton, who was a cousin of Darwin, was the founder of eugenics and argued for improving the human species through selective breeding. The 'feeble-minded' were seen as a major social problem in contributing to racial degeneration and moral collapse. It was Herbert Spencer, the founder of English sociology, who coined the phrase "survival of the fittest" (not Darwin, as is commonly believed), and he applied the concepts of biological evolution to society. The Nazi 'final solution', among other factors, has changed modern attitudes towards eugenics and social Darwinism. However, the relationship between eugenics, social Darwinism and the Nazi holocaust remains a subject of controversy.

Cilento focused upon the issue of living conditions for white Australians in the tropics, specifically the sugar plantations of north Queensland, publishing in 1925 his major work in a book entitled *The White Man in the Tropics*.[161] Curiously, he denied that the tropical sun caused skin cancer in whites, but then he himself was plagued by skin cancers in later life. He was also strongly opposed to miscegenation, and continued to defend the 'white Australia' policy as essential for white survival as late as 1959 in his Elkington oration, which was a time when Australian attitudes were changing so these views were considered unpalatable by liberal opinion. Other important conditions for successful white survival in the tropics, according to Cilento, were good hygiene and housing standards and lack of exposure to a large native population with a high burden of disease.

After 1930, the Institute was transferred to Sydney as the School of Public Health, so Townsville was without an academic institution for tropical medicine until James Cook University opened a new centre for Tropical Medicine and Health in 1986, which was named the Anton Breinl Centre in his honour. Cilento was knighted in 1935 for his pioneering work on tropical health.

The historian AT Yarwood from the University of New England has accused Cilento of elitism and white supremacist views.[160] This is based upon inappropriate comments in his correspondence, and his work as Director of the Australian Institute of Tropical Medicine on establishing that whites could live and work safely in the tropics as part of the, now discredited, 'white Australia' immigration policy. Yarwood ultimately condemns him for his racist and elitist attitudes, which are certainly evident in his correspondence in which he supported Mussolini, Rhodesia and the Australian League of Rights.[160] These chauvinistic attitudes and pro-eugenics views were not all that atypical at the time, but Cilento continued to express these views publically in later life. It is certainly true that he was elitist, pro-British imperialism and anti-communist. His discredit as a racist seems unfair, and he made important contributions to:

1) tropical medicine (for which he was knighted),
2) government regulation of Queensland doctors (which gained him the ire of the conservative Australian Branch of the British Medical Association), and
3) the United Nations Relief and Rehabilitation Administration after the Second World War.[162]

From his work with Palestinian refugees after the war, he became strongly anti-Zionist, without being anti-Semitic, but showed genuine humanitarianism towards the plight of refugees. Ironically, despite his right wing views, when he was Director-General of Health and Medical Services of Queensland he came into conflict with the conservative British Medical Association representing private medicine whereas he was promoting public salaried medicine against the vested interests of private practitioners. Proud of his Italian heritage, he was described by his biographer as "too articulate, too clever and too publically involved in a broad range of activities outside medicine for completely unqualified acceptance by his colleagues."[163]

John Cumpston

Dr Cumpston was the first Commonwealth Director-General of Health of Australia, occupying the position from 1921 until 1945. He was described as enthusiastic, energetic, hard working, and a strict disciplinarian, but he had difficulty delegating tasks to others. Cilento, who was his deputy for a few years, described him as "a remarkable organizer who felt short of personal greatness by a streak of resistance and mean spiritedness amounting to ruthlessness whenever he met resistance."[164] (p2) Cilento may have been referring to his decisions against the 'tropical frontier' plan and to transfer the Institute to Sydney in 1930, but the financial constraints imposed by the great depression may also have been a factor in his dogmatic approach.

Cumpston, Cilento and Elkington were key figures in Australian public health, and played an important role in wrenching control of medicine away from private vested interests so it could be regulated by the state in the national interest of improving public health by a scientific elite of bureaucrats. Until then, public health had largely been consigned to quarantine and vaccination, but under Cumpston and Cilento it evolved into state-imposed prevention of infectious diseases, and water and sanitation projects.

As we have seen, another major concern of public health was how to make tropical Australia safe for the white population, so they could work productively and remain in good health. In keeping with this 'tropical frontier' strategy, Cilento was sent to New Guinea and later became Director of the Australian Institute of Tropical Medicine in Townsville. Thus, not only did tropical medicine have a profound connection with colonialism, it was also one of the sparks for Australian governmental racism which engendered the infamous white Australia policy. Alison Bashford states that:

> public health and infectious disease control have been part of the legal and technical constitution of 'undesirable' and prohibited entrants: an under-recognised means by which individuals and certain populations have been specifically classified and excluded from the territory and body politic of Australia.[165]

Cumpston and Cilento were among the early architects of this unfortunate Australian legacy.

Similar to Montague and Lambert's plan for a unified Western Pacific medical service, Cumpston promoted the idea of an even wider tropical medical service for Queensland, Northern Territory, New Guinea, Solomon Islands and New Hebrides at the 1923 Pan-Pacific Science Congress in Sydney and 1926 Western Pacific Congress in Melbourne. Cumpston also recommended to Heiser that the Rockefeller Foundation should carry out nutrition surveys in Pacific populations to complement their hookworm studies. He was concerned about world population pressure forcing the South Pacific to be a haven for migration, so wanted them free of disease in preparation for these migrants. This was a bizarre outlook for the Pacific islands—far from Gordon's original vision for the native population, but at least it was better than the view that with population decline, the native populations would become extinct.[12]

A Critique of Tropical Medicine

Donald Denoon at ANU's School of Pacific Studies has been very critical of tropical medicine, writing that tropical medicine training of doctors in London and Liverpool was "the origin of the worst disaster to befall

Melanesians."[140] (p20) He sees two general views of the role of medicine in a developing country, those who focus on standards and see any divergence from Western standards as undesirable, and those who stress standards appropriate to the local situation and see Western standards as inappropriate. The medical course is seen by Denoon as an appropriate blend of both perspectives with an emphasis on community medicine without threatening the ability of graduates to pursue postgraduate qualifications and fellowships in Australia or further afield.[140]

As we have seen, the first medical research centre in Australia was the Australian Institute of Tropical Medicine (AITM) in Townsville opened in 1911, and directed by Anton Breinl and then Sir Ralph Cilento, and then transferred to Sydney in 1930. The focus of the research at AITM was on making the tropics a safe place for Europeans, and the main health threats were seen as the indigenous population and migrant labourers with endemic diseases and poor hygiene. As with the London and Liverpool tropical medicine institutions for British doctors, the AITM became the training centre for doctors going to the Pacific from Australia.

Denoon alleges that tropical medicine blinkered doctors' humanity and competence by focussing them on the delight of technical solutions of narrowly defined problems.[140] He insists further that "it was the Townsville version of tropical medicine which influenced medical policy in New Guinea and Papua through the training of doctors to serve the dependencies, and through research collaboration."[166] He cites William MacGregor as an exception to this trend. His criticism of tropical medicine is mainly aimed at its focus on quarantine and racial segregation instead of instituting public health measures to control diseases of poverty in the native populations.

Denoon blames tropical medicine for causing "the diversion of medical practitioners and planners away from the real causes of infection, towards the diseases falsely defined as tropical."[140](p24) In his view, the Townsville version of tropical medicine was more racist than in London and Liverpool, partly due to the influence of Sir Raphael Cilento. He acknowledges that Australian public opinion and the views of settlers shaped the nature and extent of medical services in the Australian Territories, but considers that the medical profession, the AITM in Townsville and the Rockefeller Foundation were the major forces in driving the tropical medicine model.

He accuses Australia of a lack of interest in the health of the native population, and the health department of being amateurish and incompetent due to insufficient resources. In his view, a reliance on public health knowledge would have served the department of health much better than a focus on tropical infections. In his view, the hookworm and yaws programmes were ineffectual, of marginal significance to the population's health and diverted resources from other more effective measures such as "regulation of diet, the provision of clean water and nutritious food, and the isolation of such non-tropical diseases as tuberculosis."[140] (p51)

Denoon also accuses doctors of being "blinkered by the mental strait-jacket of tropical medicine, which specified only a limited number of diseases and complaints which required the attention of tropical doctors."[140] (p52) Thus, for Denoon, tropical medicine was fixated on exotic conditions, and the diseases which it could treat in New Guinea and Papua were either cosmetic or trivial. It led tropical doctors down the path of intellectually stimulating but therapeutically marginal activities, ignoring the more important conditions which would have responded to more mundane approaches.[166]

In other words, tropical medicine was disease-based instead of being health-based. This is a criticism which is frequently heard about indigenous health in Australia, that 'the biomedical model' has failed and there should be a focus on 'the social determinant of health'. Although Denoon's criticisms are not unfair comments, there is a little of 'being wise after the events' about them. In fact, the pioneers of tropical medicine in Australia such as Cilento, Cumpston and Elkington were strongly public health orientated, so their orientation was very much to population health, not just on tropical diseases.

The yaws and hookworm programmes did have a significant impact, although it as true, as we saw in chapter 6, that some areas had a low hookworm densities and the continuing low hygiene and sanitation standards resulted in only transient benefits from hookworm treatment. However, Rockefeller's hookworm campaigns did attempt to institute sanitation programmes, but the funding of these was left to local Ministries of Health, rather than being funded by Rockefeller, as discusses above.

Another important point in response to Denoon's critique of tropical medicine is that we have learned from recent research just how difficult it is to change health behaviours, particularly in a foreign cultural setting. Probably one of the few success stories has been the anti-smoking campaign in Australia (with the notable exception of the indigenous population in the north), which was only successful when it abandoned preaching the risk of lung cancer and focussed on marketing sexuality ("kiss a non-smoker and taste the difference") like the advertising industry does. Indeed, this has now become the main focus of health promotion. So it is not obvious that a more health-promoting policy to improve the living standards of the native Pacific populations would have had much success at that time.

Despite enormous resources having been expended more recently, there has been minimal success in promoting hygiene, sanitation and dietary change to improve child growth in the developing world, or indeed in promoting diet and exercise to combat obesity in Oceania. So would it have been feasible and successful for colonial powers at the time to have spent more of their health resources on nutrition, hygiene and sanitation programmes? Perhaps, but certainly not at the expense of ignoring the pressing need for basic health services and the few effective medications available, including arsenicals for yaws.

Malaria was another of the tropical diseases, which was absent in Fiji and Polynesia, but decimated the first Europeans to visit New Guinea. One of the first descriptions was by the Russian scientist Mikloucho-Maclay, who was conveyed to the north coast in 1871 and describes his fascinating experience of first contact.[167,168] He survived, but many later missionaries and gold prospectors died of malaria and dysentery.[140] The health status of Papuans around Port Moresby (e.g.

Hanuabada) was abysmal with high rates of malarial splenomegaly, yaws, TB lymphadenitis (scrofula), bacillary dysentery and anaemia in children. The TB prevalence of disease was thought to be 18% in adults in Hanuabada, and malaria was equally an endemic problem. The under-5 mortality for Papua and New Guinea was extraordinarily high, even for the time, at around 400 per 1,000.

As we have seen in chapter 6, the Rockefeller Foundation commenced its hookworm and yaws treatment program with oil of chenopodium and arsenical compound injections, respectively. In 1925-6, there were 49,518 hookworm treatments and 12,643 yaws treatments, the former having a high failure rate and both infections a high relapse rate due to reinfection.[140]

The focus of the post-war health effort was on disease control campaigns, particularly against malaria, TB and leprosy. A number of technical advances and new knowledge acquired during the war made this possible, such as in malaria prophylaxis, mosquito control, new drugs, and especially well organised programmes from the central administration. For example, the war had revealed the efficacy of malaria prophylaxis with existing drugs such as quinine and atabrine, whereas previously they were avoided in natives due to concerns about interfering with natural immunity, which was poorly understood. Similarly, mosquito control and residual DDT spraying of homes had proven effective in Sardinia. DDT was employed, not to kill mosquitoes, but to shorten their life span after biting, when many species of anopheles mosquitoes repose on walls, which if sprayed with DDT ensures that they do not survive the approximately two weeks (variable) required to transmit the disease with another human feed.

The availability of new sulphonamides and penicillin antibiotics provided effective treatment for bacterial infections such as pneumonia, and made quarantine much less important. For TB, there was the BCG vaccination (which was not new), the new drug streptomycin and chest surgery, with 700 operations performed between 1956-66.[140] TB was an introduced disease, with about 2,000 new cases of disease per year in the 1970s, but since then the disease has been completely out of control up to the present. With the recent emergence of HIV/AIDS and multi-resistant TB, its control appears increasingly difficult.[169]

In 1945 when *kuru* was identified in the highlands by one of the refugee doctors from Hungary, Dr Vincent Zigas (who wrote a most entertaining book about it),[170] Gunther tried to limit the research to Australians and the Walter and Eliza Hall Institute in Melbourne.[159] But Carleton Gajdusek from the American National Institute of Health insisted upon access on the basis of New Guinea being a UN Trust Territory, eventually revealing the cause and gaining a Nobel prize in Medicine. Gunther later acknowledged in interviews and a manuscript his mistake in opposing his involvement in the research.[140,159] Warrick Anderson has recently published an interesting account of the kuru story,[142] which is outside the scope of this book.

The Papua New Guinea Medical Journal began publication in 1955, and commenced publishing reputable studies on the health problems of PNG.[144,152] Heywood and Hide reviewed the impact of cash cropping on nutritional status and found better growth in cash cropping families in PNG highlands, compared to traditional subsistence farming.[171]

The author carried out a similar study in Solomon Islands in 1986-87 in 6 urban, rural and remote villages in collaboration with agriculturalists from the University of New England. Like the PNG study, we showed that child growth improved with the better income from cash-cropping, although it might take a few years before the growth benefit was seen in the young children. But even peri-urban families were relatively protected from the effects of inflation and economic recession by still having access to a garden to grow food for consumption. Sadly, this study was never published due to the non-cooperation of the agricultural collaborators, who made it difficult to access to their data for publication despite having agreed to collaborate. The author had similar difficulties in Samoa and the Northern Territory of Australia, because child nutrition is such a sensitive area of research, like sexual health and substance abuse. These are some of the issues that make research difficult in the region.

University of PNG

Not only did the training of indigenous medical practitioners come late to PNG, but a local university was not established until 1966. This was partly related to prevailing attitudes amongst colonial Australians that there was little point in educating natives who were only suited for manual labour in the plantations. This view was not only expressed by the New Guinea Planters' and Traders' Association in 1928, as might be expected, but was given academic credibility by a historian at the University of Sydney who later became Vice-Chancellor.[157] (p11) The Rabaul strike in 1929 confirmed the views of many whites that education of the natives was not only wasteful, but was even dangerous.

A more enlightened perspective, however, was taken by FE Williams, who was the government anthropologist in Papua. He pointed out that this racial prejudice was based upon poor communication due to the language barrier, so the solution was improved English literacy for the native population. Even the enlightened long-serving governor of Papua, Sir Hubert Murray, opposed higher education for natives whom he saw as inferior to whites, and therefore discouraged the emergence of an indigenous educated elite. Although Christianity did invest in schools, some missions were more orientated to saving souls than educational advancement of natives, operating in the vernacular without teaching English.[157] These views were also shared by Cumpston and Cilento, as discussed above, which contributed to their refusal to send students to Central Medical School in Fiji in 1928.

With the advent of PMC Hasluck as Minister for Territories from 1951 to 1965, education of natives achieved higher priority and the budget for education increased from 3.6 to 10.4% of government expenditure and the number of government schools increased from 76 to 417.[157] However, universal primary education was still a long way off as only 10% of children attended school. Thus, in 1947, PNG students were finally sent to Central Medical School in Fiji for training in medicine and dentistry with a total of 20 graduating. In 1960, the

Papuan Medical College in Port Moresby, which had previously trained nurses and medical assistants, commenced a rather innovative four year medical course with a focus on behavioural sciences and three months rural health training in Goroka in the final year. Its first graduating class of three students was in 1964. Under Dr John Gunther, the Public Health Department pursued a vigorous policy of indigenous staff development, aiming to localise all medical positions by 1984.

From 1962, with the critical Foot Report of the Trusteeship Council, the issue of Australia's neglect of higher education in PNG became a key political issue for Australian politicians, the press and the UN.[172] The idea of an ANU-sponsored university college in PNG was strongly promoted, so Hasluck appointed three distinguished commissioners to report on the issue of higher education in PNG. They were Sir George Currie of UWA, Dr John Gunther in PNG and Professor OHK Spate of ANU.[173] The Commission still encountered strong public scepticism about the readiness of PNG for tertiary education in view of the lack of basic education. Nevertheless, the report came out strongly in favour of a university with 172 major recommendations, including the creation of an autonomous University of PNG with the Papuan Medical College as its Faculty of Medicine and a bridging preliminary year after secondary school.

Hasluck had been moved to another portfolio in 1963, and the new Minister for Territories, CE Barnes, and his Secretary, GW Smith, were Country Party politicians who considered the report a radical document. While the government was prevaricating, pressure came from anti-colonial groups who portrayed Australia as preventing PNG from developing an educated elite to delay independence. Finally, in March 1965 the Cabinet approved the establishment of the University.[156]

From 1957-66, Gunther was appointed Assistant Administrator, and later became the foundation Vice-Chancellor of the new university. Despite being an Australian nationalist, he pushed strongly for PNG's independence and was esteemed as the greatest of Australia's post-war colonial public servants by many of the leaders of PNG at independence.[159] In 1962, he wrote that "Australia has met the challenge in New Guinea, and let us be proud of what has been done."[174] (p415)

A dispute erupted between the Minister for Territories, CE Barnes, and UPNG in 1969 regarding the Faculty of Medicine. As this concerned the upgrade of the Papuan Medical College Diploma to University Degree, it has interesting parallels with the FSMed—USP issue in Fiji. The Currie Report had recommended that the Papuan Medical College should remain under the Department of Public Health until 1966, so the University made arrangements to transfer it to the University with the agreement of the Director, Dr R Scragg, following the terms of the Maddocks Report, by Dr Ian Maddocks, who was Dean of the College and was to join the University as Dean of Medicine.

Once again, Minister Barnes procrastinated until December 1969 when he decided to block the merger. The reasons given were financial (it would increase costs) and a denial of university autonomy, but there was also personal animosity towards Gunther. This provoked a hostile reaction from the medical profession, the press and from medical students (denied a degree), so eventually under pressure, Barnes agreed to leave the decision to the Administrator's Executive Council (AEC), which was the embryonic PNG Cabinet, and promptly agreed to the University merger. Maddocks was named the Foundation Dean and Scragg the Professor of Social and Preventive Medicine, which helped reduce friction between Health Department and University.

With the opening of the University of Papua New Guinea, there was a proposal for the Papuan Medical College to join the university with a proper degree course as a Faculty of Medicine. Although the Australian Minister for Territories rejected this as too expensive and too high a standard of education, the reaction in PNG forced him to reconsider and a degree course at the university commenced in 1971. Hence, a medical college offering a Diploma made a successful transition to a Degree course within the University in PNG.

There is an obvious parallel here with Fiji, as—unlike PNG—the new regional university (USP) failed to incorporate the Fiji School of

Medicine around the same time for reasons that are discussed in chapter 11. But the Minister's fears of cost blowouts and lower student numbers proved accurate. The Maddocks Report estimated an annual cost of $9,800 per student, whereas the real cost was $13,000 by 1973. The Papuan Medical College had granted 34 Diplomas between 1965-9, whereas the Faculty had only granted 13 MBBS degrees by 1975, including to 5 expatriates.[157]

Gunther's period as Vice-Chancellor of UPNG was characterised by conflict with the Australian administration over the issues of autonomy and maintaining international academic standards, which Gunther saw as crucial for the university. This early phase of the university also helped transform PNG society, breaking down many of the sex-race taboos, such as mixed marriages to white women, students drinking with white faculty, and an end to 'whites-only' clubs.[157] By promoting greater political awareness and challenging the norms of colonial society, the university helped prepare the way for independence. With self government, a key recommendation of the Gris Committee—one of many reports on higher education—was to cut the tie with Australian academic salaries in 1973. This was designed to help control the costs of higher education and accelerate localisation of academic staff, but it also transformed the characteristics of expatriate staff (e.g. 'missionary' instead of mercenary).

Gabriel Gris was a PNG graduate of FSMed's Assistant Dental Officer programme in 1963, after which he pursued a postgraduate degree in health education at an American university, before being appointed as the head of dental training in the Department of Public Health in Port Moresby. He had participated in a number of influential committees and boards, before chairing the first Gris Committee on academic salaries. Another member of the committee was Ron Crocombe, who was seen by Sir Michael Somare as a critic of Australian colonialism. Crocombe, who died in 2009, was a renown writer on Pacific affairs.[175-177]

The Committee went beyond purely salary issues to recommend a reduction in Australian staff, a denunciation of elitism and 'the hidden curriculum', which in this case was referring to the isolation of students from the realities of PNG. This report engendered a hostile response from academic staff, who were also critical of Crocombe's ideological views and acceding to government wishes in unfairly penalising academics.[157] This resulted in political tensions with militant unionists, whose claims were eventually dismissed by the Mathews Tribunal in November 1974.

In 1974, the Cabinet took a further step by appointing an Academic Salaries Review Committee, although the university did retain some control over salaries through the Office of Higher Education. By way of contrast, up until 2008 the University of the South Pacific in Fiji was still struggling with the issue of academic salaries, and had still not delinked them from those of prestigious universities in developed countries. At the time of the Gris Committee, Crocombe was on the academic staff of USP, which was still supplementing expatriate salaries with inducements, so his anti-colonial rhetoric was seen by some as hypocritical. On the other hand, due to its regional nature and Council structure, USP arguably did manage to maintain greater autonomy than UPNG, where the Cabinet exercised more direct control to ensure it followed national objectives.

The Second Gris Committee (Committee of Enquiry in University Development) included an impressive array of PNG university graduates, and its report emphasised the importance of study-work integration, outreach (extension activities), meeting human resource needs and amalgamation with other tertiary institution to form a truly national university.[157] However, the two Gris Committees and Oldfield Committee in 1973-4 were influential in UPNG taking a different track from USP in avoiding ivory tower elitism and making it more responsive to national objectives outlined in an Eight Point Plan.

The mid-1970s were characterised by student activism and strikes against the Somare government, which was largely seen by the PNG public as an abuse by a privileged group. Somare set up a Commission of Inquiry to investigate the causes of student unrest in 1978. The White Report was a comprehensive review of the University, but on student militants it concluded that they had exploited national politics as part of the Somare-Okuk rivalry, which only encouraged the government to exert stronger control over the university. There was also a strong academic nationalism movement which was pushing for localisation of academic staff. Gris took over as the first local Vice-Chancellor from 1975-77.

The reason for dwelling on this issue of UPNGs experience is as a contrast to Fiji's university experience with USP, particularly in terms of medical education. Of course, there is the obvious difference of UPNG being a national university (although UPNG does have many Solomon Island medical students) whereas USP is a regional multi-national institution. Another difference is the length of the medical course which is four years in PNG *versus* 6 years in Fiji. Although PNG medical students do have a foundation science year at the university prior to commencing medicine, it is really the equivalent of Fiji's Form 7 before high school matriculation. Further, on a population basis, Fiji trains far more doctors than PNG, but PNG does better at retaining them. But an important difference which needs to be underlined is that—in spite of migration of doctors from both countries to Australia and New Zealand—PNG has managed much more successfully to localise both its health services and medical school staff than Fiji. The three key reasons for this difference have been:

1. Greater migration of doctors from Fiji due to the coups
2. Security issues in PNG making Port Moresby an undesirable posting for expatriates
3. Strong promotion of indigenisation of the Health Department and University by the PNG government.

Despite the limitations of the health services in PNG, this policy appears to have worked successfully. On the other hand, Fiji has much better health indicators than PNG as well as a better functioning health service—both public and private.

The Pacific Basin Medical Officers Training Program

Let us now turn briefly to an experiment in medical education in Micronesia. The US-Associated Pacific comprises about 2,100 islands spread over an enormous area of the western Pacific—as large as the continental US—between Hawaii and the Philippines. It includes the three US Territories of Guam, American Samoa and the Commonwealth of the Northern Marianna Islands, and the three 'Freely Associated States' of the Federated States of Micronesia (FSM), Republic of Palau and Republic of the Marshall Islands with a total population in 1994 of 426,923.[178]

Medical students from the Pacific Basin had attended both Fiji School of Medicine (FSMed) and John A Burns School of Medicine at the University of Hawaii. The first Central Medical School medical graduates from the US Pacific had been from American Samoa (1938) and the Trust Territories of the Pacific Islands (1951), but there were none from Guam. There had been a total of 55 medical graduates at FSMed from Micronesian countries up to 1980, but only a few had graduated in the 1970s.[179]

By the 1980s, there was an acute shortage of medical officers in this region, and most of those trained at FSMed were nearing retirement. The educational standards were low, exacerbated by the best students going to the US for secondary school, but even among students accepted into medical school in Hawaii or Suva, there was a high failure rate and successful Hawaii graduates tended to stay in the US. It is probably also true that FSMed had instituted higher academic standards from the 1960s, so there were fewer Micronesian students who were successful.

The first high level attempt to address the serious Micronesian staffing shortage was by Dr Terrence Rogers, Dean of the Hawaii medical school and Dr E. Pretrick, Director of Health of the Trust Territory of the Pacific Islands in 1981, who decided that the best solution was a Micronesian medical programme similar to FSMed's.

So in 1984, the US Public Health Service confirmed the shortage to the US Congress, who funded a 10-year programme under the auspices of the Hawaii medical school due to the strong support of the indigenous Hawaiian Senator Inouye. Apparently the US Surgeon General attempted to transfer the funding to FSMed, but Dr Pretrick convinced him that FSMed had not worked for Micronesian students over the last decade and the program needed to be based locally.[180]

The two initial challenges were the tyranny of distance and the need for a curriculum adapted to local needs, as well as consistent with the low literacy and numeracy skills in the region. An innovative primary care, community health-oriented curriculum was developed with a focus on problem-based learning and self-directed learning with the support of the University of Newcastle, Australia. Students spent half of their time in a supervised clinical setting, but with a focus on dispensaries rather than hospitals.[181]

The five year medical course commenced in January 1987, and the first 15 medical graduates were in 1992. Another innovative aspect of the programme was that the Year 4 and 5 students trained 13 Community Health Assistants for Pohnpei. By 1996 when the programme ceased, there were a total of 68 medical graduates, 81 Assistant Medical Officers (3 years) and 12 Health Assistants (1 year). Students were recruited by local admission boards in each country with an obligation to employ them on graduation, and a total of 160 candidates were selected of whom 140 were enrolled. The 68 medical graduates came from FSM (44), Palau (11), Marshall Islands (6) and American Samoa (7), with none from Guam.[180] Much of the credit for the success of the programme goes to the Director, Dr Greg Dever. He had important support from Jimi Samisoni, Rex Hunton, Jan Prior, Joe Flear, Sitaleki Finau, May Okihiro and Joji Malani, who all joined FSMed subsequently.

With the closure of the Pacific Basin Medical Officers Training Program, the US Institute of Medicine recommended in 1998 that U.S.-Associated Pacific Islands promote training of the primary health care workforce. Consequently, the Hawaii medical school established in

2001 an Area Health Education Center (AHEC) at Palau Community College which coordinated postgraduate and undergraduate courses in General Practice and Public Health taught by the University of Auckland and FSMed's Department of Public Health. The aim was to address the primary care training needs of Micronesia's remote and isolated health workforce.[182,183]

'Off-Shore' Medical Schools

This chapter is about other models of medical education in the region, so would not be complete without mention of private medical school ventures in the Pacific Islands designed to attract fee-paying students, mostly from developed countries in North America, Europe or Oceania. The off-shore model of medical education was initiated in the Caribbean in the 1970s, when the author was a volunteer doctor in St Lucia. It was aimed at the American market of wealthy students who could not gain entry into an American school, so the curriculum was very didactic and oriented to the American examinations.

The market for such schools has expanded exponentially in recent times and is highly competitive with well-informed applicants. There are currently at least 20 off-shore Caribbean medical schools in operation, with China and India also having entered the market more recently. Many reputable universities are also competing for these students, and all Australian medical schools accept up to a third of their students as overseas fee-paying students at a cost of A$35-50,000 per year.

Probably the best established off-shore medical school in the Pacific Islands is the Oceania Medical University in Apia, Samoa.[184] It commenced operations in 2002, and has struggled to get accreditation for its programme, so students are prepared for the Australian AMC or American USMLE exams. It now offers both graduate-entry MD (4 years) and undergraduate MBBS (5 years) programmes. Although it has accepted some Samoan students and pays lip service to producing doctors for the region, it is mostly oriented to Australia, NZ, North

America, Malaysia and the Philippines. In 2009, it inaugurated an electronic Samoan Medical Journal.[185]

The website under Caribbean off-shore medical schools mentions the Pacific Basin University Medical School, PBU-SOM (Federated States of Micronesia which offers a 9-semester MD degree program.[186] Judging from its poor use of English and its dysfunctional website links, it is not likely to be as successful as the earlier Pacific Basin school had been. There have been a certain number of other attempts at setting up off-shore medical schools—notably in Cook Islands and Vanuatu—at least some of which have been criminal scams. With big players now fully engaged in the market and the massive increase in medical students in Australia and New Zealand recently (described by some as a Tsunami), it now makes little sense to use the Pacific Islands as a site for an off-shore medical school.

Chapter 9

The School and its Graduates

Central Medical School after the War

In his presentation on medical education at the Seventh Pacific Science Congress in New Zealand in 1949, Hoodless supported the appropriateness of training native Assistant Medical Practitioners (AMPs) for the Pacific Islands against the prevailing European view that it took 5-6 years at colonial medical schools for the local population to be trained as doctors, such as in Senegal by the French and in Indonesia by the Dutch.[187] He took the example of the Gilbert and Ellice Islands where there were 14 AMPs supervised by a single European doctor, pointing out how no other model would work for such dispersed islands. When Hoodless was asked whether NMPs trained at the School would eventually be able to replace doctors, he replied that:

> the medical training of a Native Medical Practitioner is limited and although very satisfactory so far as it goes, it does not pretend to be a complete medical course. The necessity for fully qualified medical men must always remain.[13]

Hoodless also touched upon nursing training at the NZ Congress, mentioning the existing schools for training native girls in Fiji, Western Samoa, Tonga, Gilbert and Ellice Islands, and pointing out the lack of native nursing schools in Melanesia. He favoured training nurses locally, opposing a central Pacific nursing school like the medical school. He also mentioned the training of native dental practitioners, sanitary inspectors, infant welfare nurses and mosquito control assistants, which was just beginning in Fiji. Finally, he commented on traditional medicine ('bush doctoring') in Fiji, stating that 60% of traditional treatments were useful despite poor hygienic practices, 30% were useless and 10% were definitely harmful. With improved educational levels and access to mass media, native customs were waning. He attributed much of the success of AMPs practice to the effective NAB injections for yaws which had commenced in 1910.[187]

In an appendix to the Congress and separate report, Hoodless provided details of the Central Medical School programme in the late 1940s.[13,187] There were 45 students in the 4 year course, twenty of whom were from Fiji. The annual cost per student for running the School had been £70 per year from 1929-35, increasing to £100 in 1940. Hoodless was the only full-time teacher, but was assisted by nine medical doctors, a pharmacist, laboratory technician and sanitary inspector as honorary lecturers. Students were accepted on the basis of entrance examinations (Fiji, Tonga, Western Samoa) or educational recommendations alone (Melanesia, Nauru, Gilbert and Ellice). They were all required to:

1) have proof of a medical examination (especially to exclude TB)
2) be of good conduct and morals
3) be aged over 17 years, and
4) have reasonable knowledge of English.

The curriculum in 1949 was divided into three parts:

a) six months of chemistry, physics and biology
b) twelve months of anatomy and physiology, and
c) thirty months of medicine, surgery, obstetrics, materia medica, public health, etc., which included mornings at the hospital.

In 1949, there were 161 AMPs in practice, including 80 in Fiji, 23 in Western Samoa, 17 in Tonga, 13 in Gilbert and Ellice Islands, 8 each in Cook and Solomon Islands, 6 in New Hebrides and 3 in Nauru.[187] The principal duties of AMPs included:

1. routine preventive and clinical work (e.g. vaccinations, NAB injections)
2. control of a small district hospital and dispensary
3. acting as auxiliary public health officer (e.g. good sanitation), and
4. enforcing quarantine regulations during epidemics.

Their salaries were divided into three grades, which had increased to a minimum of £120 and maximum of £300 per annum plus free quarters. It was intended that each AMP would be visited several times a year by a European Medical Officer to supervise his work.

In terms of later developments at Central Medical School, Dr Frater was Principal of the School from 1946-53. He was also a Presbyterian minister and had been in a prison camp during the war. In 1952 he decided to divide new admissions to the School into two groups, a 5-year course for those with School Certificate and a 4-year course for those from regional countries. This running of two separate curricula, however, was impractical, so was replaced by a Preliminary Course of English, mathematics and basic sciences which brought regional students up to the level of the School Certificate. In its first 12 years, the 5-year course had 119 graduates, including the first 4 women graduates, who were all Fijians.

Dr AR Edmonds became Principal from 1954-64. The number of hospital consultants involved in part-time teaching increased from two in 1946, to four in 1953 and to ten by 1966.[136] The name of the School was changed to Fiji School of Medicine in 1961, which is dealt with in Part III. To give more of a perspective about the School, we will now recount some of the interesting stories which have been documented about graduates of the School.

Stories of School Graduates

Graduates of the School were a link between European medicine and native culture.[187] This friction between European and indigenous traditions was a stumbling block for some, as they were intermediaries between two worlds, with a foot in each camp.

NMP Geoffrey Kuper, for example, graduated from the School in 1937. He was a Solomon Islander from Santa Anna whose father had been a German trader and his mother a chief's daughter. He served as a coast-watcher during the war, for which he earned a medal, and was appointed to the Advisory Council and became Master of the Melanesian mission ship *Southern Cross*. In 1960, he retired to his community at a relatively young age and entered local government politics. However, despite his wealth and education, he failed to become a traditional 'big man' because he was not a good organiser and never really identified himself as Melanesian, referring to locals as 'natives' and refusing to uphold the traditional way of life.[188] Thus, Kuper illustrates the tension of NMPs assimilating Western biomedical knowledge while retaining traditional cultural credibility, although in his case his half-caste status made it even more difficult.

This intermediate status of NMPs between European and native culture was often tenuous and difficult. Annie Stuart has carried out a case study of one of the NMPs which illustrates some of these issues, so is worth recounting in some detail.[87] Mesulame Taveta was a Fijian from Lau who attended high school at Queen Victoria School and graduated from Central Medical School with the gold medal in December 1931. According to Stuart, he received a high commendation from Lambert as 'the next thing to a qualified physician' and 'knows how to act like a gentleman'. Lambert recounted an incident in which Taveta defeated a Tongan 'about twice his size' in a boxing match. He was a good rugby player, joining both for the school team and also the all-Fiji team. But there was another side to Taveta, as illustrated by an argument with an Australian nurse at CWM Hospital which offended his pride, because he was in the right but 'natives' were not expected to stand up to Europeans.

After graduation, he was sent to the island of Malekula in the New Hebrides. This colony of many small islands and languages had been administered jointly by Britain and France since 1906 in a Condominium with parallel administrations of health and education, which was usually referred to as 'Pandemonium'. There had been a previous Fijian NMPs in Malekula in 1925, named Malakai Veisamasama, who had so ably assisted Lambert in his hookworm project. His posting was due to British concern about depopulation, so he worked at a medical centre for plantation labourers.

The French side of the Condominium was less concerned about this as they had recruited labourers from Indochina (referred to as 'Tonkinese'), many of whom were treated very badly by their French employers. In any case, Malakai found his role difficult and was not given proper support as an NMP, so resigned after 18 months of a 3-year contract. Although promises were made to him about improving the situation, he developed severe malaria with blackwater fever, so returned to Fiji. In addition to helping Lambert for three years, Malakai had also replaced an alcoholic European doctor in Gilbert and Ellice Islands for 6 months, so there was little doubt of his capability. However, the French used this episode as another reason to keep New Hebrides' students from training as NMPs until later. In view of Malekai's difficulties in New Hebrides, both Lambert and Fletcher, the Western Pacific High Commissioner, had advised the British Resident Commissioner in New Hebrides of the need for friendly supervision and warned of the danger of ridicule by European doctors.

Taveta commenced his posting in the capital, Port Vila, with morning rotations to the French hospital and afternoons at the British hospital so both sides could assess him before going to the district. He was rated very highly by both nationalities, with the French CMO, Dr Morin, describing him as an excellent auxiliary doctor of high competence and eager to learn. There were also highly appreciative reports of his medical activities in rural villages, including one tour where 3,604 yaws injections were given as well as many hookworm treatments.[87]

In spite of this auspicious debut, Taveta started drinking heavily with an increasing number of incidents of unruly, inebriated behaviour. It was due to a combination of predisposing factors, including the difficulty of being an islander yet a foreigner in New Hebrides, of still being treated as a native by the British community and of being allowed to drink with French nationals, which was a source of conflict between the dual administrations. Of course, alcoholism was a major problem for isolated Europeans in the Pacific too, but when Taveta was drunk, he lost all inhibitions and became abusive and aggressive.

The French doctors on the island of Malekula, Ortholan and Laporte, were disdainful of Taveta and prevented him from doing his job as a NMP, including activities such as fieldwork, administering drugs and even treating natives. There was ample evidence of racism and contempt from European colleagues, not appreciating that he was also in a foreign country. He was clearly a very capable medical practitioner, but coping with disdainful or contemptuous attitudes is very difficult for anyone. However, correspondence at the time shows that senior colleagues and administrators in both Fiji and New Hebrides were sympathetic to his plight. Clunie in Suva concluded from this that further secondments of NMPs outside of their own country should cease. Lambert subscribed to the view that the danger of alcohol was islanders' lack of 'immunity' to alcohol, which hardly explained the alcohol problems of 'immune' Europeans in the region, as Stuart has pointed out.[87]

The dénouement of the Taveta story is tragic. He was severely reprimanded and punished for his binge drinking, and tried to reform his ways. After finishing his three year contract in January 1935, he planned three months leave on Norfolk Island followed by postgraduate training in Suva. However, his leave was postponed and then he was asked to visit a European patient with severe malaria in a remote part of the island, contracting malaria himself during the three day walk. He treated himself with quinine and rum, leading to blackwater fever. On his return, Dr

Ortholan assumed he was drunk rather than ill so did not admit him to the hospital. He became delirious and died several days later.

Although Ortholan was clearly negligent in his duty of care to a patient and colleague, a French investigation exonerated him, essentially blaming the victim. Taveta's case illustrates the difficulties of NMPs adjusting to being away from their own family and community supports, combined with undermining of their role by European doctors and the peculiar political colonial context of the Condominium. As Stuart elegantly puts it:

> [Taveta] reacted to the tensions and ambiguities of his singular situation—a young inexperienced, lone, Fijian NMP, suddenly exposed to the gamesmanship of rival European powers with different professional expectations and inherently incompatible attitudes to native and colonised people.[87]

Another illustrative example of a later graduate of the School as Assistant Medical Practitioner is Filipe Vulaono. Originally from Lakeba in Lau province, he attended Queen Victoria School and graduated from the 4-year course at Fiji School of Medicine in 1943 as AMP at the age of 21 years.[189]

His first medical posting was in Matuku in southern Lau province in 1944-5, where in addition to a busy medical practice he had to grow his own crops and catch fish for subsistence since his salary was only paid once the district commissioner came on tour. He described giving a blood transfusion for a difficult obstetric delivery, which he had done before in Suva, but it was a first for Matuku. From there, he was posted to Lomaloma in northern Lau from 1945-6, where he describes using the new sulphonamide drugs, which required 4-hourly administration at the time.

His next posting was Naitasiri province on the main island of Viti Levu, where a different dialect was spoken. He found the people very unfriendly initially because of a rumour that he had been promiscuous with the young girls in Lomaloma, so they would not help him prepare the house or clear the ground with a cane knife. But it did not take him long to establish a reputation as a good person and capable medical practitioner. He also carried out a Tuberculin survey using the skin test which had just become available.

From 1948-51, Vulaono was posted to Macuata province in Vanua Levu with an increase in salary to £300 per year. The people of Macuata are renown for house building, but in ancient times there was a tradition of human sacrifice in constructing the chiefly house. Although the practice of *ai vakasobu ni duru* or 'burying a man with the house post' was no longer current, when a chiefly house was ordered to be built for the new doctor, people were still wary, as they had heard too many rumours. Since he had a large district to cover, he resorted to doing house calls and outreach visits on horseback.

In one incident, Vulaono had to remove a tumour from the skull of the paramount chief. In Fijian culture it is strictly forbidden to touch the head of a chief or shed his blood, a very tricky situation for the young Fijian AMP. However, the operation was a great success, and was followed by a traditional ceremony which exonerated him and presented him with a *tabua* (whale tooth).

His next posting was Bua province, also on Vanua Levu, where he stayed from 1951-55. He now had 10 years experience as a qualified doctor, and his salary had risen to £504 per year. But he still had financial worries due to four children with expensive school fees. However, he grew food in the garden, and benefitted from the Fiji custom of giving gifts of food, although this also placed upon him a reciprocal obligation.

He described his visit to Suva in 1953 to see the new Queen, which was a major event for Fiji. From 1956-60 he was posted to Lakemba Hospital in his home province of Lau, returning to Central Medical School in 1961 to do the new Certificate in Public Health. His next postings were in Nadi from 1961-3, on the island of Rotuma from 1964-7 and to Tailevu province in Viti Levu from 1968-76. He planned to retire in 1976, but due to a staffing shortage was sent back to Lakeba to be in charge of the whole Eastern region. His career and multiple postings were fairly typical of graduates at the time.

The Burden of Disease

Both the practice of medicine and the pattern of disease were very different in the Pacific Islands at the time of the Central Medical School from today, so let us consider what medical practice and diseases were like in this setting at the time. According to CMO Montague, the chief causes of morbidity and mortality in Fiji in 1929 were: enteritis and bronchopneumonia of young children (often complicating influenza or whooping-cough), TB, typhoid, pneumonia, dysentery, yaws and filariasis.[42] (Annex 4, p94) Although many of those conditions still occur in the Pacific Islands, there were of course no antibiotics, vaccines or intravenous infusions available to treat them at that time.

Montague's key health objectives were to:

1. prevent the entry of malaria, plague, cholera, typhus and yellow fever
2. provide sanitary latrines
3. reduce fly infestation
4. control hookworm and yaws (for which there were effective treatments)
5. isolate infectious cases of pulmonary tuberculosis
6. apply European medicine to the Fijian and Indian populations, and
7. reduce Fijian infant and child mortality through educating mothers about child welfare.

The Fijian infant mortality rate was still high in 1925 at 172.2 per 1,000 live births. The research priorities were the discovery of a curative treatment for filariasis and the investigation of tertiary yaws, including its relationship to syphilis.

Yaws (Fig 12), which was also called *framboesia*, was described in Cook's 1773 voyage, so it was present before European visits and not due to syphilis.[190] One of the earliest Fijian reports on yaws in the medical literature was in 1901 by an assistant medical officer, who described the features of secondary yaws affecting long bones and the mucous membranes with highly destructive ulcerations, resembling secondary syphilis.[191] This report attributes a high infant mortality and miscarriage rate to yaws, but recognised the cross immunity and clinical differences from venereal syphilis. Montague also reported the high prevalence of yaws, pointing out the consequent rarity of syphilis in indigenous Fijians, but not in Indians.[192] At this time, the treatment of yaws was iodide of potassium, which was only slightly effective against the serious manifestations of the disease, compared to the later salvarsan (NAB) injections.

Lambert also reported his experience in treating yaws in 1929, claiming it was the 'greatest cause of infant mortality'.[132] Yaws was still highly prevalent in Fiji in Lambert's time, affecting 50-75% of the native population and accounting for 18% (329/1825) of hospital admissions in Suva in 1905-7, and 25% (2167/8819) of admissions to provincial hospitals.[193] Although a medical officer in Gilbert and Ellice Islands claimed that both yaws and syphilis were common there, he was clearly confusing cases of secondary yaws and syphilis.[194] So it was considered that yaws protected Fijians from venereal syphilis, although the protection may not have been complete since there was a case report of a Fijian male in Labasa contracting syphilis from an Indian women despite clear evidence of scars of past yaws infection.

The advent of salvarsan for treatment largely eradicated the severe manifestations of yaws. The Rockefeller-supported programmes of mass treatment of yaws virtually eradicated the disease from Samoa in 1923-6, so eradication was initially the aim in Solomon Islands, Vanuatu and Fiji until it was appreciated that treating only symptomatic cases missed the reservoir of latent yaws cases who developed disease later. Since blood tests for yaws were expensive, Lambert recommended treating all children and adolescents up to age 17 years with two doses of salvarsan (NAB solution) at a weekly interval and only symptomatic adults, so the aim changed from eradication to disease control.

Filariasis was another highly prevalent disease in the Pacific Islands. In 1912, Bahr found a prevalence of 27.1% (microfilariae in blood) and another 25.4% affected by the disease but without blood microfilariae, giving a total prevalence of 52.5% among indigenous Fijians.[195] Unlike filariasis in other settings, there was no periodicity of the microfilariae in Fiji. Filariasis affected Indians much less with a microfilariae rate of only 1.4%.[196] The prevalence in 1949 had fallen to 19% with microfilariae, but varying from 12-30% between regions, although the rate of elephantiasis disease was low at under 1%.[197] Although the new drug Hetrazan was available, it was still felt that mosquito control and public education were the mainstays of disease control.

Fijians had a much higher prevalence of TB than Indians, since 40 percent of Fijian deaths in people aged 3-64 years were from TB. This gave them a TB mortality rate of 137 per 100,000 population compared to only 30 for Indians.[198] There were 170 beds for TB cases at Tamavua hospital in 1949, but it was estimated that up to 350 were needed. In 1947, two AMPs were sent to Great Britain for TB training in an attempt to control the disease as only 661 of 1,828 deaths (36.1%) were attended by a doctor or AMP in that year.[198] Although specific treatments such as streptomycin were becoming available, the declining mortality from TB in Europe was related more to improved living standards than to drugs.

There is no unequivocal evidence that leprosy was present in the Pacific prior to the arrival of Europeans. However, by 1891 there were of 400 cases in Fiji, mainly affecting Fijians with an estimated 1% of the population infected. Since the cause was entirely unknown, segregation was the only means of control of the disease at the time. An isolation station was established near Suva Hospital in 1899 for non-Fijians, and then in 1909, the government paid £10,000 for Makogai island, 29 km north-east of Levuka, which was then Fiji's capital.

The establishment of Makogai as a leprosarium for the South Pacific had its origins in the first International Leprosy Congress in Berlin in 1897. One of the resolutions of that congress was that isolation of leprosy sufferers must be practised as far as possible to prevent transmission of the disease. The new Central Lepers' Hospital opened in November 1911 with 40 patients, but by 1919, there had been 423 Fijians and 532 Indians admitted. By 1947, there were 429 cases from Fiji and 274 cases from other Pacific Island countries at Makogai, but the very advanced lepromatous cases with severe crippling were no longer seen due to earlier detection.[199] Western Samoa had also established a small leprosarium, but it transferred all 52 cases to Makogai. Fear of the disease was so great that the colonial government in Fiji ultimately asked the Roman Catholic Church to run the hospital due to resistance within the health services.[200] A medical superintendent was appointed along with two NMPs and some ancillary staff. NMPs also played an important role in detecting leprosy cases and transferring them to Makogai.

The treatment of leprosy at the time involved injections of chaulmoogra oil and camphorated oils with resorcinol, as initiated by Dr VG Heiser in the Philippines.[201] After 2-3 years of twice-weekly injections, some improvements were noted, but no return of sensation in affected nerves. Sulphone drugs became available in Fiji in 1948, and had a dramatic effect on the disease.[202] Makogai offered an ordered, hygienic life with physical activity and a good diet. Heiser visited the leprosarium in 1916 and called it the best leper colony he had seen. But Heiser did not want the Rockefeller Foundation's resources to be used in a campaign against leprosy, because it did not lend itself to scientific progress in the way that hookworm, yellow fever and malaria did. Over 4,500 patients were treated at Makogai with 1,500 deaths. Thus, the Makogai leprosarium was a model for Pacific cooperation within the health services, one which Lambert promoted and wished to extend to other areas but encountered great difficulty in doing so.[12]

Typhoid fever was the most serious acute specific fever in Fiji. There was a 1925 epidemic with 358 cases and 27 deaths, related to an infected Suva water supply. As a consequence, a vaccination programme was commenced which vaccinated about six thousand people a year against typhoid.

Diphtheria occurred periodically but there were no major outbreaks of severe disease despite high carrier rates. However, during the Second World War, soldiers in the Pacific became infected with cutaneous diphtheria, which caused tropical ulcers, but toxic nasopharyngeal infection was rare. It was concluded that children were exposed to the organism cutaneously and acquired immunity to diphtheria, but the slow absorption through skin with attenuated immune response did not lead to the severe manifestations of nasopharyngeal infection with paralysis and myocarditis (heart failure).[203] Epidemics of whooping-cough, however, did account for many deaths among Fijian children.

Of the minor diseases, *Tinea imbricata* was probably the most troublesome and prevalent. It is a kind of chronic ringworm rash caused by the organism *Trychophyton concentricum,* with characteristic concentric and lamellar plaques of scale (Fig 11). It is still highly prevalent on the humid weather coast of Guadalcanal. The treatment at the time was sulphur fumigations, which involved placing patients in a body box with the head protruding, and fumigating it with sulphur. This treatment was cheaper and more effective than iodine and ointments, so was provided at rural hospitals for treatment by the NMPs.[19,193]

A Unified Medical Service

Following the success of the Central Medical School and Makogai Leprosarium, Lambert turned his attention in 1936-39 to his goal of reorganising the medical services in Pacific Islands in order to improve the quality of colonial medical officers. He believed that a central authority for recruitment and management of the health services would be able to attract good doctors to more long-term careers in the region.

Although Fiji had about twenty doctors at the time, the other Pacific groups struggled with usually less than 4 doctors, none of whom had much training in tropical medicine. These were hardship posts due to their remoteness, the loneliness and discomfort, which led to either a rapid turnover or 'burn out' for those who stayed. Lambert's idea was that amalgamating the medical services under a central authority would improve recruitment, training, career prospects and morale. This amalgamation scheme was supported in principle by the smaller states. Although Lambert had the initial support of the Foundation, it was looking to withdraw from the Pacific by 1936.

There were examples of similar schemes in other British colonies in Africa and the Caribbean. It was not a new concept for the region either, as he and Montague had first proposed it in 1923, and Cumpston in Australia had proposed unifying health services in Melanesia and tropical Australia. The issue had no doubt been discussed, at least informally, at the Pacific Islands Health Conference in 1925 and the International Pacific Health Conference of the League of Nations in 1926 where agreements were reached for better coordination of health services such as quarantine and disease notification. In addition, since the establishment of Central Medical School, Fiji's CMO had headed the Central Medical Authority of the Western Pacific High Commission.[12]

Given Lambert's political experience and excellent reputation in the region, one would have supposed that he would also be successful in this venture. However, he encountered strong opposition to centralising regional health services due to vested interests, bureaucratic territoriality, misunderstandings and practical financial difficulties. Stuart suggests that Lambert underestimated the difficulties and by this time had provoked animosity from some key players in Fiji, including Hoodless, McGusty, MacPherson and the new Governor who had replaced Fletcher.[12]

Probably one of the main stumbling blocks to agreement was the controversial issue of private practice and doctor's remuneration. Governor Fletcher opposed private practice by medical officers, including fees from the Colonial Sugar Refining Company, because it reduced state control over medical staff, limited their time for district visits to supervise NMPs and generated professional jealousies. In wealthy areas near the sugar mills, it might increase doctors' incomes by up to £600 per year, so they were not going to give this up without a fight. In compensation for the loss of private practice, the proposal improved the terms and conditions of medical officers, but this raised the ire of other branches of the administration.

By 1934, the proposal had become increasingly controversial due to professional and territorial issues as well as other practical difficulties with the details of the scheme. For example, Lambert was baffled by the complexity of negotiations with Tonga's constitutional monarchy, the New Hebrides condominium, New Zealand's colonial territories, the Rockefeller Foundation in New York, the Colonial Office in London and the Fiji administration in Suva.[12] He was assisted by Montague, who had been appointed CMO in 1922 and continued to work closely with Lambert. Stuart describes it as:

> in some ways a surprising collaboration in that the two men came from quite different backgrounds. Lambert was a forthright, energetic, vocal and pragmatic American in the pursuit of his objectives, whereas Montague was an English colonial public servant who was retiring, unswerving, principled and parsimonious. Nevertheless, together they set about instituting these 3 projects: the central medical school, centralised leprosarium and centralising the Western Pacific medical services into a unified medical service under a director based in Suva.[12]

Lambert presented his proposal for a unified regional medical service in 1923, but he failed to get adequate support from the Governor of Fiji, the Colonial Secretary in London and the Rockefeller Foundation. With the outbreak of another war in Europe in 1939, once again the region faced a severe shortage of doctors. Fiji was left with seven vacant medical officer positions out of 22, and the financial constraints imposed by war meant that there were fewer students in medical training in Suva. With Britain fully occupied with the war, Fiji looked more towards New Zealand for help in the health area.

In July 1945, a conference was held in Suva for New Zealand and Pacific medical administrators, followed in September 1946 by New Zealand, Fiji and the Western Pacific finally signing the agreement that inaugurated the unified South Pacific Health Service. Ironically, this was just four months before Lambert died, and 23 years after he had first suggested amalgamating Pacific health administrations.[12] It followed a New Zealand report by Dr MH Watt, Director-General of Health and Miss MI Lambie, Director of Nursing.

Finally, the Legislative Council of Fiji established a joint Public Health and Medical Service for Fiji and the Western Pacific under a Director-General.[204] It consisted of a Directorate of Public Health and Medical Services in Suva, a new Teaching Hospital in Suva, an enlarged Central Medical School and Nurses Training School, the Central Leper Hospital at Makogai, research laboratories and a joint medical and nursing service with the participation of New Zealand. The main purpose of the South Pacific Health Service was the coordination of health policies and activities, particularly in relation to staffing, research, quarantine and disease reporting.[205]

At the first meeting of the South Pacific Board of Health, the name of Native Medical Practitioner (NMP) was changed to Assistant Medical Practitioner (AMP) for all graduates of Central Medical School. The enlargement proposed for the medical school was an increase from 46 to 80 students, with a capital cost estimate of £56,000. From the perspective of the medical school, the main contribution of this Service was the establishment at the School of the Department of Preventive Medicine which was opened in 1959 by Dr HB Turbott, Director-General of Health in New Zealand. This initiative was co-sponsored by the Fiji Government and Nuffield Foundation, and the new Department offered the 6-month Certificate in Public Health from 1960-69 and a course for Assistant Health Inspectors. Since there was no need for three international health agencies (including SPC and WHO), the South Pacific Health Service ceased when Fiji became independent.

South Pacific Commission

The South Pacific Commission (SPC, later changed to Secretariat of the Pacific Community) was established in 1948 by Australia, France, Netherlands, NZ, UK and USA as a consultative and advisory body for the economic and social development of the non-self governing territories.[205] The Secretariat included a Secretary-General, a deputy and three Executive Officers (later Programme Directors) for health, social and economic development. Health responsibilities included coordination of projects (especially surveys of nutrition and disease), research and technical advice. The Commission also organised meetings of Directors of Medical Services in the region along with technical experts, which proved a useful forum for discussion of regional issues, and these meetings continue to the present in partnership with WHO (WPRO), at which the FSMed Dean has observer status.

Nutrition was one of the early SPC priorities with a focus on weaning foods by their nutritionist, Sheila Malcolm, who carried out dietary surveys and developed food tables for local foods. The newly appointed Inspector-General of the South Pacific Health Board, Dr JCR Buchanan, published a nutrition guide which included tables of food values for local foods, including *palusami* (taro leaves and coconut cream), *vaisalo* (coconut with tapioca), banana soup (banana, coconut and tapioca) and other local weaning foods. The guide was intended for Central Medical School students, who were increasingly called upon to safeguard the nutritional status of Pacific Islanders.[206] As the celebrated Australian geographer Sir Greville Price observed in 1935, " . . . the briefest examination of tropical literature brings home to the student the importance of diet."[207] The Service also promoted nutrition by appointing Susan Parkinson as nutritionist to carry out field work, nutritional education and training of dieticians, which was eventually formalised with the construction of the Department of Nutrition and Dietetics at the FSMed campus in Tamavua, which opened in 1966.

Another priority of SPC was mosquito-borne diseases, with the malariologist Robert Black from the Sydney School of Public Health and Tropical Medicine publishing several SPC monographs and Dr JM Kerrest and later Dr MOT Iyengar in charge of filariasis research. Other early priorities were health education, leprosy, maternal and child health, environmental health and epidemiology. Due to funding constraints, most of the recommendations of these reports were not able to be fully implemented.

Another important role for SPC was promoting regionalism. It organised the first South Pacific Conference of Pacific Island representatives held at Nasinu, Fiji, in April-May 1950, which was one of the first examples of Pacific Island regionalism and was seen by European officials and observers as an 'experiment' in regional cooperation.[208] It was also an attempt to promote regional unity between the diverse cultures of Melanesia, Micronesia and Polynesia and there were low expectations from leaders of these 'undeveloped' societies. It was also an 'experiment' in the sense of being seen as promotion of trusteeship or 'native welfare' principles, a way of promoting self-determination and the demise of empire, and promotion of a sense of regional solidarity among Pacific Islanders in an attempt to keep the region free from Communist influence.

The conference was attended by high-ranking islanders, including Indo-Fijians, and confirmed that Samoans, Tongans and Fijians were much more advanced educationally and in political sophistication than the peoples of Papua New Guinea, Vanuatu and the Solomons. Not only did the conference start to develop a regional identity among islanders who had had hardly any contact until then, but it also showed the European colonisers that islanders would soon be able to run their own affairs. Thus, it was an important debut in regionalism, at a time when the only long-standing regional organisations had been Central Medical School, Makogai leprosarium and some of the Christian missions.

Chapter 10

The Biomedical Model

In chapter 7, we saw the changes to the curriculum with the establishment of Central Medical School in which under Rockefeller influence, basic sciences and laboratory medicine were added to the new course. In this chapter, we will attempt to explain the background developments in medical education which led to these changes. We have called these changes 'the biomedical model', following its use by social scientists and philosophers, who tend to use the term pejoratively in contrast to humanistic or holistic medicine. However, it is an accurate description of the paradigm change in medicine which was occurring at this time.

How did the international developments in medical education affect the School in Fiji? William MacGregor of Fiji was unlikely to have had any exposure to the innovations of the biomedical model when he started the native medical school in Suva because it only started in Glasgow in the 1870s. Similarly, MacGregor's successor at the School, Bolton Corney, would have had even less exposure, as he never attended university at all, only completing a diploma by the apprenticeship model at the traditionalist St Thomas's Hospital in 1874. As discussed in chapter 7, Central Medical School had to wait until 1931 before its new laboratory was constructed with Rockefeller Foundation assistance. Undoubtedly, there had been gradual innovations in what was taught at the old school with the arrival of new colonial medical officers, but the new school brought radical changes to the curriculum. Thus, it was only under the American influence of Lambert and the Rockefeller Foundation that the new biomedical model of medicine, with proper physical examinations, basic sciences and laboratory medicine, was introduced with the new curriculum at the opening of Central Medical School in 1928.

Scientific Laboratory Medicine

As we saw in chapter 4, it was 19th century French medicine which led the developments of examining for clinical signs and making clinico-pathological correlations. Following the Franco-Prussian war in the 1870s, however, the lead was taken on by the new German science which was based upon laboratory medicine. Christopher Lawrence attributes this new development to Germany's idea of the research university, just as France's predominance in clinical signs had been due to the French system of large teaching hospitals in Paris with access to good clinical cases attracting many students.[98]

However, it was German laboratories that took the lead in this transition because medical education was almost exclusively in the hands of university professors rather than medical practitioners. The rise of laboratory medicine had important implications for medical education. Just as the focus on clinical signs had demanded that hospitals invest in facilities for surgery, dissection and anatomy; now the need for laboratories for microscopy, chemistry and bacteriology was an expensive investment, making it difficult for small medical schools to provide facilities for this new kind of scientific medicine. Another important effect of the rise of laboratory medicine was the decreased time available for bedside teaching due to the need for lectures on basic sciences and practical skills in microscopy and biochemistry laboratories. For example, between 1869 and 1901 there was a 52% decrease in time with patients for candidates for medical licensure in Germany due to the focus on laboratory methods.[98]

Modern readers may not appreciate how much resistance there was to this new German and American emphasis on laboratory science in medicine among doctors in Britain early in the 20th century. At the time, there were strong traditions in the medical profession in clinical medicine, and the laboratory was only a minor resource for use in patient management. This was partly due to professional conservatism and aristocratic traditions, but there was also a basic mistrust of the potential erosion of individualism and of American mass production as a result of this new science. Thus, without the direct intervention of the Rockefeller, it is likely that Central Medical School would have had to wait much longer for the biomedical model changes under British colonial influence.

This reticence was especially manifest towards the Rockefeller Foundation's promotion of laboratory medicine as a key element of clinical practice, including the appointment of clinical professors to head academic units. British doctors saw their medical schools and teaching hospital as having rich traditions which should be preserved against these foreign innovations. Lawrence refers to these elite hospital practitioners as 'patricians', and their concerns were not just about medicine but extended to the popular culture of mass consumption, the mass media and decline of the influence of the aristocratic intelligentsia.[98] But this rise of academic medicine and introduction of laboratory sciences into medical practice was part of an extensive reorganization of society which was occurring with industrialisation and commercialisation. In America, medicine was increasingly viewed as a business, and hospitals were compared to factories.

Bonner argues that the reason that neither France nor Britain led the way in laboratory medicine was that university medical schools were too detached from hospital clinical practice.[90] Despite the considerable contributions of scientists such as Claude Bernard, Louis Pasteur and François Magendie in France, none of them had an appointment to a faculty of medicine. In Britain, leading scientists such as Charles Lyell, Charles Babbage and Sir David Brewster (an ancestor after whom the author was named) had called for drastic changes in the teaching of science, following the German methods. However, there was considerable resistance to change delaying the reception of laboratory teaching due to doubts about the utility of laboratory instruction in improving medical practice and resistance by clinicians to basic science teaching in the medical curriculum. The delay in introducing courses in practical chemistry or physiology was due to the additional expenses of equipment, such as microscopes, laboratory space and reagents for student use.

The first medical schools in Britain to take an interest were Edinburgh and University College, London. Britain's industrial revolution made laboratory training more affordable, so students were encouraged to gain practical experience in the laboratory as well as from the wards. This commenced the argument over the ideal balance between basic science and clinical medicine, which resulted in considerable changes to the curriculum.[90] But the industrial revolution also led to poverty, squalor and occupational diseases, resulting in a renewed interest in public health. The recognition of the vicious cycle of poverty and disease due to environmental factors rather than moral decline (e.g. laziness, vice) led to movements for social reform, with the introduction of public health regulations and legislation.[88,97] The comparative history of medical education shows remarkably similar parallel developments and regulatory approaches between Europe and North America, which even influenced medical schools in distant colonies such as Fiji.

Lawrence discerns four major changes in medical education over this period of laboratory medicine:

1) Surgeons and other craft-oriented practitioners in guilds joined with physicians to become a more unified medical profession
2) Medical education became more academic with a combination of university lectures in basic sciences followed by practical training in hospitals
3) The new scientific focus moved from attacking medical superstitions and religious healing to objective observations, laboratory investigations and the experimental method, and
4) State interest in population health led to greater regulation of medical practice with consequent changes in medical school curricula.[209]

Flexner Reports on Medical Education, 1910-12

Abraham Flexner was an American non-medical academic who spent a year at the University of Berlin, which firmly convinced him that German universities were the best in the world.[210] Upon his return to the United States, he wrote a critique of American higher education in 1908, which called for more attention to intellectual matters within colleges and less to extracurricular affairs. This book caught the attention of the Carnegie Corporation, whose philanthropic foundation was about to initiate a major study of medical education in the United States and Canada, so it asked Flexner to carry out the study. It was perhaps no coincidence that his brother Simon was Director of the Rockefeller's Institute of Medical Research, which also had a keen interest in medical education and whose President was Sir William Osler.

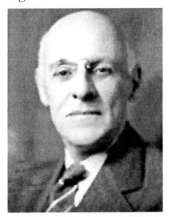

Fig. 27: Abraham Flexner

After two years of extensive research which included site visits to all 155 American and Canadian medical schools, Flexner published a detailed and highly influential report with shocking findings which recommended the closure of 120 of them.[211] His main criticisms related to inadequate facilities, outdated curricula, inadequate admission criteria leading to low standards and unscrupulous proprietary practices aimed at maximising profits. Just as the Russian Sputnik was a wake-up call for American science and the start of the space race in 1957, so Flexner's report acted in a similar way for medical education in America in 1910.

Flexner also reviewed medical education in Europe for the Carnegie Foundation in 1912 and was critical of clinical teaching, promoting a university model with close interaction between medical science, research and clinical practice.[212] After many years with the Rockefeller

Foundation General Education Board, Flexner was appointed head of the new Institute for Advanced Study at Princeton. He argued that the professions needed creative thinkers, promoting conceptual research and curricula of a more intellectual nature instead of a focus on mere job training. He continued to favour the university as an elite 'ivory tower' or 'a community of scholars' which takes a critical approach to the *status quo*, eschewing the predominant focus in America on practical research and training.[210] This concept had its roots in Greek philosophy and Medieval scholasticism rather than German academia. It was briefly popular in certain quarters at universities in the 1960s, but has been overtaken by the commercial orientation of universities at present where 'ivory tower' is clearly a derogatory term.

An important conclusion of Flexner's report on Europe was the absolute dependence of professional teaching in medicine upon the general educational system of the country. He recommended the need for a sound and well conceived system of elementary and secondary schools as a necessary precondition for good professional training. This has reverberations on the situation in the Pacific islands 50 years later, when educational levels and English language skills were major constraints for the regional medical school (FSMed). Medical students required a good educational background which taught them how to think, observe and apply. This also anticipated the current focus on deep learning as opposed to rote learning or factual recall in medical education. But Flexner was mainly arguing for a strong educational background in basic sciences prior to commencing medical school.

Another important recommendation of the report was that the country doctor should be the best trained, because he is far from specialist advice, often without hospital facilities, and works on his own. So he should have a broad and thorough training. Finally and most importantly, Flexner recommended that students entering medical school must to be motivated by the ideal of service rather than by financial gain.[212]

In terms of British medicine, Flexner noted that for a population of around 37 million, there were 27 medical schools with an average annual registration of 513 doctors per year or only a mean of 19 per school. He saw this dispersion of the student body among a large number of medical schools (as in America) as weakening the good institutions while enabling weak schools to survive. He lamented the state of scientific education in England and Scotland, compared to Germany, calling for centralised teaching laboratories of medical science. He gained support for this from the famous Canadian academic, Sir William Osler, who had recently moved from Johns Hopkins to Oxford as Regius Professor of Medicine, and had called for "an invasion of the hospitals by the universities".[90] The Flexner report strongly promoted the Johns Hopkins model of full-time salaried positions for academics at medical schools which would free them from private practice in order to undertake research. This also became the model for the Rockefeller Foundation.

The rise of academic and laboratory medicine in medical education was delayed in Britain as well because clinical teachers depended upon private practice for revenue, which is inimical to research. But, the influential Haldane Commission of 1910-13 gave momentum to the German and Johns Hopkins model of academic medical education in Britain, although it took some time before full-time medical professors with hospital positions were appointed. Soon, universities were seen as appropriate for obtaining a liberal and basic scientific education, prior to commencing clinical training at teaching hospitals. Nevertheless, traditionalist clinicians continued to resist these American-led changes.[117]

The support for this Hopkins model by Rockefeller following the Flexner Report had enormous influence on medical education globally by using their grants to fund laboratories and allied teaching hospitals with full-time medical academics involved in clinical teaching and research. However, this was not a viable model for the many small commercial medical schools in America, nor for the smaller hospital-based schools in England. Medical education became a priority issue for the Foundation when in 1919 they established a Division of Medical Education headed by Dr Richard M. Pearce. As discussed, he was elitist and refused on that basis to fund the Central Medical School in Suva. However, this Division of Rockefeller did support other medical schools in developing countries.

It established the China Medical Board in 1914 which bought the London Missionary Society's medical school in Peking and developed the Peking Union Medical College along the lines of the Hopkins model, which opened in 1921 with 140 students and 67 faculty at a cost of US $11 million as a 'Centre of Medical Excellence'. However, this expensive model of medical education was largely a failure in China and other developing countries where it was introduced. Improved health of the population did not 'trickledown', large urban teaching hospitals consumed most of the health budgets and the school system could often not adequately prepare students for these elite medical schools. At the Peking College, for example, only 166 doctors had graduated by 1937 and only 10 graduates were still in practice in 1942 when Japan invaded and destroyed much of China's infrastructure.

It was these failures of the model in developing countries which led to the focus on primary health care by WHO in the Alma-Ata Declaration of 1978, with a 2-tier medical education scheme, including fully-trained doctors and many primary care practitioners with public health and practical clinical training to meet the urgent health needs of the populations in the developing world.[12] As we will see in the next section, this had a direct influence on Fiji School of Medicine after the 1987 political crisis when the School commenced the Primary Care Practitioner programme with support from WHO and under the leadership of Ian Lewis and Jimi Samisoni. We will also explore the reasons for the failure of this primary care model in Fiji in chapter 11.

In conclusion, following the Paris School's revolution in clinical medicine, the German medical laboratories and microscopes further transformed medicine into the biomedical model, which allowed investigations into the causes of illness. Flexner, who was greatly influenced by German universities, then transformed the model of medical schools into that of Johns Hopkins with full-time professors actively engaged in biomedical research, clinical practice and teaching. The influence of this academic and biomedical model extended as far as Central Medical School in distant Fiji.

PART III

FIJI SCHOOL OF MEDICINE
1961-2010

Chapter 11

The Politics of Transition to a Degree

Fiji School of Medicine

In 1961, the School was renamed the Fiji School of Medicine, which was abbreviated FSM, but was later changed to FSMed to differentiate it from Federated States of Micronesia. Many were unhappy with the new name because it downplayed the School's regional role and was symbolic of the change to a more insular and nationalistic outlook. Nevertheless, FSMed continued to broaden its training activities in paramedical subjects in order to meet the increasingly sophisticated health needs of Fiji and the region.

Dr Archibald Roy Edmonds was Principal of the School from 1954-64, so oversaw the name change. The medical diploma (DSM) had been increased to 5 years in 1952 and the name for graduates changed from Assistant Medical Practitioners (AMPs) to Assistant Medical Officers (AMOs). Recent changes to the course curriculum had been aimed at:

a) providing a stronger basic science foundation
b) placing more emphasis on the social and preventive aspects of medical practice (including environmental sanitation), and
c) better preparing students for later postgraduate studies.[213]

According to Edmonds, the entry requirements for the School were much lower and more variable than for university entry. Very few applicants would have had a suitable academic record for entry to a university medical course in Australia or New Zealand at the time. In Fiji, the minimum entry requirement was the Senior Cambridge School Certificate, and some regional students from the larger islands had five years of high school. However, many of the entrants had received little or no secondary education, and their learning capacity was untested. Many from smaller territories with a limited educational system and poor English language skills entered FSMed after only two years of high school. Those with even less than that could sometimes still enter medicine if they passed a basic entrance examination in English and mathematics. Most students from outside Fiji were required to do a preliminary Foundation Year before starting the medical course, when they studied English, mathematics, physics, chemistry and biology.

The first year of the medical course focused upon the three basic sciences of chemistry, biology and physics with an orientation towards the scientific method in medicine. Although still below the standard of university medical schools, it was a challenging year with a high failure rate. The second year curriculum dealt mostly with anatomy, physiology, histology and biochemistry. Years 3-5 were clinical years as in other medical schools, but there was a greater emphasis on social and preventive medicine at FSMed. In the final year, there was an extensive project on a health survey and final examinations in the clinical disciplines and preventive medicine.

With the opening of a regional University of the South Pacific (USP) in 1968, medical students at FSMed did their Foundation year at USP, which included chemistry, physics, biological and behavioural sciences. This greatly improved the academic standard of students entering second year at FSMed, and this arrangement continued until 1990. However, with the higher standards came a barrier for students from small island states, such as in Micronesia, which ultimately led to the Pacific Basin Medical Officers Training Program in 1986 (chapter 8).

Dr Ken Gilchrist was a Scottish surgeon in Fiji between 1946-49 and 1952-70, and was Principal of the School from 1963-69. During this time at the School, he also taught anatomy, histology and surgery, and was also responsible for the School's first dissecting room. One of his responsibilities was to embalm corpses, which he obtained initially from unclaimed bodies at the hospitals, but later he purchased embalmed bodies from Australia. As there was no air-conditioning of theatres at CWM Hospital, Gilchrest recounts how unpleasant it was in October to November for long operations when he would lose 700g per hour from sweating, sometimes totalling 2 kg weight loss from sweating for a long operation. Gilchrist also visited Makogai Island leprosy station when the treatment of leprosy was still only chaulmoogra oil made from trees grown on the island. There were many advanced cases there, but he did not attempt surgery on deformed limbs.

Gilchrist was also involved in occasional outreach visit to other islands ("mercy runs") by inter-island ships or using the two Medical Department auxiliary ketches, named *Vuniwai* and *Makogai*. Often there was poor communication about the case, so a surgeon was sent as he was more versatile in dealing with either a medical or surgical problem. Since the voyage often took several days, patients had often recovered or died by the time he arrived. Later, when air travel became feasible, it reduced such delays. Gilchrist recounts the story of one trip to Fanning Island in the Gilbert and Ellice Islands to see a European trans-Pacific cable operator. As it ended up being a medical condition, the patient was transferred to Canton Island where he caught a Pan-American flight to Australia.

Gilchrist saw a number of shark bites with teeth embedded in the femur as well as barracuda bites, frequently due to the practice of hanging a string of caught fish around the waist or neck which attracts sharks. One day a pregnant shark entered Suva waterfront and was caught by an old Chinese fisherman who donated the 16 baby sharks to the School for biology class dissections. He recounts another anecdote to illustrate the local sense of humour. It was his habit on ward rounds to wash his hands in a bowl of water with soap and a towel pushed around the ward by the sister. One day he plunged his hands into the bowl only to discover that the water was boiling hot. When he looked up, he found all the patients were under the bedclothes and giggling. He also burst out laughing and there was general mirth at the incident.

Fig. 28: Operating Theatre CWM Hospital.[13]

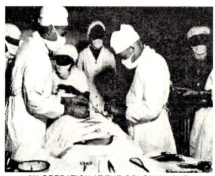

AN OPERATION AT THE COLONIAL WAR MEMORIAL HOSPITAL.
A FINAL-YEAR STUDENT ASSISTS THE SURGEON WHILE AN N.M.P. ACTS AS ANAESTHETIST

There was a strong earthquake in 1953 with a *tsunami*, which struck while Gilchrist was about to commence an operation. As usually happens with earthquakes, everyone tried to run out of the room, including Gilchrist, whose recent war experience made him panic. From the hospital lawn, there was a good view of the tidal wave coming into Suva harbour which caused a few deaths from drowning and left fish stranded in Albert Park, which were quickly picked up for dinner. However, upon returning to theatre, he found the anaesthetist and patient under anaesthesia stuck in the side-room covered with plaster dust from the ceiling.

Gilchrist also recounts several incidents of witchcraft, one form of which is referred to as *vaka draunikau* or casting an evil spell on someone, which usually resulted in deterioration and death. In one desperate case of a Solomon Island woman, he resorted to covering the patient with a horribly smelling bright yellow ointment from head to foot, convincing her that this potion was more powerful than the spell. She went on to recover from an otherwise hopeless prognosis. Interestingly, Gilchrist labels his use of this 'placebo effect' as unethical, and some bioethicists would no doubt condemn any deception of this sort, but most utilitarians (which includes the majority of bioethicists in Western countries) would feel that the end justified the means. Medical practitioners have often resorted to the placebo effect to benefit patients, although generally avoiding confrontational trickery.

A Canadian doctor who visited the School in 1962 described Principal Edmonds as follows:

[He] has boundless energy to concentrate upon this project [the School]. Physically he is of the wiry, energetic type, and from his talk one can readily appreciate the keen interest he takes in the school . . . Dr Edmonds' desk is that of a busy man with a neat docket for his various departments. With a certain pride, he conducts his visitors over the school, which is clean and well kept.[214]

He went on to describe Gilchrist, in the following terms:

Even to his well-trimmed iron-grey beard and open-neck shirt, Dr Gilchrist appears well poised, in love with his work and with life.

Assistant Medical Officers (AMOs)

By 1970, there was a ratio of 36.4 medical practitioners (including AMOs) per 100,000 population for the region (excluding PNG and French territories), based upon an estimated 444 doctors for 1.22 million population. For Fiji alone, the ratio was 41.3 (217 doctors for 526,000 population). But in 1972, there were 48 vacant positions for doctors in the Fiji Ministry of Health and there were only eight new Fiji graduates from FSMed. The staff of FSMed at the time consisted of 17 full-time teachers and tutors, and another 16 part-time hospital consultants to teach a total of 218 students, including 117 in medicine, 22 in dentistry, 14 in dental therapy, and 65 in paramedical sciences (e.g. radiography, laboratory technology, physiotherapy and dietetics). Although only 7% of paramedical students were regional, the majority of the medical students (62%) at this time were from regional countries outside of Fiji.

From 1959-1965, FSMed broadcasted a weekly radio programme of continuing professional education for its AMO graduates, which could be heard in most of the islands, although the quality of sound was poor in some isolated regions. The first broadcast in May 1959 included talks by school tutors on the use of penicillin, environmental hygiene and perforated peptic ulcers. Most of the talks were by expatriate tutors, but the first one by a local graduate was AMO Maciu Salato on health education and school health in August and November 1959. In inaugurating the broadcasts, Fiji's CMO stated that postgraduate training for AMOs would be a priority, including both the new Certificate in Public Health in Tamavua and speciality training in Australia and New Zealand. That year there were eight new Fijian AMOs, bringing the total number in practice in Fiji to 132.

Many of the broadcasts recounted interesting anecdotes. For example, the story is told of a patient at a district hospital who was admitted in a coma following a severe head injury. Upon regaining consciousness after several days, the doctor asked for his notes and became exceedingly angry at the inability of the hospital staff to find them—until the patient in the next bed explained that the patient had used them as tobacco for smoking. The broadcasts were generally well received by AMOs, who asked a total of 43 questions in the first year. By 1960, there were two Fijian-born full-time tutors at the School, namely Ram Singh and Jimi Samisoni, although soon both had taken up positions in Australia. The School lacked an aggressive recruitment policy to attract Pacific Islander academic staff. This was expressed with bitterness by Samisoni, who later returned to a position in the region at the Pacific Basin Medical Officer Training Program, rather than to FSMed. This was a common complaint at developing country institutions during and even after the colonial period, when expatriates received supplemented salaries unavailable to locals.

Another important theme of the broadcasts was tuberculosis (TB). Following 18 months of study in Europe, AMO Panapasa gave a talk in which he pointed out that there were 648 TB notifications that year in Fiji, 74% of whom were indigenous Fijians. AMO Peni Vuiyale gave a talk on miniature chest radiography for TB screening in Fiji, with 90,000 mini-chest films done between 1954-60 in adults over 40 years of age, with a positivity rate for TB of 5%. Following 6-months of training in ophthalmology in Melbourne, AMO Seni Buadromo gave a talk on eye conditions in Fiji.

One of the tutors, Dr Bookless, gave a talk on diphtheria, pointing out that there had never been an epidemic recorded, but there were records of 40 sporadic cases with 8 deaths between 1955-1959. He makes no mention of cutaneous diphtheria as it was not always recognised as a cause of superficial leg ulcers. However, in response to a question about immunisation, Dr Hawley pointed out that "little clinical diphtheria occurs in the Southwest Pacific, probably because of frequent subclinical cutaneous infections." The author experienced an epidemic of limb ulcers in Samoan high school students in 1979 following the cessation of penicillin injections by nurses due to a death from anaphylaxis. Initially assumed to be yaws, the correct diagnosis was only obtained after biopsy of the crater surface in one case, revealing sheets of *Corynebacteria diphtheriae* on microscopy.

New Programmes at FSMed

In 1958 the Nuffield Foundation granted a sum of money to the Fiji Government for the building and equipping of a Department of Social and Preventive Medicine at FSMed's Tamavua campus in Suva. This was opened in June 1959 with three members of academic staff; namely, a lecturer, an AMO (graduate of the School) and a nurse. The outpatient clinic in Tamavua was called the Nuffield Clinic, and final year medical students and postgraduate students were attached to it for training. The Department was also responsible for a dispensary in a low rental housing development in 'Nabua Fijian Settlement' where they taught child welfare, did home visits and implemented domiciliary treatment of tuberculosis. In 1960, the first class of eight AMOs completed the six-month course for the Certificate in Public Health offered by the Department of Social and Preventive Medicine. AMOs for this course were paid a full salary during their studies, as were clinical postgraduate students based at CWM Hospital. This

Public Health certificate became a very popular postgraduate course for AMOs, and there were also refresher courses and special clinical discipline courses available for graduate AMOs.

Since the School's Diploma in Medicine and Surgery (DSM) was not accredited as a medical degree, many FSMed graduates pursued speciality training overseas in order to gain accredited qualifications. However, since most of them did not return to Fiji at the end of training, there was an incentive for the School to introduce its own postgraduate training in clinical disciplines—a Masters Degree in Medicine (MMed)—in an attempt to stem the tide of migrating doctors. For example, among Fiji graduates with DSM in 1988 there were 13 with postgraduate Diplomas or Masters and 16 with Fellowships or Memberships of a College, but only 14 of the 29 were still in Fiji and 41 medical practitioners (15% of the medical workforce) were overseas pursuing postgraduate studies.[215,216] This illustrates that the issue of migrating medical officers dated from at least the 1970s.

An MOH Memorandum in 1972 expressed concern about the number of Indo-Fijian AMOs who were going to India to complete a condensed MBBS instead of continuing with the Ministry. This was clearly a prelude to migration, since there was a lot of dissatisfaction with the administration of the health department. There were eight new interns in 1972, and since paediatrics was done only as part of medicine, Dr Hawley suggested expanding the internship training to two years so other speciality areas could be covered. Although there were 234 medical positions with the Ministry, there were 45 vacancies, meaning only 189 doctors were actually employed, including only 11 consultants and 8 interns.

The Assistant Physiotherapy course started in May 1960 with only three students initially. A new sanitation building was completed behind the Nuffield Clinic in Tamavua in preparation for a new Health Inspectors course in 1961. Students were involved in doing village health surveys every year, but these were often hindered by the villagers' hospitality and expectation that after working hard all day, the student surveyors would dance all night.

Although FSMed had been delivering pharmacy education since 1944, it was not until 1991 that the emphasis changed from pharmacy technicians to pharmacists. There was an anomaly in pharmacy training at FSMed where graduates of the 3-year Certificate course were not allowed to practice as pharmacists in the private sector. However, by 2006, the FSMed Diploma in Pharmacy was held by 46% of pharmacists active in the private sector. However, ten of 68 Fiji pharmacy graduates (15%) had migrated from Fiji between 1993 and 2006.[217]

Table 4: FSMed Teaching Staff, 1972

Principal:	TG Hawley, MB ChB (NZ), DPH (Eng)
Anatomy:	JB Senilagakali, DSM (Fiji)
Biochemistry:	S Reddy, MSc (Otago)
Clinical Medicine:	B Pathik, MB BS (Bombay), MRACP
Dental Surgery:	D Narayan, DSD (Fiji), BDSc (UQld), DDPH (Sydney); Celia Ross, BDS (Birm)
Hygiene:	C Prasad, MRSH, AAIHS PC Qasevakatini, MRSH
Nutrition and Dietetics:	JE Macpherson, Dip HSc (Otago), Cert Diet (NZ)
	S Tikaram, Dip HSc (Otago), Cert Diet. (NZ)
	SV Parkinson, Dip HSc (NZ), MNSc (Cornell)
	R Robinson, BSc, Dip Nutr (London)
Obstetrics and Gyn:	Mary Schramm, BSc, MB BS (Melb), MRCOG
Physiology:	JR Masarei, MD (West Aust), FRCPA
Surgery:	L Goodman, MB BS (Lond.), PRCSE
Social and Preventive Med:	JA Kay, MA, BM, BChir (Oxon), DTM&H, DPH (Lond)
	Laisa M Naivalulevu, DSM (Fiji)

Between 1961-69, the total student enrolment at FSMed increased from 138 to 207 students, and the medical course from 78 to 113, two-thirds of whom were regional students. An increasing proportion of students were women, rising to 20% by 1969. The first four Fijian women had started in 1956, with the first Indo-Fijian women a year later and the first woman in the dental programme in 1967. The female student accommodation in Tamavua was initially very poor, but improved when the former nursing quarters opposite the Tamavua campus became a FSMed dormitory. Distinguished visitors to the school in 1962 included the Lancet editor, Sir Theodore Fox, Professor Bradford Hill of the London School, and Dr Lindsey Davidson from Rhodesia.

There was an interesting incident of mass hysteria in 1968 among 18 adolescent girls at an Indian school near Labasa, manifested as hyperventilation with induced carpo-pedal spasm (tetany).[218] Medical officers investigating the outbreak had little success, but identified the trigger girl and closed the school temporarily, advising parents to keep their daughters at home. The Hindu parents refused to accept medical advice because they believed that their children had been possessed by hostile Fijian spirits of a sacred pool on the edge of the school playground that had been damaged by an Indian bulldozer operator who later died. After being taken to Hindu healers, a Muslim healer with Fijian-derived powers and a Fijian ceremony of appeasement at the pool (including a kava ceremony), the girls eventually recovered. This was a notable incident because the Indian and Fijian communities combined their beliefs and rituals to appease the spirits and, despite an accurate diagnosis, Western medicine was futile.

The USP Fiasco

With the establishment of the new University of the South Pacific (USP), a Committee of three medical academics was asked to assess the following four issues:

- a) the future health training needs in the region
- b) the role of Australia and New Zealand
- c) the FSMed-USP relationship, and
- d) the cost of a proposed university medical school.

This 1971 international mission was chaired by Professor ROH Irvine of Otago, with the two other members from Jamaica and New

South Wales.[219] The Irvine Report made 17 recommendations, which included ceasing the existing DSM diploma after the 1972 intake, and commencing a "new type of medical school" with a 6-year programme leading to the MBBS degree. Although this new course would "benefit from the experience gained in more than 80 years of pioneering work by the Fiji School of Medicine" and would retain its regional focus, there was a clear assumption that FSMed would be phased out and that the new degree course starting in 1973 would be granted by USP via a new School of Health Sciences, which would take over all FSMed assets from the Ministry of Health.

For the period 1970-79, the report recommended a total of 40 medical graduates per year, with 20 from Fiji and 20 from the region, which was reminiscent of the numbers proposed for the founding of Central Medical School 43 years previously. Other important recommendations were for:

a) a 2-year bridging course to upgrade those with the diploma to a degree
b) a new 3-year course for health officers (similar to PNG's Health Extension Officers),
c) an assistant pharmacists course, and
d) an upgrade of dentistry to a degree course.

USP's reaction to the Irvine report varied from apathy to frank hostility. The powerful University Grants Committee expressed the view that no USP funds should be expended on the medical school initiative. The USP Council appointed an *ad hoc* committee which never met, but eventually the Council acquiesced to appointing a WHO consultant to advise on implementation of the report. This eventually became the Boelen Report and WHO Master Plan of 1985.[220]

Basically, USP was reluctant to embark upon a new expensive course without guarantees of substantial additional funding. A Memorandum of Understanding (MoU) between the Government and the University was eventually signed after a decade of procrastination since the Irvine Report, which agreed to an *external* 5-year MBBS degree granted by USP but run by the School, so that USP would not have any financial responsibility. The MoU made no mention of any eventual amalgamation between USP and FSMed.[221] FSMed staff had the option of retaining their position in the Fiji Public Service.

This 1981 MoU included the recommendations of the Conjoint Committee, which had included five USP representatives and four government representatives, including the Principal of FSMed, Dr B Pathik, and the Permanent Secretary of Health, Dr Jona Senilagakali, who had previously taught anatomy at the School. The university's two chief concerns were the need for improved academic standards and more resources for the upgrade to a new university medical degree course. Although there was an implicit understanding in some quarters that FSMed would ultimately become part of USP, this was not officially sanctioned and both parties seemed reluctant partners for amalgamation.

The Conjoint Committee had specified that the 5-year degree was to be external to USP, but require the USP Foundation Year or equivalent. The initial MBBS intake in 1982 included 36 students, of which only nine were regional students (25%), which was a significant reduction in the regional proportion from the 1960-70s. The administrative structure of the School was to include a 15-member Advisory Council, an Academic Board and a Conjoint Council with university and government representatives. The Principal (later Head of School and then Dean) of FSMed was responsible to the Advisory Council, but reported to USP Senate on academic matters and to the Permanent Secretary of Health on administrative matters. Thus, the School remained part of the Ministry of Health, and it would take another 15 years before it would finally gain autonomy. The report also required external examiners to be appointed in consultation with USP, and expressed concern about the inadequate staffing and facilities at FSMed for a new degree course.

The 5-year curriculum for the new MBBS degree was prepared by the Principal and approved by the Curriculum Review Committee.

It envisaged teaching medical sciences in years 1-3 and clinical medicine in years 4-5, and—although not particularly innovative—it did strengthen behavioural sciences in the early years and include 6 weeks of community medicine and 16 weeks at Lautoka Hospital in the final year. But a new curriculum had to be drafted in 1987 (Table 5) by the new Head of School, Professor Harry Lander, and Chair of the Curriculum Committee, Dr R Gyaneshwar, when the MBBS Degree was increased to 6-years on the advice of David Newble and the Biddulph Report.[179]

Table 5: MBBS 6-year Curriculum, 1987

Year 1
Semester I: Biology, Chemistry, Physics, Statistics, Psychology
Semester II: Anatomy, Biochemistry, Physiology, Human Development

Year 2
I: Anatomy, Biochemistry, Physiology, Social and Preventive Medicine
II: Anatomy, Physiology, Social and Preventive Medicine

Year 3
I: General Pathology, Microbiology, Immunology, Epidemiology, Pharmacy/Pharmacology Behavioural Science
II: Systemic Pathology, Microbiology, Immunology, Epidemiology, Community Health Pharmacology, Introduction to Clinical Skills

Year 4
3 Blocks (12 weeks each) of Medicine, Surgery, Paediatrics

Year 5
3 Blocks (12 weeks) of Psychiatry, Obstetrics and Gynaecology, Primary Health Care and General Practice

Year 6
Clinical attachments to various hospitals (5 weeks each): General Out-patients Department, Medicine, Obstetrics and Gynaecology, Paediatrics, Pathology Laboratory, Primary Health Care and General Practice, Psychiatry, Surgery (including ENT, Anaesthesia)

The Biddulph Committee was appointed at the request of USP Senate to investigate the academic standard of the proposed MBBS to be offered through USP and generally the USP-FSMed relationship. Dr John Biddulph was Professor of Paediatrics at the University of PNG Medical School and was joined by two other academics from Auckland and Hawaii.[222] The report concluded that the new MBBS degree must be increased to 6 years and required additional funding to meet basic international standards, as USP had been arguing all along. The staffing restrictions imposed by the Ministry of Health on the School was at odds with the 1981 MoU and had seriously hindered the development of the teaching programme.

The report was particularly scathing of the control of recruitment and conditions of employment by the Ministry of Health and Public Service Commission. There were numerous examples of inappropriate and incompetent recruitment practices, such as when candidates were interviewed with no clinical colleagues on the panel and long delays in the appointment process and in obtaining visas and permits. The heavy demand on teaching made staff development activities and research impossible. Additionally, the lack of university affiliation made it difficult to recruit high quality academic staff. The Committee recommended that USP take over from the Ministry of Health the financial, administrative and recruitment responsibilities of the medical course as soon as possible, which was reminiscent of the Irvine Report of 14 years ago and the equivalent had already happened at UPNG.

In terms of academic standards and the quality of the students, Biddulph felt that their knowledge of the pathophysiological basis of disease was weak. The evidence for this was 12 failures out of 36 in the basic sciences exams in 1983 and repeated comments about this by external examiners from 1982-84. Although examiners had commended the practical skills of the students and the high quality of some students, they considered many students very weak with great variability in the standard. The report called for more clinical exposure in the initial 3 years of the course, and stated that the current 4th year class would not reach the standard required by the MBBS degree by the end of 5th year. It also recommended that the new 6th year students should be paid an allowance for their clinical responsibility, but this was never implemented.

David Newble was Reader in Medical Education in Adelaide, and was asked by FSMed to advise on curriculum issues for the new medical course, with visits in October 1984 and August 1985. He made a number of important recommendations, including that:

a) FSMed be incorporated into USP as soon as possible,
b) a curriculum committee with student membership be established,
c) a problem-based learning approach be adopted,
d) the number of clinical appointments be increased,
e) an assessment working party report back on examination processes, and
f) student admission selection policies be reviewed.

Admission criteria were specified as a C grade in chemistry, physics, biology and communication and study skill of the USP Foundation Programme or 250 out of 400 in the Fiji 7th Form examination, including English and at least 60% in biology, chemistry and physics. Tuition fees for the MBBS were FJ$5,107 which included $1,905 for board and lodging. Fiji students were bonded by the Public Service Commission for 5 years, but were not guaranteed a government appointment on graduation.

In March 1986, the South Pacific Commission (SPC) held its 11th meeting of heads of health services in Noumea on the subject of training of health professionals in the South Pacific. The report strongly recommended that postgraduate training should be carried out as much as possible in the region to ensure training was appropriate and staff were retained in the region. Its recommendation #14 specifically endorsed the amalgamation of FSMed and USP with upgrading of staffing and facilities. It also recommended rationalisation of dental training by "largely confining" it to the University of PNG. This would certainly have avoided a lot of later hassles, if it had been implemented (see chapter 15).

There was some opposition to the upgrade to a degree course. In a speech at a Regional Medical Education Conference for the Western Pacific in 1988, a Fijian doctor opposed the new 6-year MBBS as an imported USP degree which no longer catered to the needs of the predominantly rural population of the region.[223] However, this was not the consensus view among health professionals.

The medical degree course was increased to six years, and the Diploma programmes in Medicine and Dentistry were phased out, but there was no action on the amalgamation issue or phasing out of dental training. Paramedical programmes were shifted to Tamavua so medical students could be near CWM hospital at the Hoodless campus. Concerns, however, remained about the high failure rate of around 40% in the basic science years in the new degree course. In December 1982 a motion in the Fijian Senate expressed concern at the high rate of failure of ethnic Fijian students at the School, requesting an investigation. In the ensuing debate several senators blamed the current Indo-Fijian Principal, Dr Bhupendra Pathik, and he was arbitrarily dismissed by the Permanent Secretary of Health. However, he appealed against the decision and was reinstated by the Public Service Commission.

The subsequent investigation exonerated him, but he was still sidelined by being sent on study leave while the Public Service Commission arranged a review of the School by a team from the University of Adelaide.[224,225] This inquiry also revealed considerable resistance to the MBBS degree within the Ministry of Health and highlighted the need for improved recruitment processes and better facilities for the School. This issue of high failure rates was a real concern at the time, but raising it in a context of ethnicity further polarised views within the School, which was not a good omen.

By 1986, there were 133 students in the new MBBS programme (years 1-5), including 34 indigenous Fijians, 57 Indo-Fijians and 7 others from Fiji. Only 26% were regional students and 24% were female. There were also 99 other (non-MBBS) students at FSMed, of which 35% were regional, which was the first time that there was a higher proportion of regional students in the non-medical courses than in medicine. Clearly, the regional commitment of the School had diminished since the days of Central Medical School or even since the 1970s, which was partly related to higher academic standards.

There were 11 full-time academic medical staff and 9 paramedical staff at FSMed. The Cole Report by three WHO consultants and medical school deans considered the staffing shortages as:

> the greatest single source of obstruction to the well-being of the staff and thus the morale of the School, and ultimately the quality of the degree. If Fiji politicians want a medical degree from their regional USP they must bravely accept that the FSM staff must be treated in a special manner, more appropriate to a university-style institution.[226]

There were also concerns about the long delays in appointments, immigration bureaucracy, spouses unable to work and the inequity of salary supplements by Australian aid funding leading to a 2-salary structure of expatriates *vs* locals. Of particular concern was the absence of 17% of local staff overseas seeking further qualifications, including Australasian Fellowships which were deemed inappropriate for the region and had very high failure rates for Pacific Islanders. Indeed, the pass rate for Australian and NZ graduates in the FRACP (physicians) written and clinical exams at the time was only around 33%, so islanders were severely disadvantaged in this competition.

Dr Charles Boelen was the Regional Adviser in Health Manpower Development at the WHO Office for the Western Pacific in Manila, and his report followed a 5-day visit to Fiji in February 1985 to develop a long-term plan for FSMed.[220] At the time, the Fiji Cabinet, Ministry of Health and Public Service Commission all accepted in principle the proposal for FSMed to join USP as a new medical faculty. This option was also favoured by the Head of School, Prof Harry Lander, as a means of improving staff recruitment, attracting external funding and improving the quality of medical education. There was also a threat that USP might withdraw accreditation of the new MBBS degree if

FSMed did not join USP, in spite of USP's refusal to amalgamate on financial grounds. As it turned out, USP seemed to lose interest in the new medical degree programme and did not even send official representation to the first MBBS graduation.

The WHO master plan for the development of FSMed was—as is so often the case with WHO documents—very strong on rhetoric, reflecting the Declaration of Alma-Ata from the 1978 International Conference on Primary Health Care.[227] The key jargon terms were: meeting the specific health needs of the South Pacific community, primary health care philosophy, community-based medical school, using appropriate educational methodology and technology, problem-solving learning, student-centred approach, and implementation of national health manpower development plans.

On a more concrete note, the plan did commit WHO to supporting the school with two long-term staff in medical education and community medicine, short-term consultants for 1-2 months per year, and strengthening of a health learning resources centre. The master plan consisted of a reorientation of the curriculum towards community health, improvement in the learning process, acquisition of appropriate learning resources and training facilities, control of students' performances, improvement in the quality of care in the teaching hospital and health centres and sharing of human and material resources with other health training institutions. The plan was welcomed by all parties.

Despite the numerous external reports and recommendations for amalgamation, the main barrier remained funding. USP was reluctant to recommend an increase in the regional governments' grants to USP for a new medical faculty. The Fiji government, for that matter, might also refuse to increase its subsidy of USP as it was the largest grant and was already funding FSMed. It did not favour a large increase in its budget for the medical school just so it could be part of USP. A figure of FJ$6 million additional funding was mooted as the minimum USP would accept to take over FSMed, although this was never made official policy.

In fairness to USP, they were under considerable financial strain at the time, and did not want a new medical faculty to be either third-rate or a financial burden. They saw little point of just taking on what FSMed was doing with no additional funding, wanting to improve medical education to a university degree standard, for which there was clearly a need. On the other hand, since the total budget of FSMed in 1986 was only FJ$1.7 million, the Fiji government was reluctant to increase funding for the School at a time when it would lose financial control, and it had a long history of underfunding health as a percent of GDP. Both the government and university hoped that an external donor, such as USAID, would come forward to fund the medical school on terms acceptable to them both. But a nationalistic feeling in certain quarters of government and within the School remained, a feeling that the School, with its long and distinguished past, was an indigenous Fijian institution that should not be relinquished to a regional institution.

Since finance was the main constraint to amalgamation, Lander contracted an American accountant for a detailed report on the operating costs of the MBBS programme alone (excluding other FSMed programmes), the monetary value of the resources provided to the program by the Fiji Government, and the predicted annual operating costs of a high quality MBBS programme run by USP.[228] He reported that the total expenditure for the 1986 academic year for the medical programme alone was FJ$1.12 million, of which 65% was salaries but only a quarter was for full-time staff. Only 17% of the cost of the 18 part-time staff was costed to MBBS since they also taught in other programmes.

The monetary value of the Fiji Government's contributions to the MBBS programme's 1986 operating costs was estimated at FJ$779,482 or almost 70% of the total cost. When the costs to USP for a high quality program were calculated, assuming an increased intake from 130 to 240 students and 52 staff, the cost increased to FJ$2,749,162 with 55% for salaries. As this proposal was still less than half what USP was apparently seeking, it did not really support USP's financial demands.

The Minister of Health, Dr Kurisaqila, for example, stated that the previous Cabinet in 1985 had approved the proposal for USP to take over the School, but since "no decision was forthcoming from the USP, the government had decided to seek assistance from WHO."[229] Following the WHO Master Plan, in September 1989 (post-coup) the Fiji Cabinet approved the "Plan of action for the development of the Fiji School of Medicine as a centre for education of health personnel in the Pacific", which envisaged autonomy for the School under a Council with equal government/health services and school/university representation. Funding for the School would be FJ$1 million from Fiji Government and another FJ$2 million was sought from other donors through the intermediary of WHO.

Between 1981-86, a total of 26 people had been sent overseas for postgraduate training to fill consultant positions at CWM Hospital and tutor positions at FSMed in five specialities (surgery, obstetrics/gynaecology, paediatrics, microbiology and pathology). Out of the 26, only two had returned, but there was confidence that, with the transfer of FSMed to USP, the rest would return to the Ministry or School within the next few years. This confidence unfortunately evaporated with the failure of amalgamation and especially after the 1987 coup. During the transition period, it was hoped that WHO would consider subsidising salaries for tutors under the master plan.

Dr Charles Engel, Associate Professor of Medical Education at the University of Newcastle, produced a long-term plan of action to assess the on-going health manpower requirements of the region and the development of the School. He consulted all of the teaching staff, and yet again recommended that the School be adequately funded. His proposals were also accepted in principle by all parties.[230]

Nevertheless, in April 1985 at the meeting of the USP Council, it was decided that if there were a Fiji Government request to take over FSMed, the University's reply would be refusal unless funding was substantially increased lest it merely exacerbate their existing financial problems. As a result, FSMed remained separate from the university and ran its own curriculum, but its degrees continued to be granted by USP with the necessity for annual external examiners and reviewers for new courses. So, in spite of all the reports recommending amalgamation with USP since 1971, FSMed remained under the Ministry of Health—which was far from a satisfactory arrangement. It remained under the Ministry until 1997, when it finally gained autonomy.

USP maintained a fairly disinterested and 'hands off' approach to the MBBS degree over the next 20 years, other than insisting upon external examiners. With hindsight, it seems likely that a compromise could have been reached if there had been political will and serious negotiations, but neither government nor university at the time was really motivated to bring about this vital change to the School. After the 1987 coup, there was even less interest on the part of government.

Poor Management at Ministry of Health

There had been great dissatisfaction with the performance of the Ministry going back virtually to independence, due to general ineptitude, deplorable standards of management and incompetent leadership (referred to as 'deadwood'). This was increasingly a problem for the School, which was a branch of the Ministry, due to intolerable delays in appointing staff, ordering equipment and allocating budgets. Many previous reports had documented these issues.[220,226,231-235]

One such review was carried out by David Coombe during his 12 month appointment as Health Administration Advisor.[235] His major findings included: overcentralisation of decision-making, chronic underfunding, inadequate training, excessive industrial union pressure compromising professionalism, lack of loyalty and the rising expectations of the public. There were 230 recommendations in his report, including health services administration training for senior administrative staff through USP or Fiji Institute of Technology, and four new positions for FSMed in psychiatry, histopathology, microbiology and chemical pathology as well as six new positions at CWM Hospital with teaching responsibilities at FSMed. CWM Hospital had opened in

1923 with 60 beds, but had increased to a 376-bed capacity with 109% occupancy by 1985 with a mean length of stay of 8.1 days.

A 1986 report proposed a plan for decentralising the Ministry into four divisional health boards.[236] This report also pointed out that half of the Ministry of Health budget of FJ$35 million was spent on urban hospitals and health centres, and that Fiji's government health budget was only 3% of GDP and 7.3% of the total government budget. Clearly, health was underfunded, and this has continued until the present. So the refusal to adequately fund a new medical degree-course at USP was part of the overall underfunding of the health sector, under which FSMed's budget was allocated.

Between 1976 and 1984, there had been a significant increase in the number of doctors and medical assistants in Fiji from 260 to 444, as well as dentists and dental assistants from 54 to 165. The total number of hospital beds in Fiji in 1985 was 1,743 (2.5 beds per 1,000 population), and now included a new 100-bed maternity unit and 60-bed children's ward at CWM Hospital. It was estimated that 93.2% of live births were delivered in hospitals and 26.8% of women of child-bearing age were protected by family planning (33.3% of Indo-Fijians *vs* 16.4% of indigenous Fijians). Despite this substantial growth of the Ministry, management had not kept up, and it was adversely affecting the School, particularly in relation to the management of CWM Hospital. This has also continued up to the present. Medical schools are obliged to work closely with their associated teaching hospitals, so this has remained a difficult issue for the School even after gaining autonomy from the Ministry of Health.

The School Centenary

As the School approached its Centenary in 1985, it could be proud of having made a significant contribution to the health workforce in the region. It had graduated 815 medical graduates, of whom about 60% had been from Fiji, but included 77 from Samoa (including 18

American Samoans), 50 from Tonga, 30 from Solomon Islands, 28 from Kiribati, 26 from Cook Islands, 17 from Tuvalu, 16 from Papua / New Guinea, 12 from New Hebrides (Vanuatu) and 54 from other islands. Out of 477 Fiji citizens who had graduated from the School in medicine in the last hundred years, 279 (58.5%) were still practicing medicine in Fiji at the time.[215]

In addition, there had been 146 dental graduates since 1946, of whom 67 (46%) were from Fiji, and an additional 168 dental auxiliaries (including therapists technologists, assistants). Since 1964, there had also been 596 paramedical graduates (90% from Fiji), including 213 health inspectors, 127 laboratory technologists, 74 radiographers, 65 primary health care workers, 50 dieticians, 34 physiotherapists and 33 pharmacists. It was a remarkable achievement.

Professor Harry Lander summarised the School's accomplishments at the centenary of its first graduates in 1988.

> Founded in 1885, probably no medical school in the world has a prouder and more innovative past. Certainly, with its graduates scattered throughout the multitude of island groups spread over 64 million square miles of the Pacific Ocean and within the metropolitan nations of the Pacific Rim—an area occupying almost one-half the surface of the globe—no medical school has exerted such a profound influence upon the health of so diverse a group of people as those who occupy the vast reaches of Melanesia, Micronesia and Polynesia. [. . . It] represented a unique move, an attempt to train indigenous 'savages' to look after their own sick in 'western' terms; and most outstandingly, in terms of prevention as well as of cure. Certainly the islanders had their own tribal healers practicing their traditional arts handed down over numerous generations in oral history, but those who came upon the islands used different techniques to look after their own and many of these were clearly superior to the host of those that existed.[179]

In fact, the Centenary of the School was only celebrated in 1988, which was a hundred years after the first graduation, because the 1985 centennial passed unnoticed. The Fiji Times published a Centennial Feature insert on Saturday Dec 10th 1988 congratulating the School at a time when it was struggling with staffing issues following the 1987 coups. A photo of administrative and academic staff indicates there were only 43 employees left in December 1988, including 5 white expatriates.

In 1988, Fiji School of Medicine commenced the 3-year Diploma of Environmental Health with WHO support and modelled on the Bachelor of Applied Science at Hawkesbury (north-west of Sydney), replacing the Assistant Health Inspector course. Planning for the course had started in 1982 with a key role played by Jim Ireland, a WHO short-term consultant in environmental health. The first group of students included seven from Fiji and four regional students. There were also plans to upgrade the Certificates in Medical Laboratory Technology, Pharmacy and Radiography to Diploma level.

In many ways, the School was at its peak of success at its 1985 Centenary when Harry Lander was Head of School. According to the annual report of 1987, there were 256 enrolled students, of whom 81 were regional students, and 152 were medical students. To teach these students, there were a total of 66 staff members, although this included technicians and part-timers. Dr Colin Tukuitonga of Niue was a significant new regional recruit to teach Community Medicine, but unfortunately he returned to NZ after the coup. The academic staff reported an impressive total of 46 publications in peer-reviewed journals that year. The School recorded the visits of 75 distinguished academics and 43 overseas elective students.

An American aid grant of US$360,000 for upgrading teaching and clinical facilities was awarded in 1987, and 29 students were flown to Rabaul, PNG on a two week elective visit to the US *Mercy* 1000-bed hospital ship. On May 14th 1987, Lander was invited to meet the new Prime Minister, Dr Timoci Bavadra, to discuss a merger between the School and the University of the South Pacific. There were good reasons for optimism. This all changed with the fateful political events of May 14th 1987, after which it was mostly downhill for the School. Sadly, this is now the story that remains to be told, which includes my time as Dean.

1987 Coup

The political events of 1987 (see chapter 14) had serious economic repercussions for Fiji and the School. Almost immediately, there was a 15% reduction in salary for government employees, a 30% reduction in budgets, a 35% devaluation, a 6% rise in inflation and an 11% fall in GNP.[237] Foreign aid from Australia, NZ, India and USA was suspended. But the main impact for the health sector was the loss of over a third of the medical practitioner workforce, which nearly resulted in closure of the School. This loss of human resources for health meant a loss of good leadership, with poorly-trained individuals placed in senior positions without management experience.

A detailed census of medical practitioners and medical assistants was carried out on March 15th 1987 (pre-coup) and March 15th 1988 (post-coup). This established that 20% of the 294 established posts for doctors were vacant pre-coup, and this rose to 36% post-coup, signifying a loss of 61 doctors to the Ministry. When the private sector is included, out of a total of 313 doctors 108 (35%) left during those 12 months, including 44% of private practitioners and 9 of 12 medically-qualified academic staff at FSMed. Another 26 Indo-Fijian doctors were in the process of leaving.[237] This loss of 108 doctors in 12 months compares to only 67 over the previous five years. Over the decade after 1984, Fiji lost 586 doctors through emigration. These losses were only compensated by 21 new graduates (18 from FSMed in the first group of MBBS graduates, of whom 17 were Indo-Fijians) and 6 retired doctors returning to active practice. An additional 21 expatriate doctors were recruited by the Ministry of Health from Burma and Philippines, with plans for an additional 10 doctors from China.

In addition to doctors, there were also significant losses of dentists, laboratory technologists, radiographers, dieticians and pharmacists due to migration. For example, the number of dentists fell from 67 to 48 after the coup.[238] Overall, official statistics showed that 5,910 people migrated in the 12 months after March 1987 compared to only 3,226 in the 12 months before with implied immigration much higher still (Fig 29).[237] Between 1987 and 2001, 8,669 professionals left Fiji including 2,728 teachers and 1,137 medical professionals.[239]

Lander recounts an anecdote which illustrates the difficulties with migration and anticipated the findings of a later a study of FSMed postgraduates.[240] In 1987 there were 5 pathologists in Fiji, 4 Indo-Fijians and an indigenous Fijian. Dr Karam Singh had been Director of Pathology at CWM Hospital and President of the Fiji Medical Association in which capacity he had been a critic of the Ministry's shortcomings. Although he had been successful in bringing about some changes, he left government service in 1985 due to these frustrations, and set up a private pathology service, apparently in a former Chinese brothel in Suva. Although this laboratory provided some important pathology tests not otherwise available in the country, the Ministry refused to use the service, preferring to send specimens overseas at greater expense. The Ministry also refused to allow him to work part-time at FSMed.

With the new Labour government in 1987, Singh was to become Permanent Secretary of Health under the new Minister Satendra Nandam, a former academic in the English Department of USP and one of Fiji's rare 'public intellectuals'. However, after the coup the former Ministry officials were re-instated and Singh's private laboratory was destroyed, leading him to migrate to Sydney. Two of the other Indi-Fijian pathologists also left and the fourth was replaced as Medical Superintendent in Lautoka, so went into private practice. This left the country with only one pathologist in government service, who was often away attending workshops and regional meetings.[241] This kind of political interference in medicine is almost always detrimental to health services.

As a member of the scholarship selection committee, Lander had become disenchanted by many examples of ethnic and sexual discrimination by the Public Services Commission as well as numerous instances of nepotism and scholarships granted with little relationship to academic ability. In his articles about 'an uncertain future' for the school, Lander issued a dire warning in the following terms:

> The future for the Fiji School of Medicine seems bleak as the country sinks into political and economic turmoil, a turmoil made worse by the second military coup in September 1987. Key expatriate staff members of the school and numerous experienced doctors throughout the health services are leaving the country and replacements will be difficult to recruit. Nor is the position helped by recent severe devaluations of the currency, a reduction in public service salaries of 15%, an across the board reduction of 20% in all budgets, and by the suspension of staffing assistance and aid funding from Australia, New Zealand, the United States, and India. The provision of two senior staff positions by the Commonwealth Fund for Technical Cooperation is also now in doubt, as is the proposal of the government of India to furnish six additional members of staff. The regional nations whose medical and paramedical students comprise 36% and 39% respectively of our total student body now seek alternative training institutes for them, particularly at the University of Papua New Guinea. The 20 final year students of the Fiji School of Medicine who graduated on 18 December 1987 may well not only be the first but also the last to gain the external MB BS degrees of the University of the South Pacific.[224]

Dr Joji Malani recounted that after the coup when Ratu Mara had accepted a position in the interim government of coup-leader Rabuka, he went to see Mara as his paramount chief to try to get A$910,000 worth of drugs and biomedical equipment donated by Australian Aid on a humanitarian basis (through an NGO) released to the hospital, which desperately needed them. A chief in his own right, Joji was humiliated and his request refused by Mara who was visibly infuriated by Australia's opposition to the coup. Mara clearly put political considerations higher than humanitarian concerns in this instance. As will be seen in chapter 13, his role in the political events of 1987 hardly places him above suspicion of collusion.

Fig. 29: Declared or Implied Migration from Fiji. [242]

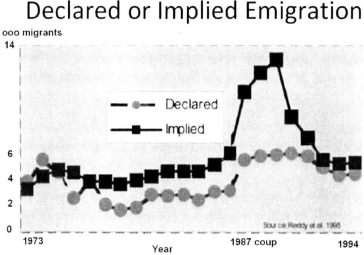

Harry Lander's position as Head of School at FSMed had ceased after the coup due to the suspension of Australian Aid which funded his position, leaving a young Canadian surgeon, Brian Cameron, in charge of the School. He reported his experience as Acting Head of School after the coup in which he stated that the future of the School "will only be assured when the funding and political resolve can be found to make the school a truly regional academic institution, with the medical course integrated into the University of the South Pacific".[243] (p835)

Lander returned to Fiji on a consultancy with Australian aid (AIDAB, the predecessor of AusAID) to help prepare an aid package for post-coup Fiji.[241] He maintained an office at the School in 1988, only leaving Fiji at the end of 1988 to take up a position as Professor of International Health at the University of Hawaii.

Before leaving, Lander's confidential recommendations to the Australian aid agency (AIDAB) included:[244]

1. Focus on replenishing the drain of skilled manpower in the health sector
2. Give priority to the following positions:

   a. Bio-medical and electronic engineering
   b. Laboratory technology
   c. Pharmaceutical and stores management
   d. Health management (within the Ministry of Health)
   e. Pre-clinical science
   f. Clinical disciplines (especially paediatrics and medicine)

3. Do not provide consumables (expensive and inappropriate) or vehicles (misappropriation by military as they had taken over 6 MoH vehicles and still had 4 of them in 1988)
4. Primary Health Care is not such a high priority for aid, especially if it involves requests for vehicles and vaccines (due to cold chain problems).

The Health Sector Report presented a list of 31 requests to Australian aid at a total cost of A$12.6 million. The most expensive items were for hospital, laboratory and X-ray equipment, including maintenance, for the three major hospitals in Suva (CWM), Lautoka and Labasa. The last item was for FSMed, namely exploration of the FSMed-USP relationship in medical and paramedical training ($125,000), but FSMed was also included in a request for additional clinical and pre-clinical staff. There was also a proposal, without the School's involvement, for a regional 12-month postgraduate Diploma in Child Health for eight students a year through the University of Queensland.

The FSMed Council recommended transferring MBBS students elsewhere due to staff shortages, but this was opposed by the Ministry of Health, and USP threatened to withdraw accreditation of its degree. Due to staff shortages, the 1988 academic year was deferred for 10 weeks until March 28th, and 18 MBBS regional students were transferred to PNG, although another 18 returned to FSMed. The School coped with the staff shortages by recruiting 11 short-term expatriates with assistance from Australia, NZ, Canada, UK and WHO. The academic staff establishment was increased by the Public Services Commission from 17 to 22 in 1989 and vacancies were advertised in the *Lancet*, resulting in 50 applicants.

It was clear from this crisis that the divided management responsibilities of the School between the Head of School, FSMed Council, Ministry of Health, Public Services Commission and USP was totally dysfunctional. It took almost another decade before this was modified by the FSM Act of 1997 which granted autonomy to the School. At the time, there was also renewed pressure on USP to take over academic and financial responsibility for the degree programmes in medicine and dentistry, but without a substantial increase in government or donor funding, USP was recalcitrant.

Professor Ian Lewis took over the Head of School position from 1989-1991, following his retirement as Dean of the University of Tasmania medical school in 1988.[245] He was a paediatrician by training, and had a genuine interest in developing country medicine as well as in Fiji. He was given a traditional Fijian welcome, and recounts the following anecdote. He knew he was supposed to clap before drinking the kava, so he put the shell on his lap to clap, and some of the kava spilled on his trousers. As he was already beyond retirement age, he was worried that guests would think the excitement had caused him to wet himself, so he gave his speech sitting down to escape embarrassment. Soon after his arrival, he called for a new 500-bed teaching hospital due to overcrowding at CWM Hospital.[246] He also called for a doubling of staff at FSMed to increase the staff to student ratio from the current 1:12 to 1:6.

He strongly endorsed the new Primary Care Practitioners (PCP) course and the focus on regional health issues, and had been greatly influenced by China's 'barefoot doctor' experience. Lewis was responsible for implementing the new 6-year primary care practitioners course with problem-based learning (see chapter 12), based on the WHO Plan of Action for FSMed. This involved three tiers of training, the first was three years of community primary care with 50% of time in health centres and a focus on primary health care.[247] Primary Care Practitioners (PCPs) were intended to be the "backbone of the Pacific Island Health Services" and from 1993 to 1996, the School graduated a total of 90 PCPs. The graduates of this first tier had to work as PCPs for at least a year before going on to tier two, hence a total of six years before being granted the MBBS degree. The second tier involved a further two years of a more hospital orientated curriculum after the rural PCP internship year, leading to the MBBS degree.

This strong focus on primary care was partly a reaction to the high failure rates of Pacific Island students in the more scientifically oriented western models of medical education, partly to migration of doctors and also a reflection of the dominance of primary care rhetoric at WHO which was predicting 'health for all by the year 2000'. This new approach was strongly endorsed by some older Fijian doctors with the Diploma as a return to the practical training of the 1950s and a way of keeping health practitioners in Fiji, both of which they approved.[248] The final third tier involved four years of postgraduate training for conventional Western specialities such as Medicine, Paediatrics, Surgery and Obstetrics & Gynaecology.

Table 6 outlines the curriculum of the PCP course, showing the strong emphasis on public health and lack of basic sciences or medical sciences other than epidemiology. The programme failed in the end because—despite primary care rhetoric of the time—both students and the public in Fiji wanted doctors rather than PCPs. The Native Medical Practitioners and Assistant Medical Practitioners of the past had been valued at the time, but now Fiji was ready for fully-trained doctors and nothing less would do in the 1990s. PCPs was a return to the NMP days for the School. By then, the world had moved on from the 1978 Alma-Ata primary health care focus.[227]

Table 6: Curriculum of the Primary Care Practitioner Programme[247,249]

Semester	Year 1	Year 2	Year 3
1	Introduction to community health and epidemiology	Communicable disease epidemiology	Epidemiology II and health information
	Maternal & child health	Antenatal clinic	Village visits
	Environmental health	Health care system issues	
2	Epidemiology concepts	Health promotion	Health management / administration
	Antenatal clinic	Occupational health	
	Environmental health practice	Elective—Pacific health care issues	

Shortly after his arrival, Lewis had to explain the new course at a cabinet meeting of the interim government which included the acting Prime Minister Ratu Kamisese Mara and coup leader Rabuka. The two main problems at the School were understaffing and high failure rate of students (30-40%). In 1991, there was a 26% increase in student numbers to 405. The Minister of Health was Dr Apenisa Kurisaqila, a FSMed graduate and Paediatrician, whom Lewis blamed for some poor decisions, broken promises and skulduggery, which were undoubtedly politically motivated. For example, Lewis blamed him for vetoing dormitory funding from Australia, France, and other donors and for proposing a 'racist policy' of an 80% indigenous Fijian student intake for MBBS places leaving only 20% for Indo-Fijians. However, when this proposal was leaked to the press, the Minister dropped it.

Lewis also managed to recruit Dr Jimi Samisoni back to the School from the Pacific Basin Medical School in Pohnpei in September 1990. In March 1991, Lewis had his contract renewed, but while on a Pacific Island familiarisation trip, he discovered in Vanuatu that he had been sacked as Head of School by the Public Services Commission, and replaced by Samisoni. Although he blamed the Minister for the sacking, other evidence suggests that Samisoni was also behind it, although not out of any personal animosity to Lewis.

There is a vitriolic letter in the School file from Samisoni to the former Head of School, Harry Lander about his brief history of the School,[23] which suggested that he had had 'a chip on his shoulder' about the School not having had a Fijian Head of School until he took up the position. In any case, the School was ready in 1991 for its first indigenous Fijian Head of School, a title which was then changed to 'Dean'. Samisoni was very enthusiastic about the PCP programme, but was concerned about the lack of good quality tutors for the programme. He was also frustrated by the bureaucratic bungling at the Ministry of Health, so pushed strongly for autonomy of the School. For example, when he sought to renew his contract at a higher level, the Ministry approached his deputy (Baravilala) to offer him the position instead. Certainly expatriates who worked closely with him, like Ian Lewis, Brian Cameron, Greg Dever, and Jan Pryor spoke very highly of Samisoni and his contribution to the School. His funeral in Fiji in 2007 was a very moving occasion.

Autonomy at Last

On 17 October 1997, an Act of the Parliament of Fiji was passed granting the School autonomy from the Ministry of Health and providing the legal framework for its operation. This Act continued the role of the Council, which met twice a year, and established its membership and powers, which included appointment of the Dean. There were university, government, professional, School, student and regional country representatives, but none from the Staff Association (union) or donors (e.g. AusAID). Another problem with the functions of Council in the legislation was that legally it was given an active management role (e.g. 'to appoint, demote, discipline and dismiss') which was impractical for a large committee of at least 19 members who met only twice a year. In practice and of necessity, it was the Dean and senior management who performed these functions, and the Council only approved the decisions after the fact. This discrepancy meant effectively that the School was functioning illegally according the Act.

There were a total of 620 enrolled students for the ten undergraduate and postgraduate programmes in 1999, which was the highest number ever. In August 1999, a payroll clerk was found to have embezzled money from the School, and these issues recurred on a regular basis due to poor financial management and accountability. On the academic side, the author was external examiner for the MBBS and paediatric postgraduate programme. He found that the written exams tended to be very didactic, testing factual knowledge instead of deep understanding of clinical medicine. The final year clinical OSCE (Objective Structured Clinical Examination), which was a recent innovation for the School, was plagued by the tendency of some staff to grill the students instead of allowing them to perform (well or poorly) the required task.

Dean Wame Baravilala reported to Council that these detailed comments were very useful for the examination process. The author was asked to return in June for two faculty-wide workshops looking at assessment and teaching evidence-based clinical practice, but this was cancelled at the last minute due to the political events of May 2000. It was unfortunate, in my view, that the final year OSCE was subsequently dropped on the recommendation of the next external examiner in 2003, as it is the only reliable and feasible way of assessing clinical competence. The OSCE needed improvement, not scrapping.

2000 Coup

The coup by George Speight in 2000 (see chapter 13 for details) had an immediate effect on the School. As with the events of 1987, there were a spate of resignations of staff after the political events of May 2000 with locals migrating and expatriates leaving. Despite the coup in May and military mutiny of November 2000, students and staff kept their composure and the examination process proceeded with minimal disruption. Wame Baravilala wrote very perceptive comments about the political events by email to 'friends of the School'. The School stayed open throughout the crisis, except for two weeks in June. The approximately six hundred undergraduate medical and paramedical students mostly managed to complete the year, but 16 of 57 postgraduate students withdrew, three staff members resigned and several others did not renew their contracts.

A NZ anaesthetist at the School, Wayne Moriss, actually documented traumatic injuries related to the coup events (unpublished report). Following looting in Suva on May 19th, there were 10 admissions with lacerations and shotgun injuries. Then, the following weekend, three soldiers were injured from rebel shooting in front of Parliament and two others from rioting, including one death. On July 4th following shooting near parliament, six rebels required urgent surgery, and then on 13th and 17th July, a total of 36 prisoners were treated (most requiring surgery) following the storming of Naboro prison, including one death. There were 12 admissions and one death on July 27th following the storming of a school. Finally, the mutiny at Queen Elizabeth Barracks, Nabua on Nov 2nd led to 29 hospital admissions and 12 emergency operations for gunshot injuries, with five deaths on arrival and three deaths in hospital. This is by no means a complete list, but does show that the coup was far from bloodless, and resulted in considerable violence.

From 2001 the MBBS programme entered a new era with the commencement of the trainee internship year that merged primary care and public health into an 18-week attachment at health centres and sub-divisional hospitals in the Western Division. Solomon Island, Samoan and Tongan students were later allowed to do this rotation in their own countries before returning for the clinical hospital rotation in Lautoka. The trainee internship programme enabled final year students to develop their roles as doctors both in and out of hospital and become more competent in clinical reasoning and diagnostic skills while remaining under the supervision of a qualified doctor. Some regional countries had expressed the wish for graduates to be able to function more autonomously on their return home and the Year 6 trainee internship was aimed at achieving this objective. The Ministry of Health strongly endorsed the programme, and the goodwill of their staff was vital for its success.

An accreditation of the MBBS programme was carried out in 2002 by an external survey team comprised of Professors Laurie Geffen and Richard Hays from Australia and Mathias Sapuri of Papua New Guinea under the auspices of the World Federation of Medical Education. The review team found that the School had met the basic standard in all nine areas and the quality standard in five areas. However, with hindsight, a weakness of the accreditation process, which is meant to assess more than just academic standards, was its failure to detect the corporate chaos which was affecting the School at the time. This shortcoming was acknowledged subsequently by Hays, and became the subject of a corporate review appointed by Council and chaired by Dr Jimmie Rodgers of SPC.[250]

It is a pity that this accreditation process missed these corporate issues, as the advantage of accreditation over the system of external examiners is precisely this more general focus on non-academic issues. The external examiner system has been criticised as an old boys' travel junket which just focused on the exam process instead of bench-marking the institution compared to similar ones. When Dean, the author pushed USP to change from the expensive annual parade of external examiners to a 3-5 year comprehensive quality accreditation process of the degree programmes, to which they agreed in principle.

In September 2002 an MoU was signed with Scripps Health in San Diego to facilitate the provision of visiting medical specialists to FSMed and CWM Hospital. Scripps is an American health care provider which includes faculty of the University of California, San Diego. Dr Lance Hendricks was the Scripps coordinator, and brought high quality specialists to Fiji to teach and work for two-week stints at no cost to Fiji except for providing accommodation.

Following the Pacific Forum Ministers meeting in 2002, the School became a member of CROP—the Council of Regional Organisations of the Pacific. CROP included regional technical agencies, SPC, and educational institutions such as USP. The School also developed academic collaboration with Australian universities such as James Cook and Curtin.

The School staff were saddened by the death of Savenaca Siwatibau in 2003. He had been first chairman of the autonomous FSMed Council, prior to becoming Vice-Chancellor of USP.

In 2003, the School requested USP for three new public health degrees, in addition to the Masters in Public Health (MPH). These were Bachelor of Public Health (BPH), Master of Applied Epidemiology (MAE) and Doctorate in Public Health (DrPH) by coursework. Dr Aileen Plant reviewed the proposals favourably for the university, but the latter two programmes failed to attract students.

More successful for public health, however, were the contracts with American-affiliated Micronesian countries to deliver courses on site by FSMed staff on 10-14 day visits. However, the absences of public health staff members on these trips did disrupt the teaching of public health in Suva and the handbook offered far too many courses for the number of students. Later, the corporate review would find that the leadership styles of the heads of both public health and oral health were taking these 'schools' on a path of autonomy to the detriment of the interests of the School as a whole.[250] These issues would re-emerge during my time as Dean.

Research

Under the capable direction of Dr Jan Pryor, a number of high quality research projects were commenced at this time, which provided invaluable practical field research experience for some of the local junior staff members. The Fiji Pneumococcal Project (FiPP) was a phase II clinical trial investigating effective and affordable combinations of polysaccharide and conjugate vaccines, along with related burden of disease studies. It was being directed by Kim Mulholland and Jonathan Carapetis of the University of Melbourne and funded by both the USA (NIH) and Australia (NHMRC).

The Obesity Prevention in Communities (OPIC) study was a community intervention trial targeting the prevention of obesity in adolescents being conducted in Fiji, Tonga, New Zealand and Australia. It was funded jointly by NZ (HRC) and the Wellcome Trust as part of the international collaborative grant programme with chief investigators at Deakin University and the University of Auckland. Non-communicable diseases, including obesity, were a key health issue for research in the region (Fig 30).

Fig. 30: Prevalence of Obesity in the Western Pacific (WHO Database on Body Mass Index, 2006)

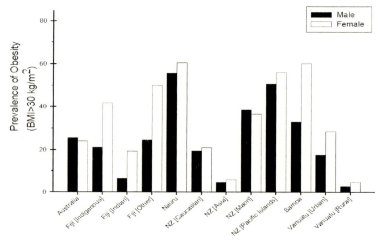

Another study funded under than programme was the molecular epidemiology of Hepatitis B virus in the South Pacific, which was researching the viral and host genetic characteristics related to "escape" from immunization and to the development of chronic infection in five Pacific island countries with the collaboration of Massey and Oxford universities.

Four additional research projects deserve mention. The Stepwise Surveillance of non-communicable disease (NCD) Risk Factors study was investigating the prevalence of NCD risk factors in the Pacific through multiple nationwide population-based surveys. It was conducted in collaboration with the World Health Organization (WHO) and the

University of Tasmania, and the School had a major role in carrying out the surveys. The Fiji Tobacco Burden of Disease project investigated the epidemiologic and economic burden of tobacco-related disease in Fiji in collaboration with the Ministry of Health, WHO, SPC and the University of Queensland. The Fiji Salmonella Surveillance Project looked into the development of appropriate surveillance procedures for Salmonella surveillance as a model for communicable disease surveillance. It was a collaboration with WHO, the US Centers for Disease Control (CDC), and Pasteur Institute. Finally, the Pacific Acute Flaccid Paralysis (AFP) Surveillance Project was a WHO initiative to develop monitoring and evaluation procedures for surveillance throughout the Pacific as a prelude to polio eradication.

In conclusion, there were a number of key developments at the Fiji School of Medicine over this time. Firstly, the numbers of graduates (Figs 31-2) and students (Fig 49) increased exponentially. Although medical students also increased, the most striking increase was in health science and public health students. For the first time, graduates in dentistry, radiography, dietetics and physiotherapy were unable to find jobs starting around the year 2000, so many accepted unpaid attachments to the hospitals for months to years before being employed or migrating.

Fig. 31:School Graduates by Discipline of Study

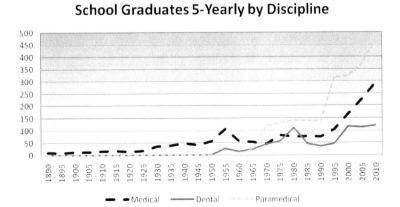

Due to the political coups, the poor management and the migration of doctors, there were still insufficient doctors, especially specialists, employed by the Ministry of Health—despite the marked increase in medical graduates. Secondly, although the School did finally upgrade to the MBBS degree in 1982 and gain autonomy from the Ministry of Health in 1997, it failed to become part of the university because of inadequate funding from Fiji government and aid donors. Although becoming part of USP might have led to a new set of problems for the School, it is our contention that it was an unfortunate missed opportunity which could have improved academic standards and procedures, corporate administration, recruitment and petty factionalism within the School.

Fig. 32:School Graduates, Regional & Total

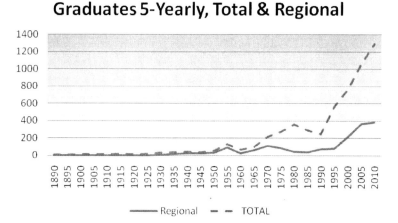

Finally, the 1987 military coup and resulting economic and ethnic crisis had a devastating impact on the School from which it has still not recovered. This is especially disappointing as FSMed was progressing so well up until that point. It is a poignant illustration of how a stable political situation with good governance is essential for a country and its major institutions to thrive.

Chapter 12

Problem-Based Learning

Problem-Based Learning (PBL) was first introduced to the Fiji School of Medicine in 1989 when Ian Lewis was Dean. This innovation was assisted by visits from George Sweeney of McMaster University and Brooke Murphy of the University of Newcastle while John Hamilton was Dean of Medicine. Hamilton had been Associate Professor of Medicine at McMaster University and Chair of the Medical Education Committee during the early days of the new innovative medical programme, which had been planned from 1965 and accepted its first group of 20 students in 1969.

The author was one of the students in the second group of 40 students graduating in 1973, so will share his experiences of this innovative approach which has had such an enormous impact upon medical education globally, including in Fiji. Problem-Based Learning (PBL) started with the recognition that acquiring a vast body of knowledge—much of which would be outdated after graduation—was less important than gaining a set of attitudes, values and learning skills which would persist throughout one's career.

PBL at McMaster

The key innovative features of the PBL approach—in contrast to a more traditional approach—were:

a) the use of small-group tutorials,
b) a self-directed or student-centred approach to active learning,
c) the use of cases (live and paper-based) to integrate basic and clinical sciences, and
d) time for independent study with the availability of flexible learning resources.[251]

Although there are variations in the PBL model, the core concepts involve student-centred learning, tutorial groups, teachers as facilitators, cases as the stimulus for learning, a focus on problem-solving skills and acquisition of new information through self-directed learning.[252] The traditional approach to pedagogy had been individualistic and competitive, demanding the assimilation of a prodigious amount of factual material (*bourrage de crane* in French), and valued competence over caring. The new PBL approach, on the other hand, was based on small group collaborative learning driven by students, which was collaborative, problem-solving and sought to inculcate life-long learning skills.

With hindsight, Neville sees the three essential elements of the McMaster approach as:

1) self-directed learning,
2) problem-based learning, and
3) group tutorial learning.

He attributes the first to the influence of the Harvard Business School, the second to a popular book by Malcolm Knowles,[253] and the third to the famous Oxford and Cambridge tutorial system.[254]

It was a very eclectic approach to medical education, but was clearly influenced by the expanding knowledge base of medicine, recognition of the importance of the social sciences and the irrelevance of much of the basic sciences and hours of anatomy dissection which involved memorisation of facts which had been forgotten by the clinical years of medical school. The main advantages of the new approach were enhanced student motivation, better retention and facilitation of deep learning. However, it did result in a definite backlash in basic science departments to the replacing of 'hard' sciences (especially anatomy) with 'soft' sciences with a 'touchy-feely' dimension, such as bioethics, communication skills and cultural competence.[255]

Two initial hypotheses for the new McMaster curriculum were that a core curriculum could be defined through problems and cases, and that a focus on problem-solving would develop generic diagnostic skills which were transferable to other domains. As it turned out, both of these concepts—the core curriculum and generic problem-solving skills—were found to be false, or at least problematic.

Howard Barrows, an American neurologist, was clearly one of the 'founding fathers' of the McMaster approach and an inspiration for early students and faculty at the School. He defined the four major objectives of PBL as:

a) structuring of knowledge and clinical context,
b) clinical reasoning,
c) self-directed learning skills, and
d) intrinsic motivation.[256]

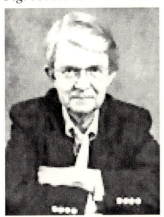

Fig. 33: Howard Barrows

PBL is fundamentally case-based, which ensures its relevance and encourages free enquiry. Barrows believed initially that from repeated case-based problem-solving, students would acquire generic skills which were transferable to new diagnostic problems. Since it was difficult to define core knowledge for medical practitioners, the solution was to make them expert problem-solvers by teasing out the generic skills of good diagnosticians. This led to a focus on research about the nature of clinical reasoning.

Clinical Reasoning

Another McMaster educational guru was Geoffrey Norman, who came from a non-medical science background, and set about researching this entity called clinical reasoning (problem—solving). He found that there were, in fact, no generic problem-solving skills. Instead, clinical reasoning was problem-specific, requiring specific knowledge about the clinical problems or what was called 'content-expertise'.[257] He contended that there were no generic cognitive skills independent of the knowledge required to solve clinical problems. Regardless of what skill was being measured (e.g. problem-solving, diagnostic reasoning, clinical skills or communication) or what assessment method was being used (e.g. simulated patients, OSCE or written exams) the correlation between performance in different cases was poor, only about 0.1-0.3 (where 0 is no correlation and 1 is complete correlation). In contrast, the correlation between measures of knowledge (MCQs) and performance (OSCEs) was high, ranging from 0.6 to 0.9. Thus, knowledge and performance are not that separable, as it takes knowledge to perform, and performance is context-specific. An important implication of these findings was that reliable assessment required multiple sampling of different problems, cases or OSCE stations.[258]

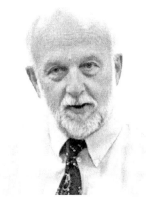

Fig. 34: Geoffrey Norman

Clinical reasoning appeared to be largely based upon the 'hypothetico-deductive' method which we popularly associate with the detective work of Sherlock Holmes. Clinicians tend to generate hypotheses early in the clinical encounter and proceed to rule them in or out from subsequent data. What distinguished experts from novices was that they generated better hypotheses, particularly for complex cases or when there were time constraints. But this expertise had nothing to do with using extensive amounts of previous patient experience or basic science knowledge, nor was it characterised by either thoroughness or extensive memory recall.

In this way, medicine differed from the mastery of the game of chess, for example. Expert clinicians have more knowledge generally, but more specifically about probabilities. Much of this knowledge is local knowledge of disease prevalence and likelihood, such as suspecting rheumatic fever in an indigenous child in northern Australia with arthritis or ectopic pregnancy in a young women with an acute abdomen in some parts of the Caribbean. These probabilities can often be calculated and combined, which are referred to as Bayesian probabilities.

In addition to the hypothetico-deductive method, clinicians also use non-analytic or unconscious reasoning, such as pattern recognition or seeing similarity to past instances.[259] This is used commonly in dermatology and radiology, for example, but many clinical problems are too complex for simple pattern recognition strategies. Borrowing from cognitive psychology, it is proposed that clinical knowledge is represented in the mind as what have been called 'illness scripts', which are clinical narratives of a typical case of the disease, or 'exemplars' from experiential knowledge[260]—a bit like Plato's universals in philosophy which purported to enable children to recognise a chair, for example, from the many different instances of chairs.

This illustrates the complexity of clinical reasoning: that there is no single optimal pathway and that experts call upon multiple knowledge representations in solving problems. The implications for medical teachers are that:

a) clinical knowledge is context-specific
b) multiple examples are necessary, hence the need for deliberate practice with feedback
c) for basic science to be useful, it needs to be integrated into clinical medicine rather than taught separately, and

d) teaching should proceed from signs and symptoms to diagnosis rather than the common practice of starting with a diagnosis or disease.[259,261]

Looking back after 40 years of PBL in 2009, Alan Neville of McMaster wrote that PBL has revolutionised the world of medical education since its introduction.[262] Although PBL started at McMaster, it was soon followed by the new medical school in Maastricht, the Netherlands, in 1974, the University of Newcastle in Australia and the University of New Mexico in the US. Within twenty years of McMaster starting, 60 medical schools around the world had adopted it in whole or in part. What makes it especially surprising that PBL has persisted, is its lack of philosophical foundation and the lack of evidence that it has actually improved educational or health outcomes.

More recently, there have been many studies comparing PBL with traditional approaches, mostly in terms of knowledge acquisition and clinical competence of graduates. The evidence that PBL is superior to traditional approaches has been dogged by confusion about what exactly constitutes a PBL approach, how to control confounding variables, what should be the outcome of interest and what effect size is expected. Generally, studies have not been able to document an improvement in knowledge with PBL, but there does appear to be a significant improvement in knowledge application.[262]

In terms of clinical performance, no significant differences have been demonstrated in studies from McMaster, Harvard and New Mexico in overall competency, but PBL groups tend to perform better in social and cognitive domains, such as coping with uncertainty, ethical issues, communication skills and self-directed learning.[262] Although results have been equivocal, they are consistent with the view that PBL increases students' intrinsic motivation to learn, better integrates knowledge and contributes to life-long learning.[263] Certainly, a potential weakness of PBL is for tutorials to avoid delving deeply into issues by glibly accepting superficial answers to questions. But PBL still generates considerable controversy between purists, eclectics and traditionalists.[264-269]

Stevens has even argued that the acceptance of PBL can be attributed to differences in national culture.[270] He explains the wide adoption of PBL in northern Europe (Scandinavia, Netherlands, UK) compared to France, Italy, Greece and Spain in terms of Hofstede's four value dimensions:

1) individualism *vs* collectivism
2) large *vs* small differences in distribution of power
3) strong *vs* weak uncertainty avoidance, and
4) masculinity *vs* femininity social roles.

Thus, medical schools in countries with high levels of power hierarchy, masculinity, collectivism and where uncertainty is threatening are less likely to adopt PBL. There are also undoubtedly cultural factors, as well as the degree of dominance of doctors in the healthcare system, and probably also the receptivity to English-speaking—or what the French call Anglo-Saxon—innovations.

Alan Bleakley and colleagues have recently suggested that the Western medical curriculum is steeped in a particular set of cultural attitudes with its emphasis on PBL, OSCE and clinical skills, so represents a new wave of imperialism.[271] This article expresses concern about the export of Western medical education techniques to developing countries, as well as the capitalist agenda in medical research such that less than 10% of funding goes to problems affecting 90% of the world's population (the so-called '90/10 divide'). The authors call for an interdisciplinary post-colonial theoretical analysis by medical educators to avoid the pitfalls of educational neo-colonialism.

This is illustrated by examples of cultural values which conflict with participation in small group discussion, student-centred approaches to learning or personal appraisal reports. In a response by Hans Karle and colleagues of the World Medical Federation, it is pointed out that migration of doctors and lack of both financial and human resources in health are a far greater concern for developing countries, and that it is medical practice which is spreading in an imperialist way, particularly private medical practice.[272] Global standards are intended to acknowledge regional and national differences, but the need for good communication and clinical skills are universal requirements for doctors. Nevertheless, whether neo-colonialist or not, it is remarkable how much the medical school in Fiji has been influenced by these global trends in medical education, from Flexner's report in 1912 to McMaster's PBL in the 1960s and Australian medical educational trends in recent decades, including assessment techniques (OSCE, blueprinting, 360-degree, etc.).

My McMaster Experience

At a personal level, there was another important innovation of the McMaster approach. It allowed humanities students into the medical school without the need for undergraduate science courses or entry exams, such as the GAMSAT / UMAT admission testing in Australia. With the McMaster programme, I ended up a doctor (intern) three years after having been a philosophy student in France. The only other viable pathway to medicine for me would have been a minimum of 6 years, including two years of basic sciences before applying to medical school.

But in addition to the attraction to medicine, my initial motivation came more from a disillusionment with philosophy, particularly the analytical and logical positivistic tradition dominating British philosophy. The history of philosophy in my first four years of university had been fascinating and exciting, but the 'nit-picking' nonsense demanded of me in graduate school was disillusioning for someone who was politically active and committed.

I had become attracted to Husserl's phenomenology,[273,274] done a treatise on Herbert Marcuse's *One Dimensional Man*[275] and was interested in Sartre's existentialist movement of commitment (*il faut s'engager*).[276] So *my* commitment changed to practicing medicine in developing countries, as a more practical role than teaching and writing analytic philosophy. I remember well when one of my respected philosophy teachers wrote in his referee's report that at least I would earn more money as a doctor, which said more about him than me as—in my state of youthful naive idealism—it had not really been a consideration.

Readers may not be aware of the extent to which universities were exciting places to be in the heady days of the late 1960s in Canada and France, and our generation of students was out to change the world. As I was overseas in France studying philosophy at the time, the McMaster admissions committee asked me to write an essay on my motivation for wanting to enter medicine, in place of an interview. As I had been writing long philosophical essays for the last 4 years, this was something I could do well. In it, I made a commitment to working for disadvantaged populations, such as in the developing world and indigenous people—which I think Figure 1 confirms that I have honoured.

My short medical degree started with six weeks of basic sciences for students with an Arts (BA) background in August 1970, before the other students arrived in September. The inaugural McMaster medical class had been only 20 students, and our second class had 40 students. I soon discovered that I was really one of the few humanities students in the course. A few others had studied social sciences or languages as undergraduates, but unlike me, they had also done some science subjects (e.g. laboratory technology) at university before applying for medical school.

We were allocated into five tutorial groups of 8 students, and I was unfortunately put into an experimental group of postgraduate students. I had studied three terms a year, so had been doing a Master of Arts degree in Philosophy but was still only 22 years of age and was a local, having attended high school in Guelph, which is close to Hamilton where McMaster University is located. The other seven students in my group were much older than me (28-36 years), and included many foreign students who had completed a Masters or PhD degree in Physics, Biology, Biomedical Engineering, Demography, Epidemiology and other medically-related subjects. They were mostly extremely anxious about this new approach to medical education, and a few soon decided that it would not work so set about sabotaging it as best they could. In this venture, they sought the collaboration of our anatomy tutor, who was also unconvinced about the new approach to teaching in which students did not spend hours dissecting cadavers, as they did at other medical schools. The highly committed 'founding fathers' at McMaster were mostly clinicians, so there was a rearguard action by basic scientists who were disgruntled about the downgrading of their disciplines and it being taught in the patchy way of integrated case-based problems.

As a former philosophy student, however, I was very much at ease with the tutorial system with which I had already had 4 (calendar) years experience, and knew how well it could work. This favourable attitude earned me the pejorative title of 'the Philosopher'. I found it extraordinary that I had managed to integrate well into Quebeçois and French student society, but was now having trouble re-integrating into my own culture. The resolution of this issue took time and sports. We established a class basketball team, which we called the 'phantom-rectums', after a surgical tutorial, and it did not take long for the other class members to see that I was a pretty 'regular guy' and some of the members of my tutorial group were a bit weird and extremely 'up-tight'. Some of them were studying together for two 8-hour shifts a day all weekend, and crying out for lectures and exams. Soon, they were the ones seen as strange and were labelled as 'the heavies' and largely ignored after that.

It is interesting to note that despite the emphasis on tutors being experts in group dynamics, none of our tutors was aware of, or ever raised with us, the strange group dynamics going on here. However, the practice of grouping postgraduate students together was not continued. In any case, by second year the class was more relaxed and everyone had forgotten about who had come from a sciences or arts background. Later studies also found no differences in performance between them as interns.[277] However, this situation also illustrates the importance of social activities in establishing a warm collegiate relationship. As Dean in Fiji, my wife and I made a great effort to create friendly relations between staff through organising social activities at the School.

In those early years at McMaster, the success of the programme was clearly related to the powerful evangelism of the founders, since the students were too anxious about the unknowns and gaps in their knowledge, and the failure of five students in our group on the national LMCC exams tended to reinforce those concerns.[278,279] From a student's perspective two other striking features of the early course, which have not been retained to the same degree, were the total absence of any written or clinical exams until the national exit exam (LMCC) and the disparagement of didactic lectures. This was fine in the early years because we were a small group and highly motivated. We had good access to world experts at the School, had good quality slide-tape shows and were often given mini-lectures during tutorials in Phase 3 (Table 7).

Another exciting feature of the new course was exposure to patients early in the course. I still remember seeing my first delivery on the labour ward during my first week of the course, which was an emotional experience and highly motivating. This was another characteristic of the course that the students were highly motivated, so assessment was unnecessary to drive learning, and in any case there was none.

Although PBL dramatically transformed the initial years of basic science teaching, it made less difference in clinical teaching as it was not all that different from traditional medical schools, which also taught using clinical cases. With the traditional approach, subjects like anatomy, physiology, biochemistry, etc., were taught by basic scientists with lectures and practical sessions, covering the entire subject from A to Z in a didactic and comprehensive manner. By the time students hit third year (graduate-entry) or fifth year (undergraduate-entry) when they were largely based in a hospital setting, they had forgotten most of what they had been taught in the early years, so could not use it for clinical problems.

Table 7: McMaster IV-Phase Curriculum in 3-Years (1970-73)

Year 1 1 September	Year II	Year III
Phase I (10 weeks) Medical community and resources Structure and function of the body **Phase II** (10 weeks) Reaction to stimuli, inflammation, neoplasia homoeostasis, ischaemia Behaviour	*(Phase III continued)* (B) Cardiorespiratory system (C) Neurological and locomotor systems Psychiatry (D) Renal, reproductive, and endocrine systems	*(Phase IV continued)* (A) Medicine and surgery (B) Family medicine Psychiatry Obstetrics and gynaecology Paediatrics (C) Elective experience
Elective		Revision
Phase III (4 × 10 weeks) (A) Blood and gastrointestinal systems	**Phase IV** (3 × 16 weeks) Clerkships	30 April

This was very evident to me both at the ancient university medical school in Montpellier, France and during my internship in Vancouver, where most of the other interns had studied medicine for eight years, as an honours pre-medical BSc followed by the four-years MD degree. In the latter setting, the other interns had forgotten a huge amount of factual basic sciences information but 'could not see the forest for the trees' when it came to discussing these issues in a clinical context. Whereas, after only three years of PBL medical training, I could at least use what I had learned better and set relevant new learning objectives on the basis of the gaps in my knowledge. So from a personal perspective, the new McMaster programme was a great success and allowed me to pursue my medical career in developing countries.

Focus on Learning

Contemporary medical education has borrowed heavily from educational theory and cognitive science in its focus on learning.[280] The change in focus from didactic teaching, such as lectures, to small group learning in tutorials has been found to increase retention because students are encouraged to establish their own learning objectives, research these objectives using existing learning resources (e.g. the web, books, articles and experts) and then present their findings to the group in their own words with group discussion. Educational theory distinguishes between superficial and deep learning, with greater retention and understanding with deep learning. Indeed, there are many different levels of cognition, such as:

1. *Receiving*: passively paying attention only, at the lowest level
2. *Responding*: actively participating in the learning process, reacting in some way
3. *Valuing*: attaching a value to some of the information
4. *Organising*: putting together different ideas and comparing, relating and elaborating on what has been learned
5. *Characterising*: holding a particular value or belief that now exerts influence on the learner's behaviour so that it becomes a characteristic

These different levels of cognitive activity lead in turn to different levels of learning, such as:

1. *Knowledge*: recall of information, recognising, memorising (e.g. list the causes of diarrhoea)
2. *Comprehension*: describing in one own words, interpreting, organising (e.g. explain the mechanism of hypokalaemia with diarrhoea)
3. *Application*: problem-solving, applying information, establishing principles (e.g. how does diarrhoea affect nutritional status?)
4. *Analysis*: separation into component parts, flow diagram (e.g. classify the causes of diarrhoea by their underlying mechanisms)
5. *Synthesis*: combining ideas (e.g. how would you develop a diarrhoeal disease control programme for Aboriginal community children in northern Australia?)

6. *Evaluation*: forming opinions, judgements, discussing controversies (e.g. discuss the proposal to ban infant feeding bottles in Pacific Island countries)

Cognitive studies on adult learners have developed the concept of 'working memory' by analogy with computers. Teaching, especially multimedia instruction, needs to be designed to maximize learning without overloading working memory. Adults process information through dual channels, namely auditory and visual. Consequently, the best way to present multimedia instruction is through visual graphics and informal voice narration, which takes advantage of both verbal and visual working memories without overloading either. Active processing engages cognitive processing such as selecting, organising and integrating. Overload occurs when the amount of essential cognitive processing required for understanding exceeds the learner's cognitive capacity, which is a function of both prior learning and IQ.

As a result of the concept of 'working memory', educational strategies have been devised to avoid overloading it. For example, the 'Multimedia Principle' states that we learn more deeply from words and pictures than from words alone, so presenting some material in visual mode and some in auditory mode can expand effective working memory and reduce overload. 'Segmenting' means breaking up the material into smaller segments and slowing down the speed of presentation. 'Pre-training' is the technique of giving an overview of the main concepts prior to the main session, thus increasing prior knowledge.[281]

The 'Personalisation Principle' is the use of conversational or spoken language, which is preferable to a formal written style for oral presentations. The 'Redundancy Principle' underlines the need to be succinct and concise, since the use of redundant material and PowerPoint 'bells and whistles' (seductive augmentation) are undesirable because they increase working memory for extraneous material and distractions. Although we learn more deeply when extraneous material is excluded, using examples is not considered redundant material as it reinforces learning without increasing working memory. The 'Split Attention

Principle' implies avoiding instructional formats which cause learners to split their attention between multiple sources of information because the need to integrate the separate material uses up working memory. The 'Signalling Principle' states that we learn more deeply when cues are added that highlight the organisation of the essential material.[281]

The implications of these principles for medical education are that complex learning is assisted by specifying learning objectives, supported by handouts and procedural information (orientation) as appropriate. Teachers should combine visual and auditory modes, but they should also:

a) circumvent working memory overload by avoiding redundant material
b) reinforce learning with examples
c) use conversational language instead of reading, and
d) organise the learning material with cues.

Teachers should also involve students actively in selecting, organising, integrating and teaching the group. The implications for medical practice are that problems with full descriptions of clinical context invite more complex cognitive processes, stimulate learning and are a better test of clinical competence. In addition, the context of clinical practice is important as questions may not be transferable from theory to real clinical problems.

Cognitive Errors

Medical educators need to be aware of how doctors make mistakes through cognitive errors, so we can focus on counteracting or minimising such errors. It is estimated that 10-15% of all patients suffer from misdiagnoses or delays in making the correct diagnosis.[282] Of course, the airline industry has demonstrated that pilot errors are frequently due to system errors—rather than individual failings—and this is also true of mistakes in the hospital setting. But education is about critical appraisal (being sceptical) and we often fail to question cogently and think deeply about diagnosing clinical problems. For example, we often use non-specific terms such as chest infection, diarrhoea, abdominal pain, and vomiting, to avoid thinking about the diagnosis. We over-investigate patients as a substitute for thought (and as defensive medicine). We tend to reward procedures over thought.

In his book, *How Doctors Think,* Jerome Groopman of Harvard has discussed at length the issue of cognitive errors causing misdiagnoses.[283] He contends that the majority of misdiagnoses are due to flaws in thinking (cognitive traps). The following are his examples of pitfalls in clinical thinking:

1. *emotional bias* occurs when strong negative feelings about the patient (often unconsciously) blur our ability to listen and think clearly
2. *framing* or labelling patients (e.g. 'a 20 yr old woman with anorexia nervosa who is non-compliant') can be a source of serious error if accepted uncritically without questioning our assumptions
3. *anchoring*, is when the doctor places too much importance on the initial data which skews his thinking
4. *availability*, is where a recent or dramatic case overly influences judgment about a current patient who superficially resembles the case
5. *attribution error*, is where stereotypes (alcoholic, non-compliant, non-organic) prejudice thinking so conclusions arise not from the actual patient's data but from such preconceptions
6. *confirmation bias* is from selectively surveying the data ('cherry picking'), and
7. *affective error* is when we get too close to patients (e.g. dealing with family members or close friends) so lose objectivity.

Donald Redelmeier from Toronto has also written extensively about errors in clinical judgement.[284-290] He states that these cognitive pitfalls are shortcuts in clinical reasoning due to the complexity of many clinical problems, so argues that they can only be minimised by clinicians becoming aware of common errors and by follow up of patients.

As medical teachers, we must inspire our students to learn to question the quality and significance of the medical history of the patient, physical examination, and diagnostic testing. Rigorous questioning demands considerable effort "to stop and look back with a discerning eye and try to rearrange the pieces of the puzzle to form a different picture that provides the diagnosis."[282] We learn from our mistakes, so the best learning experience is when you are proven wrong, and realise that wrongly ignored key information is at odds with your presumed diagnosis or that you failed to consider in your use of Occam's razor that the patient had more than one condition causing his symptoms.

We often rely upon clinical algorithms—which may be useful for run-of-the-mill diagnoses by inexperienced staff, but are little use when symptoms are vague, complex or confusing and tests inconclusive. They discourage doctors from thinking independently and creatively, and often constrain our thinking. A good example of this was encountered by the author when examining Masters students in Paediatrics at UPNG in 2009. The use of the standard treatment protocol was introduced by John Biddulph and Frank Shann in the early 1980s, and was a major asset in ensuring proper treatments by inexperienced junior staff. However, at the postgraduate Masters level, the obsession with standard protocols appeared to have constrained critical thinking, which is expected for this level of training. For example, instead of reflecting upon the true likelihood of TB, candidates would only consider whether the TB protocol had been followed, without critically appraising other possible explanations for the child's signs and symptoms.

This trend is exacerbated by proliferating Clinical Guidelines and Evidence-Based Medicine. It has also led to the move to decision analysis which assigns utility values to decision trees using Bayesian probabilities. But there are too many complexities and unknowns in the clinical situation for a quantitative approach like decision analysis to improve on clinical judgement with all its failing. As Groopman puts it:

> medicine is truly an art and a science that requires doctors both to decipher the mystery and illuminate the meaning of the body in health and disease.[282]

We need to insist that our students get patients to tell them their story in their own words, while trying to avoid being overly biased by the presumptive diagnosis or other labels attached to the patient. They also need to question the patient's use of medical terms such as shock, dysentery, nephritis, etc., to ascertain what they are based upon. A common trap for students is jumping to conclusions too quickly before thinking of other possibilities (the closed mind). 'Red herrings' can also mislead such as a prior trivial injury, so it is important to ask whether the incident was important at the time or did it only assume importance with hindsight. On the other hand, 'alarms bells' are symptoms which lead to the consideration of a less common diagnosis, such as paroxysmal coughing, changing a cold to whooping cough or choking changing asthma to a foreign body (e.g. peanut) aspiration. Students also need to be aware of the possibility of deception, such as in child abuse or drug addiction. The challenge is to get students to increase their powers of observation so they notice subtle features of patient's disposition, behaviour or demeanour. A further challenge is to get students to examine patients properly, as this appears to be increasingly neglected in settings where sophisticated investigations are readily available.

Assessment

Assessment of students is an important role for medical schools as they have a serious responsibility to society to produce graduates who are safe practitioners, clinically competent, empathetic, good communicators and team players. In Fiji– as in Australia—this responsibility lies with the medical school as there is no state licensing examination as there is in North America. In addition, 'assessment drives learning' so is a powerful tool of the curriculum. It identifies borderline and failing students who may not be safe practitioners. It is drawing the line between borderline pass and fail students which necessitates adequate sampling in order to ensure a reliable assessment.

Assessment needs to use questions which test deeper knowledge such as comprehension, analysis and evaluation as well as factual recall. It also needs to sample the curriculum adequately by the technique of so-called 'blueprinting'. In terms of assessing clinical competence, assessments should test the application of knowledge, should adequately and representatively sample the domain of competence, should not reward thoroughness of data gathering, and should focus on the key steps in the resolution of a clinical problem. In terms of formative assessment, the long case and mini-clinical examination (mini-CEX) are suitable, but for summative assessment the most reliable tool is the OSCE (Objective Structured Clinical Examination) with at least 20 stations.[258,291]

Summative assessments used for high-stakes decision-making— such as deciding which students will graduate from medical school—must have a high degree of validity and reliability. The four broad areas to consider are:

1) *blueprinting* to ensure content validity
2) selection of best *test formats* (MCQs, short-answer)
3) applying strategies to achieve adequate levels of *reliability*, and
4) instituting appropriate *standard setting* and decision-making procedures.[292]

Testing competences across a large sample of cases has to be done before a reliable generalisation as to student performance can be made. Incidentally, it was my insistence upon the blueprinting and standard setting of exams in Fiji which allowed copies of the exam to be leaked to dental students (Chapter 15), but they are essential to ensure the exam samples the curriculum fairly and the pass mark is at the right standard. The OSCE demands well-defined training regimes for examiners and simulated patients, regular feedback to examiners and detailed statistical analyses of scores. There is an increasing consensus that the assessment of a student's academic performance in OSCE stations should be based largely on a faculty member's subjective judgements of the student's analytical skills, rather than their ability to recall memorised information. Consequently, marking checklists for OSCE stations have been simplified so as not to reward obsessive thoroughness, and global rating scores by the examiners have been found to be more discriminating—provided that the examiners have content expertise, experience of the expected standard for such students, and have had OSCE training. Any form of 'trap door' criterion (such a student who fails 2 stations fails overall) results in an enormous loss of information, so averaging and aggregating scores is much better than having multiple barriers. This was an issue at the School because some faculty members insisted on putting up such unreliable barriers which students had to pass.

The traditional assessment of clinical competence has been the long case or *viva*, which is an oral clinical examination on a case (e.g. history, exam, presentation, answer questions). Although it has high face validity (it is what doctors do), the inter-rater reliability is only 0.5-0.75 and the correlation between cases for the same student and examiner is only around 0.35. The solution to increasing its reliability would be to do ten cases per student, but since a *viva* may take up to an hour, this is not feasible. However, the mini-CEX is increasingly being used for in-training assessment, when following an encounter between a student and the supervisor (e.g. on a ward round, outpatient consultation or case presentation), the supervisor completes a brief rating on a single 7 point scale with comments. The reliability of such assessments after 8-12 such assessments is 0.7-0.8. This is much higher than for supervisor ratings of 6-12 week clinical rotations which have an inter-rater reliability of only 0.1-0.2 because of poor recall by the supervisor (especially for average students) and because examiners are more comfortable giving negative feedback on a defined task ('you did that poorly') than in general terms ('you are no good').

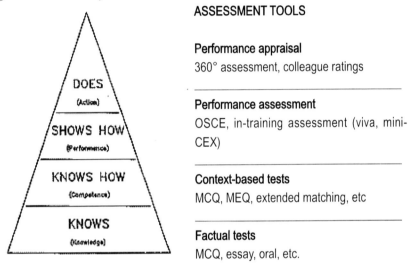

Fig. 35: Framework for Clinical Assessment[293]

ASSESSMENT TOOLS

Performance appraisal
360° assessment, colleague ratings

Performance assessment
OSCE, in-training assessment (viva, mini-CEX)

Context-based tests
MCQ, MEQ, extended matching, etc

Factual tests
MCQ, essay, oral, etc.

In addition to written and clinical exams, medical schools are increasingly assessing student's actual performance by multisource ratings. This has been adapted from professional appraisals in the workplace, completed by colleagues, peers, patients, nurses, allied health workers and administrative staff (360° appraisal). There are cultural and other constraints to this form of assessment since it requires confidentiality and trust or it could undermine people and have destructive effects. Nevertheless, we introduced it in Fiji with considerable success, despite concerns about cultural inappropriateness (see chapter 15).

Another innovative means of assessment is the use of portfolios in which students write comments on their activities (log book) and personal / professional development. These can work well for formative assessment, but are difficult to mark for summative assessment.

Other areas which have proved difficult to assess are professionalism, teamwork, ethics and cultural competence.

The Hidden Curriculum

In addition to the formal curriculum, medical sociologists have described a number of other informal curricula, such as hidden, overt, operational, null, etc., illustrating the multidimensional nature of student learning.[294] The hidden curriculum refers to the organisational socialisation or culture of the institution, such as how new students 'learn the ropes' or 'manipulate the system' in the student subculture. It refers to processes, pressures and constraints which fall outside the formal curriculum.[295] So it is about how the system actually works, as opposed to the espoused values of the formal curriculum. Students often spend far more time and energy 'learning the ropes' in their clinical rotations than they do on clinical skills.[294]

Sociologists have underlined that medical education is a system with the potential for institutions to pay lip service to one set of values in mission statements, but then behave quite differently in practice.[296] In America, role models tended to be powerful white male doctors, referred to as the 'old boys' network'. The lack of culturally appropriate role models for non-white students was a barrier. In Fiji's case, this is exacerbated by the institutional values espoused largely reflecting expatriate (Western) culture, whereas the informal curriculum also encompasses local Pacific Island or Indo-Fijian cultures.

Role models function as sources of tacit learning in the hidden curriculum, in contrast to mentors, where the school make role models explicit in the formal curriculum. Thus, medical students view the formal curriculum differently from faculty, and create a subcultural hidden curriculum which may even sabotage or manipulate the formal curriculum. For example, the formal curriculum teaches students about professionalism, which promotes altruism and dedication to patients' interests, but then students are exposed to clinical settings in which they see conflicts of interests and greed determining behaviours. Such disingenuousness and conflicting messages can result in students becoming 'ethical chameleons'.

The conventional medical school curriculum was characterised by a key distinction between the pre-clinical basic sciences and clinical phases. A key feature of medical socialisation within the traditional pre-clinical phase was anatomy dissection of cadavers, a kind of rite of passage which helped to depersonalise patients by seeing their bodies as machines. With the more integrated curriculum of PBL, this rite was replaced by learning anatomy from computer images, prosected cadavers and in the operating theatre. So PBL students did not have to experience this before being exposed to live patients, which was a major shift in the practice of medical education.[297,298]

However, it has been found that even in innovative, integrated curricula, students continue to focus on competence and learning facts, while suppressing caring attitudes, so reform may have been ineffective because it targeted the formal curriculum while ignoring the hidden curriculum. It may also be that values are formed prior to entering medical school, so rather than trying to change students' values, the focus should be on admission criteria which select desirable ethical qualities and awareness in students. However, this would be difficult to assess in practice at interview as students learn quickly what the interviewers want to hear.

The hidden curriculum has emerged as a key theme of contemporary medical education to explain student behaviour as a shared understanding of 'how to play the game' and conforming to a model of professional behaviour observed in their seniors. Any attempt at curriculum reform requires recognition of this hidden curriculum and a focus on the behaviour and attitudes of students and teachers.

Medical Professionalism

The medical sociology and medical education literature have increasingly placed emphasis on the concept of professionalism. The first two classical studies on medical student socialisation focussed upon the process of developing professional attitudes by gradual assimilation through contact with doctors, patients and other students and by surviving the process of medical training.[299,300] This involved acquiring the ability to be emotionally detached from patients and to tolerate uncertainty. But these early studies were conducted during the 'golden age' of medicine before the absolute authority of doctors had waned.[301]

> Only once the newcomers have complied with all the unwritten rules and practices, in other words completed their rites of passage, will they be rewarded by being accepted in to the magic circle of the medical profession and obtain their legitimate professional identity and privileges.[295]

Whereas professional values were implicitly inculcated from clinical exposure in the traditional curriculum, newer approaches treat them as explicit topics of socialisation.[297] Many papers in the recent medical education literature have focused upon this issue, particularly *Academic Medicine,* due to concerns about the crass commercialism (health care as a commodity) which has overtaken the profession, including the concern about increasing trend of medical litigation.[302,303]

A highly influential and critical book about medical practice was *Medical Nemesis: The Expropriation of Health* by Ivan Illich, published in 1975, which asserted that the process of medicalization of life by the medical profession had become a major threat to health, reflecting a loss of trust in doctors.[304] Illich suggested that a fifth of medical interventions actually caused harm to patients and that medical paternalism created dependency. Later, medical scandals such as the British inquiries over Dr Harold Shipman and Bristol heart surgery, and Australian media frenzy over an Indian surgeon in Bundaberg further tarnished the image of doctors and ensured that they would be held to account for their performance. Nevertheless, doctors and the profession have strongly opposed political interference by the government to improve the quality of health outcomes as weakening professionalism.[295]

There has also been an increasing focus upon the social determinants of health with the recognition that many factors outside of the health sector affect health, such as poverty, disadvantage and non-adherence to treatment, so it is futile to try to fix social problems with high technology medicine.[305] Calman refers to these defects of the medical profession as 'mural dyslexia'—an inability to see the writing on the wall.[94] (p385) The history of medical education reveals how the profession has been unable to change and adapt to new knowledge and changing circumstances. I certainly encountered this as Dean of Fiji School of Medicine—a resistance to change.

The advent of postmodernism in social science has resulted in cultural relativity, the view that truth, or truths, is largely culture-bound. Such views are apparently widespread among medical students, but are still anathema to most biomedical scientists.[306]

Medical Ethics

One consequence of these concerns has been a renewed focus on medical ethics in the curriculum of medical schools, both in research and in clinical practice. Initially, the main focus of teaching ethics was on the four principles:

1) beneficence (do good)
2) non-maleficence (*primum non nocere*)
3) respect for persons (autonomy), and
4) justice,

which acted as a kind of simple checklist.[307] In addition to the principles, there were three requirements for applying these principles to medical research, namely:

a) informed consent (autonomy)
b) assessment of risks and benefits (beneficence and non-maleficence), and
c) selection of subjects (justice).

Recent philosophers such as John Rawls and Amartya Sen have defined the concept of justice in terms of fairness, freedom or reasoned impartiality. The perspective of ethical 'principlism' has been enormously influential in bioethics, although it has been criticised as reductionist (simplistic) and vacuous in failing to offer guidance in resolving conflicts and quandaries.[308] The teaching of bioethics to students has mostly involved case discussions of ethical dilemmas, invoking principlism to try to resolve the dilemma. Assessment of bioethics has proven more difficult, since testing knowledge about ethics is perhaps less important than evaluating ethical behaviour. Some regard the 360° evaluation by peers, nurses, patients and paramedics as optimal in capturing this component of medical education.

There are at least three popular theories of normative ethics which underlie these principles and are relevant to medical practice:

1) *consequentialism:* from the utilitarian tradition of John Stuart Mill
2) *deontology:* based upon duties or obligations from Immanual Kant, and
3) *virtue theory:* which emphasises the character of the moral agent in the tradition of Aristotle, providing insights into moral character with a blend of reason and emotion.[309]

However, it has proven difficult to interest medical students in ethics, who are more focussed on learning practical knowledge and skills for their internship, and its assessment has proved even more difficult. The three dimensions of medical professionalism are competence, caring and social responsibility. The special form of caring which we call compassion transcends self-interest, and has largely yielded to the technological and commodity transformation of medicine. Consequently, there is a renewed interest in the humanities (philosophy, literature and history) in medical education as part of the focus on professionalism and ethics, partly as a way of improving communication skills, reducing exploitive commercialism, limiting litigation and improving the performance of doctors. This emphasis upon bioethics, reflecting a general societal concern, has meant that other non-clinical disciplines, such as social sciences which focus on the social context of illness, have been pushed out of the crowded curriculum in some schools.

This new focus on bioethics has also led to an appreciation of how difficult it is to change behaviour in adults, so the focus has changed to the admission process to weed out candidates with undesirable attitudes. A multiple mini-interview—like OSCE stations—has even been developed to improve the admission process.[310] The reality of bioethics teaching and knowledge is that it does not necessarily ensure ethical behaviour. Medical Councils are also playing an important role in licensing and re-licensing on the basis of mandatory continuing professional education. It has led to a renewed commitment of medicine to:

> serve the community by continually improving health, health care and quality of life for the individual and the population. This is accomplished by understanding disease, promoting health, preventing illness, providing treatment and care, and making effective use of resources, all within the context of a team approach.[94] (p347)

The medical humanist movement stresses good communication with patients, empathy and the importance of understanding patients' individual concerns and values.[311] This is a reaction against the traditional paternalistic role in which doctors told patients what to do without any consideration of their wishes or culture. The loss of consideration of the patient as a person is often considered at the heart of the quality-of-care crisis in American medicine, due to medicine as a commodity, super-specialisation by body parts, high technology investigations and a lack of time to listen to the patient's concerns. Another characteristic of medicine in developed countries has been the change from dealing with the truly sick to 'the worried well'.

Humanistic or humane medicine has been a response to this crisis, which focuses on the wellbeing of the whole person and the medical narrative of illness experience, not solely on the disease. James Marcum, a philosopher of medicine at Baylor, sees humanist or patient-centred medicine as incompatible with—indeed the converse of—the biomedical model or evidence-based medicine (EBM).[308] But his portrayal of the latter is inaccurate, since both the biomedical model and EBM (see below) have accommodated the need for good communication, empathy and accommodating patient values.[312] Medical professionalism means that doctors should always act in the interests of their patients, free of any self-serving personal or other vested interests. The profession in most developed countries has been unable to clearly identify and avoid conflicts of interest with the pharmaceutical industry, and its reputation has suffered as a consequence.[313] However, the requirement for cost containment in health care and application of the business model to public hospitals are also having a detrimental effect upon the performance of doctors, particularly in the changing balance between communal and market aspects of motivation with the resulting loss of collegiality, teamwork and goodwill.

In the words of an ancient French saying, the role of the doctor remains to:

- *guèrir quelquefois*
- *soulager souvent*
- *consoler toujours.*

(sometimes cure, often relieve, always console.)

For the future, the medical profession needs to take the lead in the process of change with regard to standards, quality of care and compassion.

Evidence-Based Medicine (EBM)

In addition to problem-based learning, another influential innovation introduced by McMaster University was evidence-based medicine, in which David Sackett played a key role.[312,314] He joined McMaster as the brash new Head of Epidemiology and Biostatistics, but realising that he needed clinical credibility to influence clinical practice, he re-trained as a physician (internal medicine). Sackett has defined EBM as:

1) the conscientious, explicit and judicious use of current best evidence in making decisions about the care of individual patients
2) the choice of interventions that do more good than harm
3) the promotion of quality in clinical practice, and
4) the supporting of good quality research findings.

Many critics of EBM focus only on the best evidence component, but EBM involves the integration of three components:

a) individual clinical expertise
b) the best available external clinical evidence from systematic research, and
c) the patient's values and expectations.

From the perspective of medical education, it means teaching students the skills and practice of critical appraisal so they can evaluate the medical literature and judge the methodological quality of studies. This new paradigm, if such it is, has had enormous influence on medical education, including at the Fiji School of Medicine.

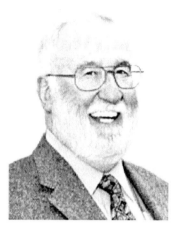

Fig. 36: Prof David Sackett

EBM also has its detractors, including Geoffrey Norman at McMaster.[315] He criticises assumptions of EBM which are open to challenge, including that methodological rigour always ensures a lack of bias, that different searches yield similar articles, and that critical appraisal skills improve clinical practice. Michael Lowe has written a critical editorial in the *Lancet* while in Fiji, pointing out the lack of available evidence which could be externally generalised to clinical problems in Pacific Islands.[316,317] Yet, EBM has been unfairly criticised as 'cookbook' medicine and only 'disease-centred', but now it clearly acknowledges the need for clinical expertise, the role of external generalisability of evidence from randomised trials, and the importance of patients' values in clinical decision-making.

So—much like PBL—EBM is shifting away from a dogmatic perspective allowing more eclectic approaches to evidence and learning. Neither has resulted in striking improvements in cognitive outcomes (PBL) or clinical outcomes (EBM), but both have transformed aspects of medical education, and greatly influenced the curriculum at Fiji School of Medicine. However, key constraints to the use of EBM are fast internet access, faculty expertise, lack of evidence and cognitive barriers due to overwhelming evidence for common conditions.[318]

In conclusion, these trends in medicine and medical education had a direct impact on FSMed, particularly through the reports of visiting academics and external examiners, and also through membership of the Committee of Medical Deans of Australia and New Zealand, which included both FSMed and UPNG as observers. Upon taking up the Dean position in 2005 at the School from a clinical Dean position at Flinders University in Darwin with links to James Cook University, I was immediately struck by the influences of Australian medical school perspectives in such areas as regulations, curriculum and assessment. With modern travel and communication, FSMed was not functioning in a vacuum, but had been highly influenced by the trends outlined in this chapter, although there was also strong resistance to them.

Chapter 13

The Aid Racket

Philanthropy and foreign aid have played an important role in the history of the School, so this chapter describes the background and gives Pacific Island perspectives on the issue.

Aims of Aid

The academic literature on developmental assistance has been quite pessimistic and critical of foreign aid. The major justifications for aid have been:

a) to assist development
b) to relieve poverty (humanitarianism)
c) to promote the political and economic interests of donor countries
d) to assist the global redistribution of wealth, and
e) as restitution for wrongs during the colonial period.

The British economist, Peter Bauer, discounts the development justification by pointing out that economic achievement occurred in many developing countries of Asia before there was any foreign aid and depended upon "personal, cultural, social and political factors, that is people's own faculties, motivations and mores, their institutions and the policies of their rulers."[319] (p7).

The United Nations target for overseas aid as 0.7% of Gross National Product (GNP) or more recently GNI (income, which includes interest and dividends) for high-income countries has only been reached by a few countries, and overall the net official development assistance has fallen from 0.42% in 1964 to a low of 0.22% in 1997 (Fig 39). However, what these figures hide is the massive increase in total aid funding to US $119.8 billion in 2008 (although still only 0.3% of GNI).

Despite such large sums of money, the evidence does not show that aid either promotes development or relieves poverty. Rukmani Gounder of Massey University examined three models (recipient need, donor interest and humanitarianism) using economic analysis and found them to be poor descriptors of the actual aid allocation process.[320] During the cold war, the granting of aid to a developing country was largely a political decision often related to foreign policy aims. So, the main reason for so little to show for the vast amounts of aid granted to developing countries is that in the context of super-power rivalries, much of the aid was spent on foreign policy and economic interests without regard to development. Even a cursory examination of the OECD aid statistics shows little rhyme or reason about how much aid per capita any individual developing country receives.

There are also destructive effects of aid, related to what is referred to as 'dumping' or unfair competition with local businesses, particularly in the food and agriculture sector with food aid. There is also the issue of rewarding governments for pursuing detrimental policies which disadvantage the most productive groups, which are often ethnic minorities.

Aid also tends to encourage corruption, as in the popular expression: 'nothing falls off the back of a truck as easily as a sack of food aid.' The old adage that 'aid transfers money from the poor of rich countries to the rich of poor countries' means that capital projects on institutions, airlines, roads and bridges benefit the rich, who profit not only from the new infrastructure but also from the purchase of supplies for the project through ownership of businesses in the country. Aid has largely failed to relieve poverty and promote economic development because donor governments' priorities have not been consistent with these aims.

Even the aim of promoting Western interest through aid has often been ineffective as large amounts of aid have often gone to regimes overtly hostile to Western interests. As a personal example, the author was involved in one of the largest relief efforts to date in Cambodia (Kampuchea) in 1980, yet the West was constantly criticised by the regime for continuing to recognise the genocidal Pol Pot regime. Incidentally, it was gratifying when Andrew Peacock, Australia's Foreign Minister, made Australia the first Western country to refuse to recognise that regime due in part to pressure from World Vision, for whom I was re-establishing a children's hospital in Phnom Penh at the time. Other examples of support for countries hostile to Western interests have included Cuba, North Korea, Vietnam and Afghanistan.

Bauer makes some suggestions about how to improve foreign aid.[319] Three of his proposals include to:

1) change the criteria of allocation so as to subsidise governments whose policies promote economic progress
2) make aid bilateral rather than multilateral so as to maintain a vestige of control, and
3) untie aid and give grants rather than subsidised loans.

But he expresses pessimism about the chances of these proposal being implemented due to powerful interest of aid organisations, bureaucracies and regional organisations such as the World Bank, International Monetary Fund, UN system and other lobby groups. However, since the Paris Declaration in 2005 (see below) there appears to be more political will for change among many donors, including Australia.

Official Developmental Assistance (ODA)

Without denying the importance of philanthropy by the Rockefeller and Carnegie Foundations early in the 20th century (including in relationship to the medical school in Fiji), ODA really dates from the end of the Second World War with the Marshall Plan for Europe. The World Bank and International Monetary Fund (IMF) were established at the 1944 Bretton Woods Conference for post war reconstruction. Following the success of this programme, it was applied to developing countries to aid economic growth. Under the leadership of Robert McNamara from 1968 to 1981, the World Bank changed its focus from the large infrastructure projects of a bank—which had failed to stimulate economic growth—to poverty reduction as a developmental agency with emphasis on rural development, housing, education, population control, health and nutritional planning.[321]

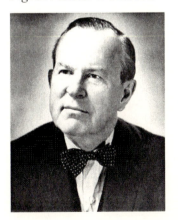

Fig. 37: Lester B Pearson

The first key UN report on ODA was called *Partners in Development* in 1969, chaired by Lester B. Pearson, the former Prime Minister of Canada and Nobel Peace laureate, which set the target of 0.7% of GNP by 1975 although 1% was considered desirable.[322] The report took a strong humanitarian perspective in favour of aid, perhaps in response to the prevailing public disillusionment about aid programmes. However, the report was criticised as lacking empirical support for its recommendations, particularly its assumption that aid was a necessity for economic growth, since this was poorly supported by the evidence. In the end, it was dismissed as a public relations exercise to promote multilateral aid.

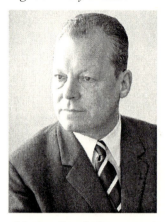
Fig. 38: Willy Brandt

Another report in 1980 was chaired by Willy Brandt, the charismatic former West German Chancellor and another Nobel Peace laureate.[323] The Brandt report called for a new international economic order on the basis of the mutuality of interests between the North (First World, including Australia and NZ) and the South (Third World) from a global Keynesian economic perspective. It argued that the North should aid the South because it is in their interest to do so, due to mutual interdependence. This report was also strongly criticised by economists for false assumptions and lacking a foundation of systematic analysis, but its failure was more related to the unwillingness of the North to grant any concessions to the South.

The World Bank has been a major aid donor and has also copped much of the criticism of foreign aid, and it has been a leader in the changing trends in approaches to aid. It is the largest financial contributor to health-related aid, contributing over US $1 billion annually to new health, nutrition and population projects.[321] Following the post war reconstruction, and large investments in infrastructure to promote economic growth in the 1950-60s, the bank turned to a 'basic needs' approach, after economic growth had not 'trickled down' as expected. Later, Western lending policies combined with the oil crisis, led to unprecedented levels of debt for developing country governments, which was then followed by the IMF's notorious structural adjustment facility and the *laissez-faire* paradigm of the Reagan-Thatcher era. The focus changed again in the 1990s with the 'Washington consensus' emphasising open markets, privatisation, good governance and institutional strengthening.

Fig. 39: Official Developmental Assistance as a Percentage of Gross National Income, 2008.

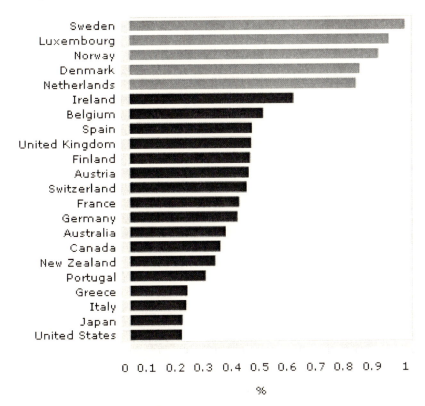

In regards to health, the Bank published a highly influential World Development Report in 1993 on *Investing in Health*, which recommended the following measures as the most cost-effective for improving health: investments in female education, empowering women, primary health care, and public health.[324] It also developed an economic indicator for health measured as DALYs (disability-adjusted life-years), and promoted user fees, privatisation and reductions in the public sector, which were much criticised.

In the nutrition field, the Bank argued that proper nutrition was important for labour productivity, so promoted nutrition programmes run by managers instead of biochemists or doctors. It went on to fund large nutrition projects, such as the Tamil Nadi Integrated Nutrition Project, involving nutrition education, growth monitoring and supplementary feeding of children. However, when its cost-effectiveness was evaluated, it was found to have had little impact due to non-intervention determinants such as low purchasing power, gender inequality and male alcohol consumption.

Devi Sridhar has argued in his recent book that the Bank's nutritional model of individual growth monitoring, behavioural change through nutritional counselling and supplementary feeding is conceptually flawed.[325] He favours a focus on structural determinants of child malnutrition rather than on detrimental caring practices. Malnutrition in India, in his view, is the result of inadequate purchasing power, gender discrimination and infectious diseases, requiring an intervention strategy of income redistribution, social protection and welfare programmes rather than growth monitoring and dietary education.

New Paradigm for Aid

The aid paradigm has again shifted, with the current focus on governance, democracy and donor harmonisation. The Paris Declaration on Aid Effectiveness in 2005 committed developed countries to specific targets for:

1) mutual partnerships with better alignment of aid
2) donor harmonisation
3) defining performance standards, and
4) mutual accountability.[326]

Amartya Sen, the Indian economist and Nobel laureate in economics has brought an ethical dimension to the aid debate, arguing that political liberties are necessary for sustainable development.[327] A strong advocate for more aid to Africa is the economist Jeffrey Sachs in his book *The End of Poverty* in which he argues for a doubling of aid to meet the Millennium Development Goals (MDGs).[328] It has been estimated that it would cost US$34 per person for countries to cover a basic package to achieve the MDGs.[329] There has also been strong support for 'glamour aid' from the educated public in developed countries as an ethical imperative, one manifestation of which has been the high profile Live Aid Concerts by popular musicians.

Recently, a distinguished African woman economist has entered the debate with her best-selling book called *Dead Aid: why aid is not working and how there is another way for Africa*.[330] Her basic premise is that aid to Africa has not worked, so there needs to be a political will to change. She documents how foreign aid has not increased economic growth in African countries due to its crowding out of financial and social capital and feeding corruption.

Fig. 40: Dambisa Moyo

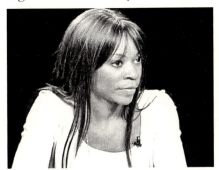

She offers a radical rethink of the aid-dependency model in the African context, using countries like Mauritius and Botswana as examples, which owe their economic success to political stability, market-oriented economies and the probity of their political institutions. Botswana, for example, has used aid wisely for the public good through sound governance and policies favouring foreign investment and equitable growth. She also points out the increasing importance of China in foreign direct investment and trade with developing countries.

Moyo sees remittances (money sent back to family members by migrants employed overseas) as a means of reducing poverty, and stresses the importance of reducing the banking costs of such international transfers. She proposes three market-based steps for turning off aid to Africa within 5 years:

1) an economic plan to reduce reliance on aid (excluding humanitarian and emergency assistance)
2) an array of alternative financing through trade, foreign direct investment, remittances, capital markets, micro-financing and savings which are harder to divert to corrupt politicians over the long term, and
3) the strengthening of institutions with accountability.

Fig. 41: William Easterly

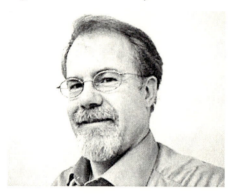

William Easterly, a former World Bank economist, is another critic of aid in his book *The White Man's Burden*.[331] He contrasts two different kinds of approaches to development. *Planners* take a systematic and comprehensive approach to issues, characterised as a global analytic perspective, relying upon expert consultants and their use of rhetoric. *Seekers*, on the other hand, adopt a more *ad hoc* or piecemeal approach taking into account local knowledge, feedback, and home-grown solutions arrived at by trial and error. He believes that development assistance has been too long dominated by a planner's mentality, whereas what is needed are seekers after truth.

Migration of Health Workers

International migration of skilled health workers has a long history, but has become a controversial issue recently with the publication of many important documents.[238,332,333] Since there is a critical relationship between migration and development, and migration of doctors has been a crucial issue for the School, we summarise briefly the issue as it relates to the Pacific islands in this section.

In terms of migration of health workers from Pacific island countries to Australia, the Australian government published a report in September 2006 for the Pacific Senior Health Officials Network on the *Health Workforce Project* with 12 recommendations about gathering information, better co-ordination and setting regional recruitment policies. The Pacific Forum also approved a document drafted by WHO and SPC setting out policies for recruitment, following an international document. But neither Australia nor other Forum governments are prepared to take serious restrictive measures against the migration of health professionals. This may change with the large increase in Australian-trained doctors, which is already making it difficult for Pacific island doctors to get training positions in Australia due to both increased competition for positions and the requirement for IELTS (English language testing). However, although most predictions of human resources for health needs have been wrong, many experts continue to predict that the need for overseas doctors in rural areas will continue for many years.

Countries like Australia, NZ, Canada, US and UK rely on international medical graduates to supply 23-30% of their medical workforces.[334] This has led to a call for these high-income countries to become more self-sufficient in medical education and training, to avoid the ethical issues of the healthcare 'brain drain' from poor countries. There have even been calls for compensation for donor countries, but Australia and NZ already compensate Fiji and PNG by their support for the medical schools in grants and scholarships. Australia has also more than doubled its intake of domestic medical students over the last decade to meet the doctor shortage.

John Connell of the University of Sydney, who has published extensively on the migration of skilled health workers, has written that 'at least as early as 1989 a medical degree from the Fiji School of Medicine was regarded by some as a 'passport to prosperity'."[238,335] So pervasive has become the issue of migration in the Pacific islands, that it has been described as 'a culture of migration' and a 'migrant syndrome'. A major motivating factor for entry into Fiji School of

Medicine has become to facilitate migration—a ticket out of the Pacific. Of course, this is not to deny the altruistic motives of many medical students.

Connell summarises the reasons for migration as follows:

> They have migrated for financial reasons, social reasons (including further education for themselves and other family members overseas) and professional concerns over the inadequacy of the local health sector in terms of the broad conditions of employment. Migration occurs because it provides higher incomes, and thus better living conditions for migrants and their families, alongside new experiences and the acquisition of superior professional expertise while migrant remittances enhance the lives of the kin who remain at home.[238]

Remittances accounted for 6% of GDP in Fiji in 2007, so migration and remittances have become central to economic development. So although an economic rationale is central to migration, it occurs in a cultural context of duty and reciprocity to families and communities, which shape the decision and share in the rewards, although this is not always without conflict. Thus the reasons for migration include five E-factors, namely: Economic, Education, Employment, Entertainment and Excitement.[238] But for Fiji, one needs to add the P-factor, for the 'Push' of politics, coups and discontent with local working conditions. There are also important motivations for not migrating, which include job satisfaction, lifestyle factors and family obligations.

Connell divides migration into three phases. The first phase was the early migration of colonial doctors, such as MacGregor and Corney to Fiji, French doctors to their Pacific colonies, and also eastern European doctors to PNG after the war until Australia would recognise their degrees and allow them to continue on to Australia. The second phase occurred in the 1970s along with the migration of other highly qualified migrants from the developing to developed world, which was first labelled as 'the brain drain', but did not yet involve many Pacific island doctors. The third phase is more complex and global, involving recruiting agencies and governments, with women (often as nurses) also involved as the primary migrants. It has also become a political issue due to the massive loss of African doctors to wealthy countries, which has adversely affected health outcomes in some poor countries.[336-339]

Connell's latest book on Pacific migration of health workers is entitled *The Global Health Care Chain* reflecting the hierarchy of migrations, for example, from Tuvalu to Fiji, from Cook Islands to NZ, from Fiji to Palau, from Fiji to the Middle East, from Fiji to Australia, from Palau to US, etc., culminating in Australia, NZ, Canada and the United States. Connelly states that:

> The Pacific is simply part of the broader structure of the 'cherry picking' (less elegantly 'poaching') of skilled workers amidst the greater selectivity of migration policies in developed countries . . . within a current global deficit of some four million SHWs [skilled health workers].[238]

This international transfer of human resources is increasingly from areas of high need and demand to the converse. Now, approximately half of all Samoan and Tongan doctors and a quarter of Fijian and Solomon Island doctors are based overseas. Consequently, the Pacific region is facing a crisis in terms of its health workforce, not just a lack of health care providers, but also skilled health administrators. Of course it is not just health workers who migrate, so over a hundred thousand Fijians and Indo-Fijians now live overseas, mostly in Australia, NZ and Canada.[238]

A recent study has documented that 652 Pacific Island-born doctors and 3,467 Pacific Island-born nurses and midwives are working in Australia and New Zealand, more than half of whom are from Fiji with significant numbers from Papua New Guinea, Samoa and Tonga as well. There are almost as many Fiji-born doctors in Australia and New

Zealand as there are in Fiji.[340] Another study of Fiji nurses working in Marshall Islands and Kiribati found that:

> the main reasons for migration in this study were . . . economic and social in nature. While international migration . . . for Fiji is dominated by Indo-Fijians and is permanent or long term in nature, this study shows an opposite effect, where intra-regional skilled labour migration is dominated by ethnic Fijians and is temporary in nature.[341]

Studies have also been carried out on migration factors in Fiji for postgraduate doctors at Fiji School of Medicine.[240,342] Although the 'pull' factors to Australia and NZ remain strong, what studies have shown is that there are also two strong 'push' factors in Fiji which have led to migration of doctors. The first is political turmoil, such as the 1987 and 2000 coups, and the other is the lack of career structure and poor working conditions for doctors in the Ministry of Health. Thus, discontent with Pacific island hospitals, health centres and health administration has been an important factor in international migration. Notably, remuneration or salaries was not considered a motive in these qualitative studies and in-depth interviews, indicating a limitation of the methodology. Another study has found that two-thirds of nurses and 46% of doctors in the Pacific were primarily motivated to migrate for income reasons.[238] It just confirms that we tend not to be fully honest when questioned about personal details such as money, sexual habits and alcohol consumption.

The consequences of the international migration of doctors from Fiji are mainly economic. Although there is anecdotal evidence of a decline in health services and outcomes, it is difficult to attribute it to migration. One crude estimate of the total cost of international migration for the late 1990s is FJ$45 million a year, with a quarter of that from the health sector, but this takes no account of compensating remittances.[343] The replacement cost for a migrating doctor is considerably more than retaining him or her. Fiji now has about a third of its doctors as expatriates, including many from Bangladesh, India and the Philippines.

There are a number of measures to combat migration, but most are of dubious efficacy or practicality. On the developed country side, there has been a strong move for ethical recruitment. However, recruiting agencies and health service organisations are unlikely to be constrained by these non-binding policies until the human resources shortages cease or immigration policies change. The greater effort for self-sufficiency in human resources for health in Australia with the dramatic increase in the number of medical students in recent years is an effective barrier to migration ultimately, but will also make it more difficult for Pacific islanders to gain postgraduate specialist experience in Australia. Developing countries like Fiji could improve working conditions, but they are not in a position to compete with developed country salaries. Bonding is another effective measure, and is increasingly being enforced compared to the past. But migrating doctors can easily pay off the bond and are still better off economically on their new salary. Stimulating the return of migrant doctors is another strategy which works in a small number of cases, which is certainly worth exploring, but most migrants are too settled to consider more than transient return visits and some who do return soon become disillusioned. Finally, the use of nurse practitioners does appear to be an effective way of meeting the doctor shortage in both developing and developed countries, provided they are accepted by the public.

Australian Aid

The Australian Aid Program has also suffered from many of the defects of ODA mentioned above, particularly excessive reporting requirements, bureaucracy, and rhetoric. The Jackson Report in 1984 chaired by Sir Gordon Jackson considered aid as a humanitarian commitment to reducing poverty, but also acknowledged its foreign policy and commercial interests, viewing aid from the orthodox growth model of development and not resolving competing priorities between humanitarianism and foreign policy.[344] Among its recommendations were to:

1) focus on education and training assistance with an increase in scholarships
2) make programs country-based rather than by sector
3) maintain 25% of Australian aid as multilateral focus on the Asia-Pacific region
4) phase out food aid except as emergency relief
5) develop special expertise on small islands states, and
6) improve the management of the aid programme.

It also placed a strong emphasis on education, arguing that it was critical for the development of human resources in developing countries.

The Jackson report was criticised for a focus on attracting overseas students into tertiary education in Australia as a policy of self-interest instead of funding primary education in their home country.[204] It was also criticised for its orientation to economic growth instead of basic needs. This was in keeping with the current trend of the World Bank away from meeting 'basic needs' to the export-led growth through a 'structural adjustment' strategy based upon neo-conservative economic policies of growth through trade. At this time, 60% of Australian aid went to Papua New Guinea, but it was estimated that 85% percent of the aid flowed back to Australia as purchases of goods and services.[320] By 1990, this proportion of aid to PNG had decreased to 34%, while it increased to 12% for other Pacific Island countries. The major priorities were human resource development, institutional strengthening, provision of basic infrastructure and technical assistance. A 1996 government report criticised the lack of humanitarian aims of reducing poverty in the Jackson report, which was dominated by foreign policy and commercial interests.[345]

A 1993 Report reiterated the commitment to the UN target of 0.7% of GNI (Gross National Income) and recommended that 7% of

Australian aid should be committed to health.[346] Australia currently gives 0.32% of GNI as aid (OECD 2009).

Although not part of official aid, direct assistance from visiting health teams in specialised areas (e.g. cardiac, orthopaedic, plastic and ophthalmological surgery as well as physician sub-specialists) constitutes an important facet of aid to the health sector. Here is a situation where Fiji benefits from elective surgery which would not otherwise be available in the country and the visiting teams benefit from the greater pathology and tourism experience. A few of the visiting specialists are doctors who had migrated from Fiji, returning regularly to give training and service to their country of origin. These specialist visits mitigate the need for many international referrals. Referral of cases for treatment in Australia is incredibly expensive and is plagued by political interference in referrals, so Fiji has resorted to sending selected patients to India where health services are much less expensive. Of course, government funding of international referrals may greatly benefit individual patients if wisely selected, but it comes out of the health budget so can limit expenditure to improve local services.

Australia, New Zealand and the European Union have adopted a good governance focus in regards to Fiji and the Pacific Islands, following the leadership of the World Bank. The basic principles are:

1. democratic system of government
2. protection of human rights
3. impartial and competent legal system
4. competent public sector management
5. market-friendly economy
6. robust institutions of civil society.

What is new about this agenda is the proposition that 'democracy is a necessary prior or parallel condition of development, not an outcome of it', which raises fundamental questions about the nature of development and economic growth. Good governance means effective administration and democratic institutions, which—it is argued—are pre-conditions for economic growth.

From his research in Kiribati, Barry Macdonald of Massey University contends that the good governance agenda "takes insufficient account of social and political processes and structures, and that reforms may well fail for this reason."[347] (p3) In the Pacific Island context, the introduction of economic conditionality as part of adjustment packages was seen as an attack on sovereignty and at odds with accountability and transparency.

The Pacific Paradox

Despite unprecedented levels of foreign aid, the prospects for sustained economic growth in the Pacific Island region are poor with little chance of achieving the MDGs for most countries. Compared to Africa and Asia, per capita incomes including subsistence agriculture are not low, yet the region receives the most aid on a per capita basis in the world. The Jackson report had acknowledged the need for aid to the region on humanitarian, strategic and commercial grounds.[344] A more cynical view is that small island states receive more per capita aid because they have the same voting rights as larger states in the UN.

There has been a strong academic critique of aid as having only marginal significance for the developing world, and coming with many strings attached such as project conditions, foreign consultants, inappropriate technology, debt and restrictions on the initiative and freedom of action of developing countries.[323] In view of the negative effects of aid, Hughes argued in 2003 that aid had failed the Pacific. She argued that 'cargo cult' expectations have been translated into a dependence on aid, concluding that "given the difficult, counterintuitive concepts of the economic theory of aid and mineral rents, an open discussion [on aid reform] in academia, politics, bureaucracies and media, . . . is essential in the Pacific."[348] (p18)

Savenaca Siwatibau, a former Governor of the Reserve Bank of Fiji and Vice-Chancellor of USP, pointed out the great diversity of the physical and economic characteristics of Pacific Island countries, with PNG and Tuvalu at the extremes.[349] He stressed the following Pacific factors:

1. the rising popular aspirations and expectations
2. the vulnerability to a rapidly changing domestic and global environment
3. the lack of political feasibility for economically sound policies
4. small domestic markets and remote export markets
5. skilled workforce shortages
6. relatively high wages
7. difficult land tenure issues, and
8. high per capita aid.

Siwatibau was quite positive about the impact of aid from major bilateral donors such as Australia, New Zealand, European Union, USA and Japan, because they have had positive impacts upon balance of payments and government budgets.

Aid and remittances constitute another important portion of revenue which maintains wages and salary levels, but which adversely affects agricultural competitiveness. Due to recent political instability in the region, there has also been poor performance in attracting private sector investment. The Pacific Forum has become the agency which coordinates regional aid, so aid is increasingly distributed competitively on a regional basis, but there are still wide discrepancies between countries on a per capita basis.[349]

The economist Wolfgang Kasper of the University of NSW saw two divergent options for Pacific Island communities in the early 1990s:

> Should they continue with tried, old ways, preserving the instinctively appealing, inherited social modes and procedures, even if this means economic stagnation,

dependency and internal civic conflict? Should valued traditions, hierarchical structures, collective solidarity and sharing *(so* typical of the 'Pacific Way') be preserved, even if this means that increasing numbers of people slip from 'low-level affluence' into 'subsistence poverty' and aid dependency? Or should a new social and economic order with more individualism and equality before the law be encouraged to evolve, one that has been successful in the outside world?[350] (p63)

He contends that an aid-claim mentality has emerged on the Pacific comparable to welfare-dependency in Western countries in which aid is seen as an entitlement. He sees the main disadvantage of aid as inflating wages and pushing up the exchange rate without increasing productivity.

Finally, Van Fossen distinguishes five viewpoints on aid to the Pacific Islands, which I will briefly summarise.[351] Those taking a *'globalist' perspective*, such as the Australia and New Zealand governments, seek to use aid to re-shape Pacific Islands politics, economies and societies to be more competitive in world markets, so oppose using aid to maintain anachronistic institutions or traditional values. On the other hand, Pacific Island governments tend to promote *the 'Pacific Way'*, so oppose aid that conflicts with 'Oceanian' ideas about culture, politics, economy and society. *'Dependency theory'* disparages aid as a means of integrating Pacific Island economies into the global capitalist system. *The 'MIRAB' model* (from MIgration, Remittances, Aid and Bureaucracy), on the other hand, sees aid as a subsidy to maintain consumption by islanders for the benefit of donors.[352] Finally, *'new ethicists'* see aid as a necessary compensation for the past wrongs of colonialism, but this viewpoint is often referred to disparagingly as 'white man's burden' or 'gate-keeping'. So there are a wide range of perspectives and vested interests in aid for the Pacific.

A 1989 Australian Committee's report on Australia's relations with Pacific Island countries expressed concern about dietary change, diabetes and non-communicable diseases adversely affecting health in the region, recommending universal low cost community-based health services. It also expressed concern about the concentration of Australian aid on infrastructure development with high recurrent costs (e.g. hospitals) instead of preventive, primary care services.

In terms of medical education, the report commented that the two medical schools in Fiji and PNG "appear to produce very good practical doctors."[353] (p111) Acknowledging concerns about the inappropriateness of Australian postgraduate training and the high loss of graduates from the region, the committee recommended that "Australia should run a program of short term, in-country post-graduate training courses conducted by staff from Australian teaching hospitals . . . [and] an increase in the number of short term specialist medical groups working in the South Pacific."[353] (p111) Following interruption of Australian aid to Fiji after the 1987 coup, aid was restored in 1988 with additional aid linked to 'political, constitutional, economic and social development in Fiji, including human rights', which put Australia in the dilemma of either endorsing the Rabuka regime or using aid to influence Fijian politics. The Committee acknowledged a certain degree of hypocrisy in this stance, since Australian aid went to much worse regimes in terms of human rights abuses and lack of democracy. With the 2006 coup in Fiji, Australia is still facing this dilemma with the 'not-so-interim' Bainimarama government, as health sector aid has continued.

The regional medical school in Fiji has a long history of dependency on foreign aid. We have already dealt with the crucial role of the philanthropic Rockefeller Foundation in the establishment of the Central Medical School in 1928. Other important donors in 1953 and 1958 were the UK Government and Nuffield Foundation, which helped fund the campus in Tamavua, where public health and nutrition were the main focus of teaching. JICA (Japan) funded the new Children's Ward at Colonial War Memorial Hospital in the 1990s, which was actually donated through the School. The European Union funded the new Pasifika campus in Suva which was opened in 2006 while the author was Dean. As the School was a CROP Agency and regional institution, and Fiji was still in the throes of the Speight coup when the grant was considered, it was channelled through the Forum as regional funding rather than as bilateral aid. The School has also benefitted from Taiwanese scholarships and funding. Although the USA was indirectly a major donor through the Rockefeller Foundation between the wars and was an important donor in the 1980s, it ceased all official aid to the School after the 1987 coup, and never really recommenced it.

But the main sources of recurrent aid for the School remain from Australia and New Zealand, who provide the bulk of scholarships for medical students, including funding for the postgraduate medical programme and annual recurrent funding. Without this assistance, the School would not be viable in its present form. Australia also funded the Lautoka Hospital student residence and classrooms, named MacGregor House after Sir William MacGregor, which was officially opened on February 20th 1998 by Greg Urwin as Australian High Commissioner, who later headed the Pacific Forum until his death in 2008. Official Development Assistance has been absolutely vital for the School to function in recent years. Despite this generous assistance, the School frequently failed to satisfy the reporting requirements of the donors, particularly Australia and New Zealand. As Dean, this was very frustrating but was largely related to administrative inexperience and incompetence by senior managers in not meeting deadlines. As one NZ official put it to me, we continue to assist FSMed despite these difficulties because 'it is the only game in town' for training doctors.

Although FSMed salaries have been generally less than USP equivalent salaries and much less than other CROP Agencies such as SPC, they are nevertheless higher than the Ministry of Health, which is the opposite of Australia where academic salaries tend to be lower. Thus, aid allowed the School to pay higher salaries to attract overseas academics from India, Bangladesh and Philippines, but was still not competitive with developed country salaries. It also enabled the School to send many local staff on conferences and for overseas study, although most of the latter did not return to Fiji. Thus, in spite of the political coups, aid has continued to flow to FSMed due to its status as a regional health institution.

Conclusions

Fiji School of Medicine is entirely dependent upon aid to function at its current level. As Dean in 2005, my plan to address the future needs of FSMed with aid funding was as follows:

1. increase the intake of medical students from 70 to 90.
2. expand clinical training in years 4-6 of the course in Lautoka and to establish a new clinical school at Labasa hospital in order to accommodate the increased intake which was too many for CWM Hospital in Suva.
3. increase the intake of the postgraduate training programmes in Surgery, Medicine, Paediatrics and Obstetrics & Gynaecology by using all three clinical sites, and
4. amalgamate with the University of the South Pacific, the regional university, in order to secure our regional institution status.

These proposals met with the approval of Fiji's democratic government of the time and were incorporated into the Strategic Health Plan. AusAID, however, did not want to support further capital projects but agreed to give substantial additional funding for the School to expand the number of medical and postgraduate students. However these changes were overtaken by political events. Despite the close connection of the Minister of Health to the School (father of the previous Dean and a member of FSMed Council), the new Interim Government after the 2006 coup was hostile to the School and also to regional issues. It blamed the School for the migration of doctors, threatened to cut funding, gave the clinical school in Lautoka to the new medical school at University of Fiji (which supported the coup), and proceeded in 2009 to amalgamate Fiji School of Medicine and Fiji School of Nursing into a National University of Fiji. This has meant not only an end to democracy, but also an end to the regional status of the School. Despite these adverse developments, AusAID has continued to fund the School and given additional funding for expansion of the school in 2008.

The Pacific Paradox is that despite unprecedented levels of foreign aid, the region has not shown the expected benefits in terms of economic development. However, there is no doubt that aid to the School has been vital for recruitment, curriculum development, scholarships, information technology support and continuing professional development of academic staff—despite migration losses. It has also definitely benefitted from the new campus and other infrastructure projects. However, there have also been numerous examples of waste, such as inappropriate 'travel junkets' for poorly performing staff members—although probably less than for senior bureaucrats in Ministries of Health in the region.

The downside of aid is that the School is now dependent upon these grants and scholarships, and their withdrawal would have serious adverse consequences. With aid dependency comes vulnerability. Neither increasing tuition fees nor the Fiji grant to the School could fully compensate for the withdrawal of AusAID and NZAID funding, so student numbers and staff salaries would fall and the School would be downsized, much as appears to have happened to USP. With the continuation of the interim government beyond 2010, this is unfortunately no longer such a remote possibility.

Finally, what should be Australia's and NZ's approach to the Bainimarama interim Government? Although both countries have been uncompromising in their opposition to the non-democratic government, aid to the heath sector has continued unchanged, including to the School. The travel bans on military and government appointees have seriously harmed the government, so have been effective, but have also caused resentment against Australia and NZ, which I felt personally as Dean.

Many Australians see the coups of Rabuka, Speight and Bainimarama in the same mould, which is entirely false. Bainimarama is strongly opposing racialist and nationalistic views by indigenous Fijians, which is extraordinary given that his support base is a military which is almost exclusively made up of indigenous Fijians. It is important to allow Bainimarama an exit strategy once he is prepared to allow a democratic government. I also believe that non-governmental organisations in Australia and NZ, such as universities, should deal directly with the Interim Government, rather than following official government policy of shunning it. However, if we are serious about good governance, freedom and democracy, then the official government policy with travel bans needs to remain.

Even from this brief historical summary, it should be clear that 'the aid racket' has come a long way from the days of cold war politics and structural adjustment. The new paradigm of donor harmonisation, working in partnership, good governance and sector-wide approaches is clearly an improvement from past approaches. It remains to be seen how much these principles will be followed by both donors and recipients. Although criticisms of aid need to be addressed, we must avoid both the heady idealism of humanitarianism and cynicism which seeks to cease all ODA. The challenge is to continue to improve aid in order to close the appalling gap in health outcomes between industrialised and developing countries.

Chapter 14

The Coup Culture

This chapter deals with the four military *coups* in Fiji between 1987 and 2006 and how they affected the School of Medicine. We aim to show that the adverse consequences of the political instability, economic decline and loss of academic staff seriously harmed the School from which it has not yet recovered. In addition to recounting the events as they unfolded, we have also widely consulted political and academic commentators for their interpretations of these events. The brevity of this account inevitably leads to oversimplifications, but it is important to understand these political events as background to the story of the School.

We will focus on three key players, namely Timoci Bavadra, Kamisese Mara and Sitiveni Rabuka—the first two of whom actually attended the School. I do hope indigenous Fijians will not see this chapter as anti-Fijian, as I have tried to be fair and honest. However, at the outset I do need to make explicit my strong commitment to political freedom, multiculturalism and democracy. As the father of a multi-racial family, including two adopted children of Indian and African descent, I have strong views against racism. But above all, I am sympathetic to the plight of Fiji citizens of both Indian and indigenous origin, for what British colonialism—my ancestors—imposed upon them, even if it was done by well-meaning men of distinction like Sir Arthur Gordon and William MacGregor.

Ratu Sir Kamisese Mara

Like Sir Arthur Gordon, Mara was born into privilege as a Lauan chief descending directly from the Tongan chief Ma'afu, who had been a rival of King Cakobau at the time of Cession to Britain. Our interest in Mara is of course due to his pivotal role in Fiji's independence and post-independence leadership as Prime Minister and President, but he is also of interest because he studied for two years at Central Medical School, later pursuing further studies in both NZ and the UK. In his memoir, he describes a significant event which affected his life:

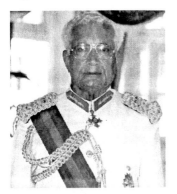

Fig. 42: Ratu Sir Kamisese Mara

"In 1931 a bacilli dysentery epidemic was passing through Fiji, and I was stricken and in hospital under . . . the Assistant Medical Practitioner in charge. After I recovered, he kept me for a week or two to help him. I went around administering medicine he prescribed, because the patients would accept it from me when I gave it to them in a spoon. This experience triggered my interest in medicine and convinced me that a medical career would be a useful one to follow."[354]

In 1937, he commenced study at the Central Medical School in Suva, where he did well enough academically to win the chemistry prize in first year and the anatomy gold medal in second year. Mara enjoyed his two years and complimented the School in his memoirs for graduating medical practitioners 'of a very high standard'. But since the School's qualification was not fully registrable, he was urged by Dr Dovi—Ratu Sukuna's younger brother—to transfer to Otago university in New Zealand, from where Dovi had just graduated. According to Mara, David Hoodless opposed this move because he felt Mara did not have the capacity for prolonged and concentrated study.

Mara claims that he learned from his medical knowledge and dissection experience the valuable lesson of equality, since chiefs were no different from others under the knife. After a year at the Marist Brothers' School in Suva as preparation for Otago, he abandoned the Methodist Church for Roman Catholicism. He did not start at Otago University until 1942, but was transferred to Oxford in preparation for a political career, so never actually completed his medical studies.[354] The decision to send him to Oxford was made by the Fijian leader, Ratu Sir Lala Sukuna, who felt that he held promise for chiefly responsibilities which went beyond the practice of medicine.[355] Upon his return to Fiji in 1950, he joined the civil service, founded the Alliance Party in 1966 and became Chief Minister the following year, leading Fiji to independence in 1970.

During the latter part of colonial times and well before independence, Fijian Indians had been pressing for political evolution towards democracy and equality with Europeans. Although the colonial government's attempt at constitutional change in 1949 had been rejected by the Fijian chiefs, there did seem to be room for a degree of self-government which would be acceptable to indigenous Fijians. The colonial political system had been racially compartmentalised since 1937 with a Legislative Council of 18 official and 15 unofficial members, representing the three ethnic groups. Efforts towards reform based upon elections were resisted by a European desire to preserve privileges out of proportion to numbers (4,594 and 6,142 part-Europeans in 1946) and indigenous Fijian fear of Indo-Fijian domination due to their greater population.

Indians did not speak with a single voice as Muslims wanted separate representation, since they constituted about 8% of the total population (20,000), which was a higher population than Europeans. As in Gordon's time, British officials tended to be sympathetic to the indigenous perspective, feeling a special obligation to protect indigenous interests. Nevertheless, Sir Ronald Garvey, Governor of Fiji, appeared not to accept the view of Fijian paramountcy on the basis of the Deed of Cession by the chiefs to Britain in 1874, writing in 1957 that:

> Surely the intention of this Deed, acknowledged and accepted by chiefs who were parties to it, was that Fiji should be developed so as to take a significant place in the affairs of the world hut, that in the process, the rights and interests of the Fijian people should be respected. To read into the Deed more them that is to suggest for instance, that the rights and interests of the Fijians should predominate over everything else, does no service either to the Fijian people or to their country . . . By their work and enterprise, the Indians in Fiji have made a great contribution to the development and prosperity of their country, and to the welfare of its people. They are an essential part of the community . . . [356] (p32)

The British were caught in the dilemma of either failing in their obligations to the indigenous population or denying the principle of universal suffrage. However, Robert Norton has re-examined the archival material and describes:

> the Colonial Office's frustration with indigenous Fijian resistance, and its eventual resignation to a transition to self—government within the framework of predominantly communal representation. At the heart of the reluctant retreat from radical reform was a fear of jeopardising security and political stability by alienating the Fijian leaders and their people . . . The only way to exorcise the fear of communal domination is to make it clear that we stand for equal rights for both communities . . . [357]

In 1959, there was a strike of oil workers in Suva and Nadi called by the union led by James Anthony, of mixed Indian and Irish descent, and a Fijian, Apisai Tora, that escalated into rioting and the imposition of a military curfew. It was characterised by the participation of both Indian and Fijian workers, and a marked anti-European sentiment, which caused great concern among Europeans that Indians and Fijians would join forces against them.³⁵⁸ In spite of the hostility generated by Indian strikes in the sugar industry with rioting in Suva, some progress was made in the 1960s towards internal self-government, but the competing claims of 'paramountcy, parity and privilege' were not resolved.

At constitutional conferences in 1965 and 1969, Indians wanted democracy whereas the other groups (including the Muslim minority) favoured communal representation. Eventually, the compromise was a complicated communal roll with cross-voting to minimise the effects of ethnic voting and a 52-seat Parliament with 22 each for indigenous Fijians and Indo-Fijians and 8 other general seats. Kenneth Bain, a New Zealander who held senior posts in the colonial administration of Fiji, stated that this 1970 Constitution:

> embraces all the conceptual protections for human rights and dignity that can be conceived *to prevent man doing evil unto man*; and it is entirely proper for Ratu Mara to take credit for being one of its principal intellectual architects.³⁵⁵ (my emphasis)

Sadly, it was not to be so.

Indigenous Fijian Disadvantage

Indigenous Fijian economic disadvantage was blamed on the disincentive of many factors, including their:

1. subsistence affluence
2. preference for a leisurely village lifestyle
3. lack of entrepreneurial instinct
4. educational disadvantage
5. communalistic values, and
6. strong sense of traditional obligation.

This was referred to as 'the Fijian question', and was a longstanding issue of economic backwardness.[359] An inquiry in 1959 blamed their communal way of life and the protective legacy of the colonial 'native policy' instituted by Gordon. Indo-Fijians were doing better in the school system than indigenous Fijians—not from being more intelligent—but due to better schools and socio-cultural factors, such as better motivation. Indo-Fijian culture favoured individual educational achievement as a means of upward mobility and migration, whereas the colonial legacy of the indigenous community was communal, rural and vocational. Paramount chiefs, such as Ratu Sukuna, had favoured technical and agricultural training over academic education, so the educational infrastructure in villages was inadequate, particularly lacking in qualified teachers. A 1969 Fiji Education Commission acknowledged the problem, and recommended a programme of positive discrimination, including in scholarships, to narrow the gap. Thus, at USP, Indo-Fijians required a mark of 261 on the entrance examination for a scholarship compared to only 216 for indigenous Fijians.

The Fijian educational issue persisted into the 1980s in spite of these positive discrimination policies. Despite a huge expansion of secondary schools for Fijians, education was poor quality due to an inadequate supply of trained teachers.[360] Indians saw education as an escape from the drudgery of sugar cane farming, whereas Fijians did not yet seek escape from village life. The constraint to Fijian education was not low intellectual capacity but decreased opportunity. Although there was good quality teaching at Queen Victoria School, the high level of supervision resulted even there in difficulty adapting to the freedom of tertiary education.

Another sensitive ethnic issue was native land leases, held by Indo-Fijian sugarcane farmers due to the shift from plantation to small-holder production. They were regulated by the Agricultural Landlord and Tenant Ordinance (ALTO) and in 1976 the indigenous Fijian-dominated Alliance government granted lease extensions of up to 30 years to Indian tenants, despite opposition from indigenous Fijian nationalists. It was one of the reasons for the Alliance's electoral defeat in April 1977. In 1966, the Alliance party had emerged from the old Fijian political party and had the appearance of a multiracial party with the support of the indigenous community but with some participation by Indian and European communities. The other major party at independence was the National Federation Party, with exclusively Indian support. New Zealand historian Ian Campbell argues that:

> the approach and attainment of independence . . . did not do away with a separate 'native policy', the hallmark of British colonialism, and Indians were . . . never to be able to direct policy.[361] (pp288-9)

Fijian public opinion was never made aware of the constitutional protection of Fijian land and paramountcy, allowing Fijian nationalists to exploit non-existent vulnerabilities and stir up minority paranoia. Historian Brij Lal summarises the independence compromise in the following terms:

> Fundamental questions about the structure and sharing of power, thorny problems of land tenure, the structure of the electoral system, and the goals of development remained unsolved. Fiji had travelled the road to independence rather hurriedly and somewhat secretively. The public were never informed, much less consulted in advance, about the agreement that took Fiji to independence. No real attempt had been made to build a solid basis of public support for the new order, the whole process being engineered from the top. Because of this, many of the problems mentioned would continue to surface throughout the dominion years and eventually consume the nation.[75] (p216)

There is no doubt that Mara and the Alliance party had made a commitment to multiracialism initially, attracting good Indo-Fijian candidates and attracting 24% of the Indian communal vote in the 1972 election in which it won 33 seats compared to 19 for the National Federation Party. Mara also made an initial effort to form a cordial relationship with the opposition leader, Siddiq Koya, but instead of providing leadership on multiculturalism, they both retreated into their respective ethnic enclaves, allowing xenophobic politicians to stir up ethnic anxieties and further polarise the ethnic divide.

The verdict of some commentators is that Mara played the statesmanship and chiefly role to the hilt, but failed to convince his community of the necessity of multiculturalism and accommodating the Indian population of Fiji. Indeed, the whole structure of Fijian administration treated Fijians in isolation from the rest of the colony, allowing them to live within their own framework virtually as a state within a state. It was an obstacle to political advancement as it dealt with native issues separately, which was a conception of native administration which had been abandoned in most other colonies by that time.[362]

Lead-up to the Coup

In the 1977 election, the Fijian vote was split between the Alliance Party of Mara and a new right-wing Nationalist Party which favoured 'repatriation' of Indians. Its leader, Butadroka, had been an Alliance minister until expelled for his racist views. With the Fijian vote split, the election was won by the Indo-Fijian National Federation Party (NFP), which was unprepared to form a government due to dissension between Hindus and Muslims, as its leader was the Muslim Siddiq Koya.

In the brief interim, Sitiveni Rabuka, the third highest officer in the military, was about to resign his commission as he refused to serve an Indo-Fijian government.[363] Similarly, three Pacific leaders refused to attend a Lome Convention meeting in Suva under an Indian leader, only coming when Mara was reinstated, illustrating the negative attitude towards the Indian community in Fiji by Pacific Island leaders.

However, the Governor-General, Ratu Sir George Cakobau, who was also Mara's paramount chief, asked him to form a minority government with Alliance and Fijian Nationalist members, who had 26 of the 52 seats. The constitution did permit him the option of appointing as Prime Minister the person who is best able to command the support of the majority of that House.[75] A new general election returned the Alliance party. These events could be seen as a warning that the principles of democracy might well be breached if Fijian power was threatened.[363] The other important lesson for politicians was that disunity disadvantaged an ethnic group, whether indigenous or Indian.

By 1985, however, the Alliance had been in power for 15 years and had come to take for granted its leadership. As Robertson described the political climate:

> [Many of the leaders] had also become corrupt. Their inability to create a Fijian bourgeoisie had resulted in the creation of a wealthy political clique allied with Gujerati, European and transnational interests, but the Fijian members of this clique depended more for its survival upon access to state perks and the abuse of land rentals . . . [They] were adept at defending their interests in the name of Fijian tradition, often arguing that privileges were necessary because of the 'backwardness' of Fijian people in economic spheres.[364]

The Alliance's response to Butadroka's nationalist threat, which had lost them the 1977 election, was a policy of economic affirmative action for indigenous Fijians to be given state-funded scholarships, and soft loans and assistance for business ventures. When these policies had little success, they resorted to a sophisticated propaganda campaign for the 1982 election campaign run by an American company. As part of a 'cold war' smear campaign, Mara accused the opposition National Federation Party (NFP) of receiving funds from the Soviet Union on the basis of—as it turned out—a forged letter. A Royal Commission was set up after the election to investigate these allegations and the foreign involvement in the Alliance's election campaign. But it was the Australian television programme *Four Corners* which exposed that Mara's election strategy had been mapped out by the American firm, *Business International*, which was alleged to have CIA links. This may also have been part of the US 'cold war' deal for Fiji to cease support for an anti-American policy for a nuclear free-zone in the Pacific, but this has not been proven. This issue could have proved to be more of an embarrassment for the Mara government, but was not pursued further in the courts. The Royal Commission report subsequently described the *Business International* recommendations as 'morally repugnant'.[108]

In July 1985, growing opposition to the Alliance party led to the founding of the Fiji Labour Party, which was Fiji's first real multi-ethnic political party, although the Alliance party had initially attracted some Indo-Fijian support. As part of its social democratic manifesto, it strongly supported a nuclear-free foreign policy for the Pacific, which—as it had for NZ—incurred the wrath of the US. In 1986, Labour joined forces with the Indo-Fijian NFP in a Coalition.

In the general election of April 1987, the Alliance was wracked by scandals. Ratu Mara, for example, had amassed a personal fortune of about FJ$4-6 million, which he could hardly have done on his public service salary.[85] On the other hand, many Fijians resented Bavadra—a Fijian commoner—for attacking a paramount chief, and felt that he was betraying his ethnic origins and serving the interests of the Indo-Fijians. After a bitter struggle on mostly socio-economic issues (not ethnic issues), the Alliance lost the election with the Labour Coalition obtaining 28 seats, including 7 Fijians, 19 Indo-Fijians and 2 part-Europeans.[365] The racial composition of the parliament was fixed by the Constitution at 22 Fijians and Indo-Fijians each and 8 general voters. Kamisese Mara, who had led Fiji for 17 years in an increasingly regal style had finally been replaced by a commoner.[108]

The new Prime Minister and leader of the Labour Party, Dr Bavadra, was an ethnic Fijian trade unionist and general practitioner. In his inaugural address as Prime Minister, he accused the Alliance government of social neglect and pledged social justice for Fiji citizens of all races.[108] Bavadra had attended Queen Victoria School, followed by 5 years at Central Medical School, graduating as an Assistant Medical Officer in 1959. He had interned at Lautoka Hospital and served in government medical service in Serua, Lautoka, Vatukoula, Lau and Rewa until 1976. He had spent the next 2 years as a medical officer in Solomon Islands followed by a year in New Zealand, where he acquired the Diploma in Public Health. He returned to medical practice in Fiji, with a special interest in maternal health and family planning.

Dr Timoci Bavadra (Fig. 43)

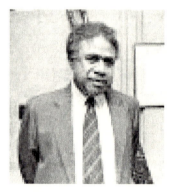

From 1981-85, Bavadra was Assistant Director of Primary and Preventive Health Services and Chair of the National Food and Nutrition Committee. His trade union and political career only commenced in 1978 when he became president of the Public Servants Association, but in 1985 he was elected inaugural president of the newly formed Labour Party and became Prime Minister on April 13th 1987. However, less than a month later on May 14th, he was deposed by a military coup led by Colonel Sitiveni Rabuka.

Here is how Bavadra summarised these events in his own inspiring words:

> The dawn of a new era came to Fiji in April 1987, when its voters exercised their democratic right through the ballot box to choose the new kind of government they wanted to administer the country. The election was a victory for a fledgling Coalition of parties over an incumbent government which had dominated the political life of Fiji since 1970. [...] More significantly, it had emerged from the seeds of a new political consciousness and unity germinating among the ordinary people of Fiji's multi-racial society.

> The outcome promised to be a long-run triumph for the vast majority of our people: the poor, the unemployed and otherwise marginal. It was these people—drawn from all ethnic communities—whom the Coalition was, and still is, pledged to serve.

Sadly, it was to be a false dawn. [. . .] Images of the brutalities, intimidation and other forms of coercion directed at so many innocent people are difficult to erase. Equally vivid is my continuing concern about the economic crisis into which our country was plunged, prompting a surge in unemployment and poverty. I was also concerned about the carefully manufactured racism which spread its divisive, and destructive, tentacles through our society and has become a central part of the institutionalised fabric of public life.[. . .] I look back on one experience with encouragement. In a bid to crush our spirits while we were being held prisoner at the Prime Minister's official residence in Suva, the soldiers tried to separate Indian and Fijian Members of Her Majesty's Government. We linked arms together—all of us—and sat on the floor. As the soldiers gradually pulled us loose, we could see the shame in their eyes. From that day our unity as a human force has never been in question. Torn loose, perhaps; but never apart or overcome. In a sense, that one event is symbolic of what our present struggle is all about—those who would separate us on arbitrary ethnic grounds will encounter a fight to the last breath, for the unity and multiracialism that must be the basis of our future.[355] (pp ix-x in the Foreword written by Bavadra)

It soon became evident that Bavadra was terminally ill, and he died of spinal cancer on November 3rd 1989. Tributes poured in from all over the world. Gareth Evans, the Foreign Minister of Australia summed up his legacy as follows:

> And in the end this was Timoci Bavadra's most enduring legacy: that he was to the last a man of faith and vision. A man of moderation and compassion who, despite the odds

against him, stood by what he believed. A leader of dignity and courage who always sought to serve all the peoples of Fiji.[366] (p362)

Sitiveni Rabuka *(Fig. 44)*

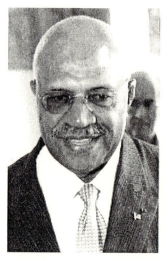

On May 14, 1987, Sitiveni Rabuka along with ten soldiers in gas masks hijacked and incarcerated the elected government of Timoci Bavadra. For Rabuka, he was allegedly protecting an elected government from the wrath of the indigenous nationalist *Taukei* Movement, which had been organising noisy demonstrations to destabilise the new government. Who was really behind the *coup d'état*? Although at the time, Rabuka insisted that he had acted alone, it is now acknowledged that elements of the Royal Fiji Military Forces, activists of the *Taukei* Movement and prominent Alliance Party members were also involved in the coup (the so-called Tovata conspiracy).

Although Mara denied any prior knowledge of the coup, according to Rabuka's biographer,[363] he had discussed it with Rabuka at an arranged meeting at the golf course, when Mara seems with hindsight to have given his blessing to a military takeover while appearing to remain aloof to maintain deniability, and he made sure that he was out of the country when it happened.[367] Although it was a 'bloodless coup', orchestrated mob violence and thuggery against Indo-Fijians followed on from the political events.[355]

Rabuka was a former Queen Victoria School (QVS) head boy who had excelled in sports, but not done well academically as he had twice failed the New Zealand university entrance examinations. QVS played an important role in his personal development. What was learned and the friendships he made at QVS had an important impact on modern Fiji, as well as on the School of Medicine, which was not always a positive influence. Much of Rabuka's political support came via the QVS Old Boys Club.

Rabuka was the first to admit, however, that he had flaws of character. Despite being a devout Methodist, he had two children out of wedlock and was demoted for irregular financial dealings and recurrent debts within the army.[363] One of his strengths as an officer, however, was that he formed close relationships with his men, looking after their interests. He served in both Lebanon and Sinai with UN missions. However, his return to Fiji was clouded by the threat of a court martial for disobeying orders in Sinai over the bereavement leave of a high chief's son. So in 1986, Rabuka applied for several positions in the civil service outside of the army, but curiously was unsuccessful despite his senior military status. His inability at the time to express himself in an articulate manner may have been a factor, since this frustration was the reason he was unable to control his temper, which often got him into trouble.[363]

After the 1987 election, he went to see the Governor-General, Ratu Sir Penaia Ganilau, who was both his commander-in-chief and his paramount chief, in an attempt to convince him to re-appoint Mara as Prime Minister, as in 1977. Ganilau was clearly a father figure for Rabuka and had helped him with disciplinary actions against him by the army. However, on this occasion, Ganilau indicated that he had already invited Dr Bavadra to be sworn in as Prime Minister. Immediately after the coup, Rabuka returned to see the Governor-General, and was very disappointed not to have his support, at least partly because Ganilau felt Rabuka had acted prematurely.

Rabuka's actions did not harm his military career as the Governor-General not only granted him an amnesty for treason—which normally carried the death penalty—but also promoted him to full Colonel, and after his second coup to Brigadier, and a year later to Major-General prior to him running for Parliament. Following his disappointing meeting with the Governor-General, Rabuka asked Mara to join the Council of Ministers with the important foreign affairs portfolio. The other members of his 15 member Council were mostly former Alliance politicians and *Taukei* supporters, but no other members of the military. Rabuka and Mara also met with the Great Council of Chiefs and gained their full support. The Governor-General then relented and swore in Rabuka as the Head of Government, against the pleas of Western diplomats and politicians.

In terms of Fijian educational disadvantage, Rabuka's post-coup administration increased further the funding for indigenous Fijian scholarships. In addition to the existing policy of reserving half of Public Service Commission scholarships for indigenous Fijians, the annual allocation to a special education fund administered by the Fijian Affairs Board was also increased. While this helped a larger number of indigenous Fijians, it did little to improve the overall record of indigenous Fijian educational achievement.[359] Rabuka's final summary for a later biography indicated no regrets over the military coup. He explained that:

> My message has always been, when the Fijians are secure the nation is secure. And you could only get the security of the Fijians if they were united. And when they are not united they deserve not to be secure and when they are not secure they make sure that everybody else is not secure, and we go back into being a real third-world country.[363]

Taukei Movement

As mentioned, many Fijians saw Bavadra and his indigenous colleagues as puppets of their Indo-Fijian masters. This led to the formation of a nationalist group called the *Taukei* movement, invoking the word meaning indigenous Fijians and calling for 'Fiji for the Fijians'. They organised protests against the government in the first few weeks after its election. The *Taukei* movement was already making arrangements to destabilise and replace the new government at the same time as Rabuka was preparing a coup on the military side, so there was clearly a joining of forces.

Within a week of the election, the *Taukei* movement with several key Alliance leaders, launched a campaign of destabilisation. It encouraged fears that Fijians would be reduced to a powerless people in their own land, using racist ideology as a desperate means of retaining Fijian political domination. Its leadership was made up of right-wing trade unionists, virulent racists, Methodist clergymen, and former Alliance government ministers who perhaps feared exposure for corruption. There were also links to the QVS Old Boy network and the Fijian military.

The Nationalist Party leader, Sakeasi Butadroka, who later joined the *Taukei*, had been jailed in 1977 for racial incitement. Robie maintains that "behind their rhetoric, the *Taukei* were less concerned with Fijian rights than using the chiefs as a prop to seize power for themselves."[108] That is certainly how they behaved after the second coup, when they were transiently granted power by Rabuka.

The *Taukei* movement also employed religious rhetoric to justify Fijian paramountcy. Even Rabuka declared his actions were ordained by God, calling them God's Truth. In fact, Fijian rights were constitutionally secure and had hardly been seriously challenged by Indo-Fijians, who sought more to end the inequalities of colonialism. However, with the violence surrounding the coup, Indo-Fijians became rather defeatist, resorting to emigration rather than struggle.

Taukei, on the other hand, adopted terrorist tactics to derail the Deuba Accord, launching a series of fire bombings around Suva which precipitated an increased military presence. A *Taukei* spokesperson even acknowledged a parallel of the *Taukei* Movement with the Nazi's in Germany.[364] However, some elements of *Taukei* were disappointed with Rabuka's reinstatement of the Eastern chiefly interests represented by Mara and Ganilau. The *Taukei* movement also played a pivotal role in the transient administration after the second coup in September.

Reactions to the Coup

There were a host of explanations offered to understand the coup. Some attributed it to the defeat of the Alliance Party that had ruled the country for the last 17 years since independence, others saw more sinister international factors related to super-power rivalries, while other still saw the rise of the Fiji Labour Party as an expression of working class aspirations against the eastern chiefly oligarchy which refused to relinquish its traditional political authority. Some even saw the coup as the inevitable result of the British colonial legacy of 'divide and rule' which was inimical to postcolonial ethnic harmony. Mara's explanation was that a disloyal Indo-Fijian majority had greedily seized power from the indigenous population, denying them a fair share of the cake.[364] Nearly all agreed that the coup had destroyed any chance for multicultural democracy.

The coup received muted acceptance by the leaders of other Pacific island countries. In September 1987 the King of Tonga was reported to have said about the Fiji coup:

> I would have acted like Colonel Rabuka, if I had been in his place. He simply had no other choice, as the Bavadra Government instructed him to maintain order, which meant that he would have had to order his Fijian soldiers to fire on Fijian demonstrators. So the only way to avoid such a tragedy and maintain peace was to overthrow Bavadra's Government . . . If I were an Indian living in Fiji, I would take my family with me and leave the country. And that is precisely what the Indians are now doing.[355]

Officially, Western Samoa expressed sympathy for the agony of Fiji, expressing confidence in the wisdom and tolerance of its traditional leadership. Vanuatu's Prime Minister, Father Walter Lini, denounced the coup, whereas PNG declared that political developments in Fiji were a matter for the people of Fiji to resolve for themselves, although this view was attacked by the opposition. The Pacific Forum's statement on Fiji expressed concern at recent events and stressed the need for reconciliation.[85] Tom Davis, Prime Minister of Cook Islands, summarised their views as follows:

> It is a characteristic of Pacific Islanders that keeping silent about a proposal does not mean acquiescence. Generally it means the opposite. In our culture, it generally means reservation or opposition, We consider it rude to openly oppose our equals or betters, Therefore, silence is preferred and should be read as such. The most vocal in the Forum were Australians and New Zealanders and it is no exaggeration to say that they verbally dominated our meetings. Our silence encouraged this domination... On the Fijian coup, our silence and attempts at verbal discouragement of intentions on behalf of Fiji was one of disagreement with them [Australia and NZ].[368] (p312)

Both Australia and New Zealand reacted strongly, with their respective Labour Prime Ministers, Bob Hawke and David Lange, harsh in their criticism of the coup. There was a widespread feeling in Australia and New Zealand that Rabuka and Mara had betrayed democracy by an act of treason with racist overtones. There was even talk of military intervention, although that seemed very unlikely. In his memoirs, Mara still sounds bewildered by their rejection of someone of his stature, presumably expecting them to have supported political developments as a matter for Fijians to resolve themselves. This was disingenuous. Both Lange and Hawke were leaders of Labour parties with close links to Bavadra's Party, and both countries had strong democratic traditions which precluded support for the military replacement of a democratically elected government. Both countries promptly suspended all planned aid programmes

The New Zealand Herald in Auckland, a city with the largest Pacific Islanders community, published an editorial entitled 'Fiji's Ugly, Race-based Military Takeover' which stated that:

> The signal now seemingly given to the world is that where the Indians were prepared to live peacefully for seventeen years under Fijian dominance, the Fijians were not prepared to suffer more than a month of the Indians . . . [355] (pp 70-71)

Also from Auckland, the Maori Professor Ranganui Walker declared:

> The coup is nothing more than a shameful use by an oligarchy that refuses to recognize and accept the winds of change in Fiji. It would appear from this distance that the Great Council of Chiefs, still living in their traditional ways, have been misled. Their land rights are secure under the constitution. But because they have not been taught their rights they are readily manipulated and swayed by demagogues.[85] (p147)

At a Sydney human rights conference, Dr Bavadra summarised the elements of the conflict:

> . . . the coup makers, in attempting to unite the Fijians against a common enemy, have left them more divided than ever. The division is political: Coalition against Alliance. It is regional: east against west. It is social: chiefs against commoners . . . [355] (p212)

Britain was in the middle of an election campaign, so left the Commonwealth Secretary General to respond to the crisis. Both the Queen and the Foreign Secretary refused to meet Bavadra when he visited London to drum up support for his deposed government. Rajiv Gandhi in

India condemned the coup as anti-Indian and refused to even contemplate the unjust repatriation of fourth and fifth generation Fiji Indians.

The American response was more measured, paying more attention to strategic 'cold war' issues. The *Wall Street Journal* blamed Libya for stirring up trouble, alluding to Rabuka's allegation that two members of Bavadra's cabinet had pro-Soviet and pro-Libyan sympathies.[85] Alluding to the NZ and Bavadra governments' anti-nuclear stance, a former US ambassador called this policy the most potentially disruptive development for US relations with the South Pacific. So Pentagon officials seemed pleased about the end of an anti-nuclear government which backed New Zealand's policy. The US had been worried for some time about Fiji favouring a nuclear-free zone in the Pacific, so had curried favour with Mara so he would drop the port visits ban of US warships, helping him in exchange with his re-election campaign, honours and with a higher allocation of aid.

David Robie details a number of suspicious coincidences suggestive of CIA involvement in the Rabuka coup, but nothing definite has been proven so it remains speculative.[108] The US also concluded a $2.6 million wheat aid package with Fiji at the time. Robie and others have also articulated a theory of tribalism to explain the coup, since the majority of coup participants were from the eastern part of Vanua Levu, which contains the Tovata confederacy headed by the Governor-General.[108] It has been alleged that a wide kinship-based network of people were involved in the coup. This theory re-emerged after the 2000 coup with allusions to 'shadowy figures' behind the coup.

From an economic point of view, the coup had disastrous effects on Fiji. The labour movement instituted a boycott in Australia and New Zealand, there was a delay in harvesting of the sugar cane crop, flights were drastically reduced with a reduction in tourism, salaries were reduced, the currency was devalued and there was mass migration of educated Indo-Fijians. Fiji's Gross Domestic Product in 1987 ended up falling by 11.2%. Property values and manufacturing output fell by 50%, and retail sales by 20%. Food prices rose 14% in June, with some items increasing by as much as 40%. Gross foreign exchange reserves dropped, obliging the Reserve Bank to devalue the currency, impose exchange controls, and adopt restrictive monetary measures.

Ultimately, the Fijian dollar was devalued by 35% and public services salaries were cut by up to 25%. Within two weeks of the coup 1,239 citizens left the country, including many skilled employees including at least 20 doctors, 92 teachers and 50 expatriate academics at USP. There was a disturbing rise in crime, including gangs of youths rioting, terrorizing families, destroying property, and looting of shops and homes, often accompanied by physical violence. Thus, the price of the coup—in addition to the loss of freedom and increase in harassment—was a sudden and substantial deterioration in general economic and social conditions.[85,365]

Second 1987 Coup

The chairman of the Fiji Constitutional Review Committee, established in the aftermath of the coup, was Sir John Falvey. The Committee's sixteen members were nominated by the Governor General, the Great Council of Chiefs, Bavadra and Mara. Heavily weighted with Alliance supporters and Rabuka himself, the review occurred during a period of continuing racial tension and political instability. Rabuka warned that there would be massive civil unrest if the Constitutional Review Committee rejected the reforms proposed by the Great Council of Chiefs.[355] In the end, the report of the Committee did endorse the Council's recommendation for a 71-member parliament with 22 Indian and 8 general seats, reserving the position of Prime Minister and key ministers for indigenous Fijians, A minority report objected that Fiji Indians would be left as disempowered second-class citizens, so urged the retention of the 1970 Constitution, which adequately protected Fijian political interests.[355]

With no compromise in sight, Mara and Bavadra had met secretly at Deuba, where they put together the proposal for a power-sharing joint party government, referred to as the Deuba Accord. This compromise was clearly unacceptable to the *Taukei* movement, who fomented mob violence yet again. On Friday 25th September, as the Governor-General was about to inform the nation about the Accord compromise, Rabuka staged a second coup accompanied by many arrests, control of the media, and declared Fiji a republic outside of the Commonwealth. As the country slipped deeper into economic chaos, Rabuka expanded the military and instituted a totalitarian regime.[108]

The role of Governor-General Ganilau during the crisis now appeared inconsistent with his supposed neutrality as the Queen's representative. After the first coup, he had initially appeared courageous in refusing to accept the coup, but now his role appeared compromised by having dismissed the democratically elected Bavadra government, granted amnesty, and sworn in the coup leader. The second coup was different as it was taken against the Deuba compromise and against the chiefs, particularly Mara and Ganilau. As the ultimate powerbroker, Rabuka finally aligned himself with commoners and the *Taukei* movement.[85] He declared a republic governed by a Council of Ministers, who were mostly from the *Taukei* movement, many of whom were hardline extremists. He also imposed martial law, and banned all commercial activities on Sunday. Over this period, indigenous Fijian nationalists complained increasingly that the government was not doing enough to help indigenous Fijians in business.[359]

But the consequences of this Military Council rule were disastrous for the country as it did not have the leadership skills and experience to guide Fiji out of its political and economic turmoil. The economy deteriorate further with even more migration. Rabuka was forced to dissolve his Council and surrender the Head of Government to Ganilau as President and Mara as Prime Minister on December 5th. Rabuka returned as Commander of the Army, now promoted to the rank of Brigadier as a 'reward' for treason.[108] Thus, 1987 was a decisive year in the history of Fiji from which further consequences would ensue and from which it could never look back.

New Constitutions

Mara announced his intention to retire from politics after a new constitution was in place, but before the next election. The new constitution clearly favoured Fijian rights and ignored the interests of Indo-Fijians, with sweeping powers to the Great Council of Chiefs and military. Due to the financial crisis, the military budget for a force of 5,000 soldiers at a cost $30 million or 8% of the total national budget became a political issue, since it was costing more than health expenditure, which only had a total staff of 2,870. The Chiefs decided to sponsor a political party for the 1992 election to unite indigenous Fijians under a new party, called *Soqosoqo ni Vakavulewa ni Taukei* (SVT). Rabuka was elected as the first president of the new party, defeating the wife of Mara, who was a high chief in her own right. The SVT party won the 1992 general election with the Indian vote split between Labour and National Federation parties. Rabuka became the new Prime Minister, but only after making a deal with Labour which he failed to honour.[367]

Almost immediately Rabuka ran into problems with scandals which showed his political inexperience. Another election in 1994 saw the Fijian vote split between four political parties, but Rabuka formed a minority government with the support of general voters and independents. However, the mismanagement and scandals continued, including sex scandals concerning Rabuka's many affairs, some of which he admitted. In addition, he failed to provide leadership on vital issues such as a revised constitution, native landholding and the faltering economy. He also failed in his attempts to repeal the unpopular Sunday bans and have the term 'Fijian' apply to all citizens of Fiji regardless of ethnic origin. The latter failure was especially unfortunate as the effort to integrate ethnic communities into a national identity was hindered by the continual use of ethnic terms.

Eventually in March 1995, a Commission was appointed to revise the 1990 Constitution under Sir Paul Reeves, a former NZ Governor-General. It included the noted Pacific historian, Brij Lal, as the opposition's nominee. Rabuka presented the SVT submission to the Commission, which represented the hard-line Fijian nationalist perspective on the future for Indo-Fijians, stating that:

> The Fijians believe the *Taukei* have a pre-eminent right to political rule in Fiji by virtue of their being the descendants of the people who have settled these islands for the last 3,500 years before the Indians and Europeans arrived. That belief may offend modern principles of equality but the Fijians have never accepted equal rights to political power as relevant to the future wellbeing of this multi-racial country.[363]

This was a particularly disappointing statement as the international exposure of Rabuka as Prime Minister had greatly moderated his ethnocentric views, partly so his legacy might be seen as a statesman instead of just a coup plotter. By this stage, Indians were no longer a majority in Fiji due to the massive emigration engendered by his coups.

The Constitutional Commission submitted its report in September 1996, entitled *Towards a United Future,* whose recommendations envisaged a free, multi-ethnic, democratic society. The key recommendations were a preferential voting system, a Parliament and Senate and retention of the political role for the Great Council of Chiefs. It was well received internationally, but indigenous Fijians were highly critical of it, particularly the *Taukei* movement. A Joint Parliamentary Select Committee accepted most of the committee's recommendations, while making a few changes such as a power-sharing multi-party Cabinet, nomination of the President and Vice-President by the Great Council of Chiefs, appointment rather than election of the Senate, and the House of Representatives to have 46 reserved seats (23 Fijian and 19 Indo-Fijian) and 25 open seats. The Constitution Amendment Bill became law in July 1997. Following his attendance at the Forum meeting and UN General Assembly, Rabuka represented Fiji at the Commonwealth Heads of Government Meeting in Edinburgh. Since Fiji had been accepted back into the Commonwealth, Rabuka took the occasion to apologise personally to the Queen for the military *coup d'etat*, presenting her with a *tabua* (whale's tooth) as a token of forgiveness.

In the run-up to the 1999 election, Fiji was facing serious economic issues. The drought was threatening the sugar cane crop, the issue of land tenancy remained unresolved, UNESCO reported that 30% of the population was below the poverty line, the government budget was overspent, the currency had been devalued by 20% in 1998, there was massive unemployment of young people, and over 40,000 people had emigrated (95% Indo-Fijians, mostly well-educated) since 1988. The election was held in May 1999 under the new Constitution of multi-party democracy with 20 political parties contesting the election, and the new preferential voting system (similar to Australia's) gave more sway to minority parties. The Labour Party under Mahendra Chaudhry won 37 seats whereas the Fijian vote was split three ways.

2000 Coup

Fig. 45: George Speight

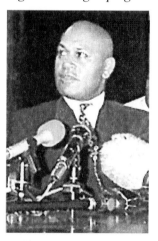

In April 2000, the indigenous nationalist *Taukei* Movement re-emerged when a small group of heavily armed men invaded parliament and incapacitated the government under the apparent leadership of George Speight, a part-European failed businessman who spouted unconvincing nationalist rhetoric. Unlike the 1987 coup, the government ministers were held captive for 56 days and the coup, disguised as a nationalist push for indigenous political control, ended up exacerbating divisions among the indigenous Fijians, when chiefs from Fiji's three confederacies were caught in a power struggle through the Great Council of Chiefs.

At the time of British colonisation, there were three large confederacies, which were the result of geographical proximity, kinship ties and conquests or military alliances. Kabuna was grouped around the island of Bau, Tovata was formed from an alliance of two smaller confederacies (Cakaudrove and Lau), and Burebasaga was grouped around Rewa. Since independence in 1970, the 'Bau/Lau' grouping had dominated Fijian politics, with Ratu Sir George Cakobau of Bau as Governor-General, Ratu Sir Kamisese Mara of Lau as Prime Minister / President and Ratu Sir Penaia Ganilau of Cakaudrove as Governor-General / President. Morgan Tuimaleali'ifano, a historian at USP, has written about the importance of the ideology of hereditary hierarchy, the *vanua*, history, genealogy and their historical struggles within traditional Fijian society on the political process in Fiji.[369]

Politically, the 2000 coup was seen as a reaction against this domination, rather than the racist nationalism expressed by Speight and Rabuka before him. Unlike Rabuka, Speight played no role in Fijian politics after his coup. There was a military insurrection which failed, and Commodore Frank Bainimarama took control and had Speight imprisoned.

Jon Fraenkel summarised the factors behind these events in the following terms:

> Many underlying tensions were exposed by the sudden removal from office of Chaudhry's year-old regime: frictions between chiefly lineages, between the younger and older elites and between the marginalised regions and the established order. Instead of proving the catalyst to a 1987-style consolidation of the country's political establishment behind the coup-instigators, Speight's *tauri vakaukauwa* proved a rallying point for deep-seated ethnic Fijian discontent, and for a concerted effort by the Bau chiefs to restore the ancient standing of their forebears. . . . They were the pawns in a revolt which ultimately served as a vehicle for restoring the political paramountcy of Fiji's indigenous elite.[370] (p308)

The Mahendra Chaudhry Labour Coalition government had only survived a year because of the backing of Ratu Mara. The 2000 crisis occurred because other indigenous Fijian groups challenged Mara's authority. The real struggle was amongst indigenous Fijians, masked by the rhetoric of a ethnic strife between indigenous Fijians and Indo-Fijians.[8] Eventually, the military intervened under its commander, Commodore Frank Bainimarama, who suspended the constitution and installed an interim government led by Laisenia Qarase, who went on to form the *Soqosoqo ni Duvata ni Lewenivanua* (SDL) party in 2001.

Fiji went to the polls in August 2001 and the election was won by the SDL party which favoured indigenous Fijian paramountcy. By 2003, Bainimarama and the government of Laisenia Qarase were on a conflict course over three proposed bills of SDL government legislation; namely, the Racial Tolerance and Unity Bill, the Qoliqoli Bill, and the Land Claims Tribunal Bill. These bills were concerned with an amnesty for the 2000 coup conspirators (so-called 'shadowy figures' close to the SDL party), control of the foreshore and marine resources by indigenous Fijians, and aggrieved indigenous landowners. Nevertheless, the SDL government was re-elected with a strong majority in the 2006 election, despite the military campaigning against them.

The 2006 Coup

Fig. 46: Commodore Frank Bainimarama

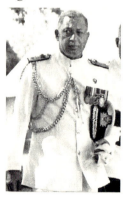

On December 5th, the commander of the Royal Fiji Military Forces took over executive authority from the Qarase government, and an Interim Government was sworn in with Dr Jona Senilagakali as Prime Minister, after Bainimarama transferred executive power back to the aging president of Fiji, Ratu Josefa Iloilo. Unlike previous coups, the 2006 coup was enthusiastically embraced by many Indo-Fijians who had disliked the ethnic-based policies of the SDL government. Indigenous Fijians, who had strongly endorsed the SDL government, felt robbed of their democratic choice and started passive resistance in the form of letters to the editor and internet blogs.

The European Union together with Australia, New Zealand, the United States and Britain applied smart sanctions with the hope that Fiji would return to democratic rule within two years. The December 2006 coup was aimed at correcting the imbalance caused by the three previous coups and to dismantle chiefly dominance, corruption, and command style structures and bring about accountability, transparency, inter-ethnic tolerance, and good governance.[367] But due to the travel bans imposed by Australia and New Zealand, Bainimarama had great difficulty recruiting high quality Ministers and other senior government appointees. He destroyed any independence of the judiciary, and expelled the High Commissioners of Australia and NZ in October 2009 for interfering when the travel bans on new judges made it impossible for him to recruit from overseas.

Additionally, since Australia, NZ and the Forum countries have opposed his interim government, he has adopted an anti-regional stance against NGOs and CROP Agencies, including USP and FSMed, and favouring the Indo-Fijian University of Fiji. On the face of it, it seems extraordinary that the head of an almost exclusively indigenous Fijian military should be able to govern against the interests of indigenous Fijians (who voted overwhelmingly for the SDL government). It is a delicate balancing act which is dependent upon favouring the military, but it is unclear what exit strategy is possible if the economy continues to decline.

Winston Halapua, a former Anglican clergyman from Fiji, has argued that the imposition of indigenous Fijian interests and rights as paramount by successive military coups has resulted in militarism, which altered the social climate so that military values and ideology dominate the behavioural patterns of the society.[371] In his estimation, this has resulted in an escalation of social ills such as domestic violence, rape, child abuse, incest and suicide. He contends that these problems have now reached a stage where they show a moral decay in the country. This seems a harsh judgement and even his evidence of rising trends in these social ills does not prove causality. These social ills are prevalent in highly religious societies—Moslem and Christian—as well as in more secular societies like Australia and parts of Europe, and the predisposing factors are multifactorial and complex. The effect of militarism in Fiji has been predominantly political and economic, rather than ethical. Like George Bush, Rabuka and Bainimarama are practicing Christians, and that certainly is no guarantee of wise political decision-making from an ethical perspective.

Conclusions

The political instability resulting from these events confirmed Harry Lander's dire prediction of an 'uncertain future' for the School.[224] The first fateful decision not to amalgamate with the new regional university had preceded the 1987 coup, and—as we have seen—was largely determined by financial considerations. Reconsideration of this decision was, of course, made more difficult by the economic crisis after 1987, and the School became considered almost a part of ethnic Fijians' birthright. As mentioned previously, my own view is that the School would have been better as a USP Faculty of Medicine because it would have allowed more academic freedom, recruitment of better faculty members, given legitimacy to its regional institution status, and improved financial management and general administration of the School. It was a missed opportunity. The 1987 coups and their aftermaths brought severe budget constraints to the School and was a major constraint for recruitment of staff, particularly high quality academics, in addition to the immediate loss of expatriates and migration of local staff. But the legacy of ethnic bitterness from the coups also harmed the School in ways that are difficult to measure directly. The Old Boys network of the Queen Victoria School was also a strong presence at the School, and the *Taukei* influence—which was still evident in my time at the School—was in the final analysis more of a liability than an asset, more detrimental than constructive, as is usually the case for old boys' networks within an institution.

On the one hand, Fiji's inheritance of two ethnic groups not of its choosing could have resulted in much worse outcomes. It avoided civil war and did not produce tyrants like Hitler or Pol Pot, nor did it follow the paths of Zimbabwe or Sudan. On the other hand, Fiji could have made a much greater effort to integrate and accommodate its two dominant ethnic groups. Arguable, the two other island states of Mauritius and Hawaii have done better with multi-ethnic communities, although there are important differences with Fiji. Mara, in particular, could have been more statesman-like in convincing the indigenous population for the need to accommodate the Indian community. Fiji has paid a heavy price politically, socially and economically for failing to do so. In the words of Pierre Trudeau, a former Prime Minister of Canada:

> Throughout history, when a state has taken an exclusive and intolerant idea such as religion and ethnicity as its cornerstone, this idea more often than not has been the very mainspring of violence and war.

Chapter 15

A Poisoned Chalice

At this point in the history of Fiji School of Medicine—from July 2005 to January 2008—the story takes on an autobiographical flavour as the author was appointed Dean of the Fiji School of Medicine. I had heard about the vacancy before leaving Vanuatu in December 2004 where I had been an Australian volunteer paediatrician at Vila Central Hospital, but had recently suffered from leptospirosis, which had required evacuation to Melbourne for management of renal failure. The condition was contracted from bats on a cave walk and river swim while on a rural clinical visit to the islands of Espiritu Santo and Ambae. The infection was transmitted at a popular tourist attraction called the Millennium Cave Walk. A young Australian had died earlier that year from the disease acquired at the same place.[372] Since the village from where the walk commenced had no warnings of the danger of leptospirosis, I wrote to the Head of Public Health in Vanuatu and to Lonely Planet. The latter did actually include a warning in their new edition, but instead of being under the walk itself, it was placed at the end of the book under health warnings. Health warnings and travel advisories for tourists are, of course, very sensitive political issues for Pacific Island countries, including after the recent Fiji coup.

Upon my return to Darwin in January 2005 to resume as Clinical Dean of the Northern Territory Clinical School, I received a further notification of the vacancy and heard indirectly that the previous Dean, Wame Baravilala, wanted me to apply. I knew the School well as I had been the External Examiner for the MBBS programme from

1998-2001 and for the Paediatric MMed degree in 2003. In addition, Wame had arranged for me to run a workshop for the academic staff on evidence-based medicine in July 2000, which was unfortunately cancelled due to the Speight coup. Some of the current and previous Faculty members were well known to me from my previous positions in the Pacific and elsewhere, including Elizabeth Rodgers (Paediatrics), David Phillips and Lester Ross (Public Health), Andrew Adjukieviecz and Joji Malani (Medicine) and Douglas Pikacha (Surgery). In addition, several of my colleagues in Darwin had worked previously in Fiji, including Alan Ruben, Michael Lowe and Jim Burrow.

My return to Darwin after a year away convinced me of the need for a change as I had been based in Darwin since 1995, the longest period of my life spent in any one place (Fig 1). My main concern about applying for the Fiji position was whether the acting Dean, Eddie McCaig, really wanted the job and, if he did, whether he was the most appropriate candidate. I was not so much worried about being unsuccessful as my application being inappropriate to stand in the way of a local applicant, but as it turned out, Eddie did not want the position or at least was very ambivalent about it. This feeling of an expatriate being an inappropriate applicant was rather reinforced by the views of my Darwin colleagues, who informed me that two local Heads of Schools were also applicants, namely Sitaleki Finau of Tonga (Public Health) and Jonacani Tuisuva of Fiji (Oral Health). Jan Pryor, the American Head of Research was the other short-listed candidate, and I was the only external applicant. In the end, I decided to 'throw my hat into the ring' and let the School Council decide, since it was made up of very prominent citizens of Fiji.

Appointment as Dean

I was called for the first interview by Faculty and management staff in Suva in February 2005. I remember being in a good humour walking from Holiday Inn to JJs in the Park, where the interview took place. I had dressed with a jacket and tie for the occasion which made me noticeable, so was accosted by a couple of tourist hawkers who asked my name and generally behaved in a friendly fashion. Before I could say anything else, my name was carved on a wooden boat for which money was extorted. I considered myself an old hand at avoiding tourist traps from years in Africa, so I was rather irritated at my naivety. Nevertheless, the interview by a panel of School staff went well enough, although it was clear to me that they supported Eddie McCaig as Dean and were also irritated by their ambiguous role in the appointment process, as it was clearly the responsibility of the Council in the FSM Act (1997) to choose the Dean.

I was informed that there would be a subsequent Council interview if shortlisted, so requested that it be done via videoconference to Darwin. This took place in April with the Governor of the Reserve Bank, other senior Fijian officials, including the recently appointed Vice-Chancellor of the University of the South Pacific (USP). My main recollection was questions regarding my track record of research, which seemed to impress some members of the panel. In the end, I was successful and travelled to Suva from July 4-25 to be oriented and sign my contract, after which I returned to Australia briefly as Royal Australasian College of Physicians Examiner for the specialist clinical examination for Paediatrics in Melbourne, Brisbane, Hobart, Sydney, Adelaide and Darwin. Consequently, I did not officially start as Dean at Fiji School of Medicine until August 2005.

My so-called 'orientation' in July was a strange affair indeed. The Registrar and Head of Personnel,—both Queen Victoria School old boys—were assigned as my 'minders' until I had signed a contract, and in a sympathetic way they seemed to want to protect me from finding out anything about the future problems which would face me. The most helpful person was my old friend Jimmie Rodgers from Solomon Islands, who was in charge of the Secretariat of the Pacific Community (SPC) in Fiji (later he was appointed as Director-General based in Noumea), and was also chair of a crucial Corporate Review of the School as a Council member. He made a special point of introducing me to key people, including Ministers and CEOs of the then SDL

Government in Fiji (before the Dec 2006 coup). There was a strange incident regarding an invitation to the French Embassy for the 14th July Bastille day reception, which was perhaps a premonition of things to come. Upon thanking the French Ambassador for his hospitality before departing, he warned me in French that I had enemies at the School because his invitation addressed to me personally had been returned with hostile comments on it.

I requested meetings with each of the Heads of School, three of whom had been applicants for the Dean position. My 'minders' were unhappy about this prospect until I had signed my contract. However, I did manage to meet the Head of the School of Oral Health, Jonacani Tuisuva, who was very pleasant and indicated his willingness to work closely with me as my counterpart so he could take over as Dean in two years. I pointed out that this would be up to Council, who had offered me a 4-year contract, but I indicated a certain willingness to work closely with him and my desire not to stand in the way of localising the position once again. However, at this stage I was still rather oblivious of the serious issues facing the School of Oral Health. I also met the distinguished Chair of Council, Savenaca Narube, Governor of the Reserve Bank.

In those early days, it is interesting to reflect back on what I saw as the key priority areas for the School:

1. Sound financial management
2. Being responsive to the health workforce needs of the region
3. Continuing professional education and in-service training for our staff and other health professionals in the region
4. High quality research on Pacific health issues with recruitment of new research-oriented staff and collaboration with regional universities
5. A strong emphasis on public health, especially population medicine and evidence-based medicine (EBM)
6. Distance learning using videoconferencing, the web and satellite technology in collaboration with USP to deliver education and training closer to home for students, and finally,

7. Improving the educational standards of our graduates: a mission to produce health professionals with compassion, empathy, integrity, competency and good communication skills, who are conversant with ethical issues, are interested in personal and professional development, understand the social determinants of health, and are focused on life-long learning rather than just memorising facts.

The Corporate Review

The first major issue facing the School was the corporate review which had been established by Council in 2004 under the chairmanship of Dr Jimmie Rodgers (a graduate of the School), due to a large deficit in the previous year and major concerns about nearly all of our corporate services, particularly finance,

Fig. 47: FSMed Management Structure, 2005

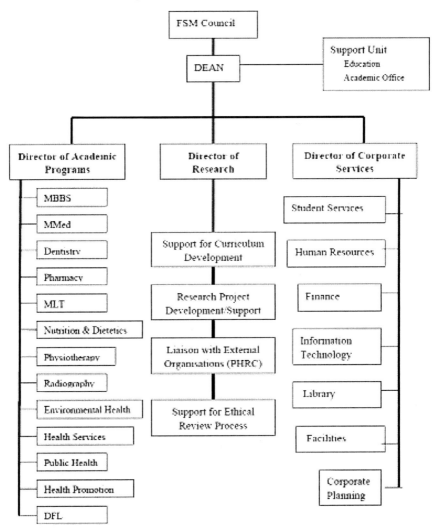

(MLT—Medical Laboratory Technology, DFL—Distance & Flexible Learning, MBBS—medical programme, MMed—postgraduate, FSM—FSMed) personnel, student services, facilities and information technology (Fig 47).

After more than 18 months of investigation, the review was presented to Council in November 2005. It was an excellent report, and went well beyond corporate issues to deal with governance and academic structure issues as well. It favoured the School joining USP so as to firmly establish its regional status as an institution, and affirmed that the four schools within the School (medical science, oral health, health science and public health) were functioning too autonomously and often at cross purposes to the overall objectives of the institution as a whole, recommending a change of structure which would strengthen the central administration and integrity of the School.

In terms of the corporate sector, the review painted a picture of incompetence, slackness and corruption which the institution needed to address urgently. Finance was clearly the main culprit, and in 2003-4, there had been a series of disastrous Finance Managers. But the School had appointed a new Finance Manager just prior to my appointment who had joined us from Pacific Theological Seminary, with qualifications and integrity which seemed beyond reproach. Indeed, the review stated that:

> at the start of the review, there was a clear perception by the key clients of the finance office that there was lack of leadership; . . . lack of training of users in finance policies and procedures; professional incompetence . . . it was like a 'black hole' where funds went into and could not be traced, making it very difficult to produce financial reports or acquittals. One of the advantages of completing the review process this late is to witness the transformation of the FSM finance office . . . to what is now an effective and responsive office that is professionally managed and putting systems in place that would help the institution deliver its financial services in a more effective and efficient manner.[250]

As I was soon to discover to my chagrin, the review was deceived and this transformation had in fact not happened. I was to discover serious irregularities of the payroll, accounts and large fines from government revenue for having neglected to pay taxes on time. But this was really the only shortcoming of the review, which was otherwise very insightful and accurate.

The review also identified major problems with the Personnel section. Particular concerns were expressed about nepotism in casual contracts, inefficiency and remnants of the public service mentality from which the School was supposed to have gained autonomy in 1997. The Personnel section seemed to be run by an administrative secretary, who made executive decisions without consultation and generally behaved in an insubordinate manner. It was not performing the way a human resources section needed to be functioning for an institution with more than 200 full-time employees.

The Information Technology (IT) section had a manager who was a previous Head of School's wife and her only 'qualification' for the position was having worked in a secretarial role for an American IT company. She was also under investigation by our external auditors for improper procurement practices from a local IT business owned by someone with whom it was alleged that she had a conflict of interest.

Finally, the Facilities Manager was also performing poorly, failing to supervise his staff and had not even arranged proper permits and insurance for our new campus. He migrated to Australia before I could start the difficult process of documenting his non-performance. Although I have not indentified these problematic corporate staff by name, it is perhaps worth indicating that three of the four positions were occupied by Indo-Fijians who all resigned and left the School within a few months of my arrival. Poorly performing indigenous Fijians, on the other hand, tended not to resign, but to remain and used the FSMEA (Employees Association or trade union) to resist change and defend their poor performance. This was hardly a coincidence as it mimicked what was happening in Fiji as a whole.

How was I to address these issues of serious corporate dysfunction? The Registrar acknowledged that he was not functioning well in his role, partly because in principle he had far too many both academic and corporate responsibilities for any one person. Consequently, he was moved sideways to the Academic Director position, and the corporate review suggested that we appoint a new position, a Corporate Director, to take overall responsibility for the business of the School. This would mean that there would be three Directors under the Dean, for the academic, corporate and research sections (Fig 47).

This model of a corporate director as business manager had worked very well for me in Darwin, both for the hospital division and the clinical school for which I was responsible because of excellent business managers. I was aware that with the existing level of corporate dysfunction revealed by the review, I would desperately need a good Corporate Director to help with the management of the School as I did not have a strong management background, especially in finance. The Council approved this new position, so we went ahead to recruit a Corporate Director in December 2005. Although we did get many applications, it was not a strong field of short-listed candidates. The favoured applicant by the Appointments Committee was the only woman applicant, an indigenous Fijian who was working for an insurance company at the time. It seemed appropriate to hire a female as our management team was almost exclusively male and we were looking for someone with corporate experience in the private sector. We checked with referees and then appointed Leba Tikoduadua.

Personnel was a more thorny issue, so we decided to recruit a new position of Human Resources (HR) Manager to oversee the section and institute a performance appraisal system. The best candidate was Ashish Chand who had previously worked for the Public Service Commission to establish their performance appraisal system. We were very concerned about how the existing Personnel and new HR Managers would work together, and with the existing personnel secretary. However, the latter resigned to take up a job with the Reserve Bank in which she only lasted for a month, and the HR and Personnel managers seemed to establish a *modus vivendi*.

A similar solution was also adopted for the IT Manager, so the existing unsatisfactory manager was confronted about the failure to follow proper procurement practices and alleged conflicts of interest, and agreed to work with a new IT Manager while these other issues were under investigation. So we went ahead and recruited a new IT Manager with the expert assistance of an IT Consultant through USP. However, our previous unqualified IT Manager then resigned and left, so we recruited Onisimo Pasikali who had previously worked for Training Productivity Authority of Fiji (TPAF). He proved to be an effective manager, and greatly improved our internet speed and IT infrastructure.

Finally, Academic Office had come under the Registrar and dealt with the sensitive issues of enrolment, charging student fees and examination security, all of which had been compromised. Consequently, the existing staff were moved sideways, and Academic Office was placed under the Dean. We recruited a new senior manager to run the office, Niraj Swami, who worked hard to re-establish the credibility and integrity of Academic Office, despite overt hostility from certain quarters.

Thus, by early 2005 we had four new senior managers for HR, IT, Academic Office and Corporate Services, the roles of Registrar and Personnel Manager had been abolished or modified, and the former Facilities and IT Managers and Personnel Secretary had resigned. So I was optimistic that with this new team it would not take long to turn things around. It was to prove much more difficult than I had thought.

My first major task as Dean was to get the School on a firm financial footing. The School had run up deficits of FJ$3.95 million in 2003 and $3.69 million in 2004, so was facing a cash flow crisis with inability to pay its bills. The following three measures were instituted soon after starting as Dean to address the financial crisis:

a) charge full tuition fees to all scholarship and private fee-paying students, without subsidising the fees of non-scholarship Fijian students
b) project funding to be managed as FSMed revenue and all projects to be charged a management fee by FSMed
c) cease holding workshops at hotels with extravagant catering costs, when they could be held on our premises for a fraction of the cost.

Thus, the corporate review was a thorough and insightful report which clearly established the agenda for my deanship. My task over the next 30 months was to implement the recommendations of this report, and I was single-minded in accomplishing this task in spite of strong resistance to change. Agents of change are often accused of being dictatorial and failing to consult, so I made a strong effort to encourage frank discussion of these issues and obtain a consensus before instituting changes.

However, I found that even after an apparent consensus, opponents tried to undermine new initiatives to which they had acquiesced. This gave the appearance of bad faith, and this form of 'white anting', as it is called in Australia, is always hard to deal with. It is not true that I was dictatorial, although I did insist upon implementation once a decision was agreed upon at senior staff meetings and ratified by Council. It may be true that too many changes were made in too short a time, but I did make an effort to consult and explain clearly the necessary changes at numerous staff forums and other meetings. However, there was one recommendation of the review which I did fail to implement. This was the proposal to join the University of the South Pacific as their Faculty of Medicine. The political will to carry this out was lacking during the democratic Qarase government and it was opposed by the later Interim Government when USP was in crisis. The Interim Government has recently amalgamated the School into the National University of Fiji, and USP has been significantly disadvantaged financially, so perhaps with hindsight it was just as well.

School Fees

The issue of subsidising school fees for non-scholarship Fiji students contributed significantly to our loss of revenue and was based upon a misunderstanding. The erroneous idea had emerged that the Fiji Government funding (block grant) was a contribution to the tuition fees of private fee-paying students from Fiji in a similar way to the USP funding model in which Pacific Island governments' contribution reduced USP tuition fees. Consequently, FSMed developed reduced fees for these students which were about a third of the full fees for scholarship students.

But our funding model was different from USP's and the Fiji Government had strongly objected to this use of its funds in a 2003 letter to FSMed on the basis that they had no control over our use of this funding, suggesting that we were essentially subsidising students' education for migration. When the School failed to respond to this warning, the Cabinet imposed limits on PSC scholarships by taking a proportion out of the block grant, essentially cutting our funding unless we ceased the subsidies. Unfortunately, the School continued the subsidies to private students from Fiji because Finance appeared not to really understand the issue. In fact, it was Jimmie Rodgers who explained this to me clearly, not our Finance section. Eventually in 2005, the subsidy was stopped for all 1st year students only.

In 2006, I instituted measures to cease all subsidies, so students (scholarship and private) would have to pay full fees which were FJ$14,500 for medicine (all paid for by scholarships), $15,500 for dentistry and $9,000 for health sciences, public health and postgraduate courses per annum. There was really little option but to make this decision as our fees had not changed since 2003, and we were near bankruptcy and had even stopped paying our bills. We also had to stop the practice of deferring fees, insisting that all debts were paid by a deadline. As a result of these measures, millions of dollars of additional revenue were raised, and it was clear than only a hard line would have been successful as many were merely trying to see whether they could continue to 'rort the system' with impunity.

Some dental and health science students objected to paying full fees on the basis that they had a contract with us for subsidised fees until they graduated, which was of course only wishful thinking.

However, for those with documented financial hardship from this measure, we had made provision for negotiation of lower fees with the Academic Director, but nearly all of these objecting private students came from wealthy backgrounds. Medical students were all on full-fee scholarships, and regional students were also charged full fees, so neither of these groups were affected by the changes. However, 55 students went to the Human Rights Commission alleging a breach of their human rights. Although I explained the situation clearly to the students, the Commission and Fiji Government in a series of meetings, the Commission ruled against us and kept threatening to take us to court. This was patently nonsense as we do not provide basic education, and it was clearly a contractual dispute (what was the human right in question?).

This prolonged legal process, which was also faintly ridiculous, was really only a form of harassment, probably with the collusion of certain staff members. I had not had much experience with legal issues, so found the litigious situation in Fiji very frustrating and stressful. This was only one of a great many issues for which I had to get legal advice, which was being exploited by the Employees Association. Rather naively, I assumed that if truth was on my side, all would go well. Instead of a frank discussion of issues and negotiated compromise, the School was faced with continuous legal harassments which were expensive and demoralising. It is sad when litigation is employed as a weapon in lieu of free discussion and negotiation of issues.

New Pasifika Campus

The official opening of the new campus by the Vice President of Fiji, Ratu Joni Madraiwiwi, was held in March 2006. It was a very colourful event with a full Fijian traditional ceremony and several hours of student dancing representing all the island groups.

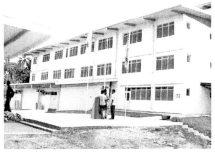

Fig. 48: The Teaching Block

In my speech, I mentioned David Hoodless of Central Medical School, and his meeting with the Vice President's ancestor as a boy, Ratu Jone Doviverata in 1921 whom he agreed to tutor. Two years later, Ratu Dovi, as he was called, was sent to Wanganui Technical College along with Ratu Edward Cakobau, eventually graduating in medicine from the University of Otago, and later returning to Fiji to supervise NMPs.

The new campus was named 'Pasifika' after a naming competition. It contained four dormitories for about 250 students, a three-storey teaching block with dental / medical laboratories and a large auditorium, a dining hall and a three-storey library and computer centre. This new campus greatly expanded our capacity for student teaching, so was a major asset. We soon discovered, however, that it was expensive to run, mostly due to the high electricity costs for air conditioning and external security lighting. I attempted in vain to get the air conditioning turned off after hours to reduce our electricity costs.

Dental School Nightmares

I have called this chapter a poisoned chalice, meaning a task which almost inevitably brings harm or unpopularity to the person who assumes responsibility for it. The Dental School (later Department) was a major component of this poisoned chalice, so we need to tell its story.

But to start on a positive note, the dental curriculum was modular and appeared highly innovative. For example, the course progressed from dental assistant (1 year), to hygienist (2 years) to technologist (3 years), to dentist (5 years) with appropriate exit points. There was a strong local flavour and community orientation to the course, with an appropriate emphasis on preventive dentistry and problem-based learning.[373-375] The teaching of research by the Department was strong, with the student presentations of their projects of high quality.

So what were the problems in dentistry? In the first instance, dentistry was costing the School much more than its revenue, so was being heavily subsidised by the MBBS fees. Dental students from Fiji were not paying the full fees due to the ill-conceived subsidy arrangement mentioned above. Since there were already too many dentists in Fiji, most of our BDS graduating students were not employed until several years after graduation, so dental scholarships had been stopped by Fiji government in 2003.

A second issue was private practice for dental staff, which had been cancelled due to corruption and abuses until such time as appropriate financial mechanisms could be developed to ensure probity, which never actually happened. A third issue was the fact that some dental staff were also enrolled as BDS students, which obviously compromised a fair assessment process of them by colleagues, and also meant their focus was more on studying than on academic excellence in teaching.

In addition, dentistry had some facilities at the new campus, but its service, clinical teaching and staff offices were still based within CWM Hospital, and this splitting of facilities was a difficulty which should have been avoided with proper planning. Finally, there was considerable long-standing tension among dental staff between the three ethnic groups of indigenous Fijians, Indo-Fijians and Europeans—more than for other Departments of the School.

But by far the most difficult issue in Dentistry, which I had inherited from the previous Dean, was dealing with the situation of the Head of Oral Health having been 'stepped down' from his position on full pay. The story had started in November 2004 at the final BDS Exams. The external examiner had been the Dean of the University of Queensland Dental School, Prof Laurie Walsh and Dr Vikash Singh was the internal examiner. Both agreed that two students should not graduate, and this was confirmed by the exam committee of the School of Oral Health.

However, the Head of School was apparently unhappy with this decision, so had it reversed by a higher committee which he chaired, at which he also proposed his favourite student for the medal. An Indo-Fijian dental staff member objected to the proposed recommendation for the student medal in a confidential letter giving reasons why this favourite student was not deserving either academically or personally for this honour.

This confidential letter was leaked to all staff and to the student himself, who then pursued litigation for defamation. Understandably, the staff member's response was to cry foul and blame the School for breaching confidentiality. This technique of leaking confidential documents to staff and the press was employed repeatedly to undermine other staff members or decisions reached apparently by consensus. As it was done anonymously, it was difficult to prove who was responsible, and it clearly raised ethnic tensions.

Following our terms and conditions of employment, Eddie McCaig as acting Dean had appointed a disciplinary committee of Jan Pryor (research), Rodney Yee (corporate) and Rajendra Singh (Employees Association) to investigate the allegations of academic misconduct. This was the situation when I commenced at FSMed, but the whole issue seemed to have been put in the 'too hard' basket with no action taken.

At the same time, there were allegations from an audit of financial irregularities in ordering dental supplies, and an investigation showed that proper financial procedures had not been followed, that we were being overcharged for poor quality materials and that this had been brought to the attention of the Department without any change in ordering having occurred. It was also clear that the proper investigation process was being undermined by some senior members of staff close to the Head of Department, so I insisted that the original disciplinary committee reconsider all the evidence and make recommendations.

To cut a long story short, the Council dismissed the Head of Department on the basis of these recommendations which I endorsed but the decision was reversed by an appeal process to a one-man Tribunal (a former labour leader). Not only was he reinstated but the

FSMEA (union) appointed him as its President. Thus, for the next 18 months, the FSMEA and its President waged a war against me personally using all of the many appeal mechanisms available in Fiji, until his contract expired and was not renewed in 2006.

Things came to a head at the Council meeting of April 2007, when the new Employee Association President presented a petition for my dismissal, accompanied by a 12 page diatribe against me which was malicious and in very poor taste. This offensive document lost the union the support of its members, so it was retracted. However, another such letter was circulated in November 2007 over the staff appraisal exercise which the union had pressured us to implement. It is easy to dismiss such letters after the event, but at the time to be called a liar and psychopath in writing and circulated to all and sundry was upsetting.

At the end of the day, were all the hassles from the union and personal stress over this issue worth it to get rid of a high status and powerful member of staff? From the School's perspective, I have no doubt that it was. He and his cronies had had their innings, and it was time for the School to move on. At a personal level, I am less sure. I am not usually 'tough' by nature, but I found that my role forced me to take a strong stance as Dean instead of either ignoring the seriousness of the issue or pretending that the well established pattern of behaviour would change. Both of my local predecessors, Baravilala and McCaig, more or less acknowledged that they were unable to deal with this issue, so I felt as an expatriate it was important to do so for the good of the institution. However, even with the sacking of the offending Head of Department, the legacy of problems in dentistry persisted, coming again to a head with the 2007 exams.

The final written and practical examinations for students in 2007 were held in early November and were organised by Academic Office, following a complete change of staff in that office due to serious concerns about irregularities when it was under the Registrar. Each Departmental Year Committee sets their exams, and then they are standardised ('moderated') to ensure that the standard of pass mark is fair (adjusting it if too easy or difficult) and 'blueprinted' to ensure that it covers the curriculum representatively and fairly, as discussed in chapter 12.

These educational activities are essential in setting exams because our standards should be criterion-referenced as we do not want to adjust marks on a Bell curve (norm-referencing). In other words, we need to compare students to a minimum standard of knowledge and competency set by academic staff rather than comparing students to each other and arbitrarily failing a fixed percentage of students, as had been the past practice. In addition, some subjects such as biostatistics and pharmacology are taught to students from multiple programmes (e.g. medicine, dentistry and health sciences), so the dental department needed to have a say about what the standard of statistical and pharmacologic knowledge should be for dental students. Consequently, a Senior Lecturer in Dentistry was asked to moderate the exams for Years 1-3 dentistry students several weeks before the exam date.

In mid-November, the Associate Professor of Pharmacology, Bronwen Bryant, contacted me about concerns while marking the pharmacology exam for 3rd year dental students. There was clear evidence from the answers and previous results of certain students that they had prior knowledge of the exam questions. Thus, some borderline students had obtained very high marks and had answered some questions with sophisticated new material which suggested preparation of the specific questions beforehand. Needless to say, I was alarmed by any suggestion of academic cheating and from past experiences did not trust an internal investigation which would be likely to conclude that there was inadequate proof or 'sweep it under the table', as had happened on previous occasions with other issues. Consequently, I decided to hire an external investigator.

The private investigator's report was based upon a thorough investigation with videotaped confessions by many students which revealed a shocking story of deceit within dentistry. Students from wealthy families without acceptable academic results were allowed into the course with payment of bribes, and then were assisted throughout their course by being given copies of exams beforehand.

The particular incident in November 2007 documented at least 4 students paying up to FJ$500 for a copy of the exam, but they shared the exam with other students and then many students studied together, so it was impossible to draw clear lines between cheating students and those who may have inadvertently been party to the cheating. Clearly the exam process had been compromised, and there was evidence that cheating had involved at least 18 exams over three years of the dental course. In the end, we decided that these exam results were invalid for these subjects, and all dental students would have to re-sit the suspicious exams in January-February of 2008, prior to the commencement of the next academic year. Fiji certainly does not condone this kind of behaviour, so the offending staff member was convicted and jailed for 18 months and some implicated dental students were expelled.

An unfortunate consequence of this sorry saga was that it received considerable press coverage in Fiji. The Fiji Sun, in particular, ran articles on it for some time, and seemed to be using it to discredit the entire School and medical profession, despite repeatedly making it clear to them that it had only involved the early years of the dental programme and one current staff member.

Project Funding

There were a large number of projects being managed by the School whose finances were less than transparent, and it seemed as if the School was subsidising them. There was no mechanism for the School to recover the management and infrastructure costs of these projects, which included research projects, consultancies for agencies such as WHO, AusAID and SPC, and educational contracts in public health for distance learning to the Federated States of Micronesia (FSM) and Palau. These latter contracts were generously funded by the USA to deliver Certificates in Public Health to graduates of the courses. Initially, these courses were partly delivered by distance and flexible learning (DFL) mode through video lectures and paper handouts, but the poor results led FSMed to resort to delivering 24-hour contact lectures normally delivered over a semester into 10 days of face-to-face didactic teaching by visiting staff.

My initial impressions of this Micronesian DFL programme were unfavourable because the educational standards were low, overtime and bonus payments (in addition to expenses and *per diems*) were being paid to staff, airfares were almost FJ$5,000 per trip via either Japan, Korea or Australia-Philippines, and Public Health staff were neglecting our Suva-based students, particularly in the MBBS programme. This latter concern was important because we had a reputation as a community-oriented medical school, but were no longer teaching community medicine in the first three years of the course because of the refusal of the School of Public Health, allegedly because they wanted additional funding for teaching medical students.

However, in May 2006 I agreed to officiate at the graduation of our students in Public Health in Palau and Yap. This was an opportunity to investigate firsthand the appropriateness of this programme, which I felt needed to be wound down, and also a chance to meet Dr Greg Dever who had established the Pacific Basin Medical School (chapter 8). Many of our academic staff had worked with him in Micronesia, including Jimi Samisoni, Jan Pryor, Joe Flear and Joji Malani. It was a great pleasure to finally meet Dr Dever, to witness his dedication and enthusiasm and to enjoy his generous hospitality. He introduced me to key politicians, and all expressed profound gratitude to FSMed, even passing an Act of Parliament officially acknowledging the School's contribution to Palau. A recurrent theme was that our courses were appropriate for the students, who remained in country, whereas when American institutions delivered courses, most of the students then left the country for the USA.

Both graduation ceremonies in Palau and Yap were moving celebrations of accomplishment, and certainly changed my mind that we should not abandon this part of the Pacific despite the tyranny of distance. Indeed, we agreed to base one of our staff in Yap to coordinate the programme and help keep travel costs down, as well as using more

DFL techniques to reduce the time spent by staff delivering didactic material instead of promoting learning, while still recognising the need for continuing face-to-face teaching. As it turned out, we were never able to fill this position.

Another important Public Health initiative had been to win the contract to manage an 8.9 million European Union aid project to Kiribati for building outer island health facilities and training health workers as part of the 9th European Development Fund. Managing an aid project was a new kind of venture for the School, especially since we were already struggling with the efficient management of our own business, but it did promise to be a source of additional revenue for the School. But it also proved to be a further source of conflict, both within the School, and with the European donor and Kiribati recipient. After some very difficult beginnings, the project proceeded mostly uneventfully, and did earn the School revenue for managing it.

Research Challenges

In view of my track record in research, I saw as a key role of the Dean to promote high quality relevant research in the Pacific. For a medical school, FSMed had a very weak track record of research with few, if any, original research papers in major clinical journals and only about four expatriate staff with PhDs and two local staff enrolled in PhDs in Australia on public health issues (AIDS and oral health). Even those few staff members with a track record in research, most had never published a study in a major journal.

Most of our research activity was consultancy reports on public health issues for WHO or other donor agencies which were never published in the scientific literature. An additional barrier to research was the total lack of research quantum, and a tax system which did not allow any deductions for professional activities such as presenting at conferences. FSMed was expected to pay all the costs of such trips, including generous *per diem* allowances, out of its funding. Although

NZ did give us generous support for professional training, but most of it went on staff seeking higher qualifications rather than increasing research productivity.

Two key players at the School in research were Professors Jan Pryor and Sitaleki Finau, who were chief investigators of two grants from the International Collaborative Grants initiative in 2005 funded by the Wellcome Foundation along with NHMRC (Australia) and HRC (NZ). The two studies were on obesity (OPIC) and car accidents (TRIP) in collaboration with Auckland and Deakin universities, respectively.

I was very familiar with this once off research initiative by Wellcome as I had spent a great deal of time in Darwin applying for a grant to set up a research institute in Timor Leste to study *Helicobacter pylori* transmission and its consequences in young children while providing basic child health services to Ermera Province. We received excellent reviews on the proposal and were short listed to the end, but then missed out on funding. Perhaps that is just as well with hindsight, as the later political developments in Timor would have made the project impossible. It was my failure and frustration with this Wellcome grant proposal, with all my efforts coming to naught, which partly motivated me to focus my efforts on medical education instead of research, and apply for the Dean position in Fiji.

The Pacific Health Research Council (PHRC), which was funded by NZAID to promote Pacific Island research, was located within FSMed and supervised by our research staff, particularly Jan Pryor. My first meeting of the PHRC Executive Council in November 2005 revealed serious conflict between the executive and Pryor, which took on a personal and antagonistic flavour. On the one hand, the executive (made up of very influential Pacific Island academics) was frustrated because the funding and supervision of the secretariat of PHRC was entirely in FSMed's control. On the other hand, Pryor had worked tirelessly and thanklessly to make the PHRC function better than could be expected under the human resource constraints.

As a consequence of this conflict, Pryor resigned from PHRC and I asked his deputy to take on the role of supervising the secretariat. I confess that I had great sympathy for Pryor, as he was our Director of Research, was incredibly hard working and productive, had been in the Pacific for some 30 years although American by nationality, and was very pro-Pacific Islander research. In addition, some of the attacks against him were expressed in clearly unacceptable terms.

Things came to a head at a very bad time for me in April 2007 while battling the Staff Association. A review committee was appointed by NZAID to report on future funding for PHRC. Their initial presentation in Suva was very reasonable, but the written draft was very negative and gave no credit for PHRC's accomplishments. This was worsened from our point of view by an accompanying commentary from the PHRC executive blaming all the failures on FSMed and accusing us of misappropriating both the funds and PHRC research staff for our own ends. Since NZAID is an important donor and scholarship provider, this was a public relations disaster for us.

The PHRC had always been requesting autonomy from FSMed, so I decided that indeed they must have it as soon as possible and we would withdraw from the organisation. The remaining question was of course whether PHRC was still viable and would continue to receive NZ funding, and indeed their funding was not renewed in 2008. It is strange how the competition for research funding leads to parochial views that only indigenous researchers should be allowed to carry out research on indigenous health, instead of judging research proposals on their merit. I had encountered similar attitudes in Australia and Africa. Basically, when the ethnicity of the researchers becomes more of an issue than the quality of the research, it is always counterproductive.

The option proposed by FSMed was an autonomous research institute based at the School in partnership with Australian and NZ Aid Programmes and Medical Research Councils (NHMRC, HRC), similar to the PNG Institute of Medical Research. The key challenges were to get a critical mass of health researchers together for productive collaboration, to attract funding and to supervise junior researchers and PhD students. Such an institute would clearly require regional legitimacy by involving Ministries of Health, and would also need to collaborate closely with WHO, SPC and USP. From FSMed's perspective, the OPIC and TRIP studies were very successful ventures because they allowed our junior staff to participate in high quality research and gain practical experience in the field.

Graduate Entry Proposal

In mid-2007, there were two positive developments for FSMed. Firstly, the Australian Aid budget was doubled by the Howard government, despite it being an election year. Secondly, several influential Australian doctors, including Prof Stephen Leeder, wrote to AusAID complaining about the lack of support for the medical schools in the Pacific region, namely UPNG and FSMed. Consequently, AusAID appointed a Committee to develop a report on the feasibility of a Pacific region Human Resources for Health (HRH) initiative. Prof John Hamilton, one of my teachers at McMaster University in Canada and the Dean of Medicine when I was on the Faculty at the University of Newcastle in Australia, was appointed to the Committee as the medical education specialist, and was a source of great moral support for me personally.

I confess to having had serious reservations at the time about HRH. I am always suspicious of current dogma, and HRH was clearly the 'flavour of the month' among aid agencies. More importantly, I did not want our development assistance funding to be wasted on fruitless manpower planning. Despite all the HRH planning in the 1990s, developed countries clearly got the need for doctors desperately wrong because the planning paradigm was to reduce doctors as the only way of controlling health care costs.

I had recently read the book *White Man's Burden: why the West's efforts to aid the rest have done so much ill and so little good* by William Easterly, which struck a chord with me about the difference between planners and seekers, and the harm of comprehensive, systematic planning in the context of development assistance.[331] But in fairness to AusAID, they saw HRH as much broader than just documenting doctor shortages in Pacific Island Countries.

In terms of strategic planning for FSMed, it was clear to me that we were not meeting the needs for doctors and particularly specialists (e.g. surgeons, physicians) in Fiji and the region. Our intake of medical students each year from high school was 70 (about 40 from Fiji and 30 from regional countries), but there were only about 45-50 graduates after 6 years. At least 15% of our graduates as doctors, dentists and pharmacists had migrated to a developed country, and clearly an even higher proportion of Indo-Fijians since the coups of 1987.[376]

Many regional countries were sending medical students to Cuba and nearly all were recruiting doctors and specialists with some difficulty from outside the region, particularly from Bangladesh, India and the Philippines. Australia had increased medical student places per year from about 1300 graduates in 2003 to potentially 3500 by 2010, including overseas fee-paying students who constituted about a quarter of all medical students. This significant number of overseas fee-paying medical students in Australia was necessitated by the 30% reduction in real terms in university funding between 1996 and 2004 by the Howard government.[377]

It was very obvious that FSMed also needed to increase its medical graduates, as well as its specialist trainees. On the other hand, it was equally obvious that we were training too many dentists, radiographers and physiotherapists as these graduates were not finding jobs until several years after graduating, accepting unpaid voluntary positions within government service until then. It may have been obvious to me, but there was considerable resistance to accepting this by some academic staff in Medical Science. There were even strong views that HRH issues were not our concern (ivory tower mentality) or that we should become more of an off-shore medical school and accept fee-paying students from out of the region to solve our budget problems.

My first attempt to increase the MBBS 1st year intake of 70 students was for 2006, but this was vetoed (the Years 1-3 MBBS Coordinator,

Joseph Flear, was particularly vehement on this and other issues) because the new campus was not yet open and there was insufficient space for tutorial groups, or so I was told. However, the next year with the new campus open, it was also vetoed due to a lack of clinical places at CWM and Lautoka hospitals, even though we still had three years to arrange for increased clinical places for years 4-6. It was clear to me that if we did not meet the needs, others would step in to do so—which is indeed what happened.

In yet another attempt to increase MBBS places in 2007, I proposed the addition of a graduate entry stream of 24 places, in which students with an undergraduate university degree would enter a special third year and then join the normal years 4-6 curriculum in 2008-10. They would still need to have a slightly modified 4th year to continue to catch up in the medical sciences, but would need to be integrated into the normal 4th year in 2008 based in Suva. This would have increased the total number of year 4-5 students by 2009 to around 175 students, depending on the number of failures and drop-outs. In order to accommodate clinical placements for these students, we would have needed to offer Years 4-5 of the MBBS in Lautoka as well as Suva, and transfer Year 6 (Trainee Intern) students to Labasa, where the hospital had just been refurbished.

This new graduate entry 3rd year would not try to cram all of years 1-3 in one year, but would be based on a digest of those years. It was anticipated that this new cohort of students (from Fiji and regional countries) would have a strong academic record and some were likely to have a background in sciences and para-medical subjects. The graduate entry students had to be integrated into the clinical years 4-5 of our exiting course to avoid the need to run a completely separate curriculum for more than a year, which would have stretched our capacity.

This proposal was based upon two essential premises. Firstly, that there were bright university graduates in the region who would be highly motivated to study medicine in a 4 year course. Secondly, that in a year they would have acquired enough knowledge to partially integrate with a clinical Year 4 students while continuing to catch-up in the medical sciences. We already know from experience in North America and Australia that a 4-year graduate entry course is feasible and the problem-based learning (PBL) approach facilitates the process of catch-up learning. Another major advantage of the graduate entry model in the setting of Pacific island countries is that medical students would need to spend less time in Suva. We were also planning to expand the programme of trainee internship rotations in regional countries so regional students might only need to spend three years in Fiji for a medical degree through graduate entry.

Although there was a lot of support for this proposal, there was also a lot of resistance to change within the Department of Medical Science. Although eventually approved in principle by Academic Board, it was postponed by FSMed Council when the Ministry of Health members spoke against it and demanded a more detailed proposal. I had actually gained approval from many members of Council about the proposal before the Council meeting, but some of those did not attend, and their substitutes were not briefed. It might have had a more receptive hearing the next year, but the Interim Government had other agendas which resulted in the loss of Lautoka Hospital as a teaching hospital for FSMed. Without Lautoka, there was no possibility of expanding student numbers for clinical training.

A Dreadful Monday

I have good and bad days like everyone, but Monday Aug 13th 2007 was a particularly bad day for me. The day started with an MBBS curriculum committee meeting. Having checked all the written exams for the School, I was very concerned that our assessments were sloppily designed with a focus on factual recall rather than the higher modes of learning. Consequently, I ran several assessment workshops for our departments to inform them about new developments in assessment and allow small group discussions on issues such as blueprinting, standardisation (moderation by criterion referencing), extended matching items, clinical competence, etc. I think these were quite successful from the feedback I received, but the small group sessions for the MBBS clinicians did not work. They essentially refused to participate and formed a large group that chatted instead of focussing on the task at hand.

It was clear to me that since assessment drives learning, we needed to focus on improving the quality of our assessment tools. Of particular concern to me were the clinical discipline blocks in years 4-5 of MBBS (e.g. paediatrics, medicine, surgery etc.), which were each marked as a continuous assessment (which had to be passed independently), a written exam and a clinical assessment. None of these on their own was a reliable assessment, yet it was a high stakes assessment as students who failed had to repeat the block or the even the year under some circumstances. In addition, there was an 'exit' written exam at the end of year 5 which was made up of discipline questions, all of a similar short answer or modified essay question format, with no standardisation or blueprinting. In a word, the problem was high stakes assessments based upon too many barriers ('must pass') and using assessments with low reliability (e.g. too few questions).

The solution was not complex and was ultimately feasible. Continuous assessment of each block should not be made an obligatory pass, but marks should be aggregated over multiple disciplines and with either clinical or written exams at the end of each block. The final exam should either be a high quality written exam using multiple modalities (multiple choice, extended matching, short answer, modified essay) of high reliability which is blueprinted and standardised, or a 20-station OSCE. If the latter, then block clinical assessments could be discontinued or made formative, and if the former, then block written exams could cease. Ideally, many would argue that we should have both high quality OSCE and written exams in the penultimate Year 5, but at least this simpler proposal was feasible without much additional work.

These recommendations were rejected as three influential members of the Committee refused to consider instituting a reliable final assessment, even suggesting that my motives were dishonest (to impress Australian medical educationalists). None of the other members of the Committee offered an opinion. It was particularly disappointing because I had patently been excluded from any involvement in the Department of Medical Science, and this was yet another slap in the face saying they were not going to accept my advice on assessment either. What was upsetting was that no arguments were offered, it was really that I was considered an outsider to the Department, provoking a defensive reaction.

The second item of bad news on Monday was in Pacific Health Dialog, which is a Journal of Community Health and Clinical Medicine for the Pacific, and FSMed is one of its sponsors. The September 2006 issue on Pacific Public Health 3 was in fact only published in August 2007 and was edited by Sitaleki Finau, who had migrated to NZ in June 2006 to take a position at Massey University. The guest editorial was a diatribe against the positive changes made in our Public Health programmes by Graham Roberts at FSMed. But most offensive and unprofessional was a personal attack on my wife as "the desperate housewife, employed by the husband on the apron string." As a matter of fact, she was employed fully by USP and has never been a 'housewife' in the 38 years of our marriage. Obviously, I was upset by this false and underhanded personal attack in a scientific journal. I wrote the Vice-Chancellor of Massey University to protest against the slur, but never received a response.

As if that was not enough for one day, I also learned that a new, junior administrative staff member had exploited our system to obtain new furniture, a printer and an air conditioner behind the back of his supervisor and in conflict with our existing policies. Additionally, I learned of evidence that someone was adjusting students marks and that a cash cheque of $750 had been paid for a simple lunch worth about $50. These were only a few of the many examples that our system was dysfunctional and was being easily and brazenly exploited for personal gain. It had indeed been an awful Monday.

Another Coup

In early December 2006, we held an important workshop at Pasifika campus to discuss our postgraduate programmes for the MMed degree. I had spent a lot of time organising this workshop because there were a number of important issues which needed wide discussion and decisions. We invited high level representatives from our stakeholders, including the Ministry of Health, CWM and Lautoka Hospitals, Public Services Commission (PSC), Ministry of Finance, WHO, AusAID, NZAID, USP, SPC, Fiji Medical Association, Private Practitioners and our senior academic staff. The key issues on the agenda were:

1) *Workforce issues*: Why are we not meeting the needs for specialists? Recruitment / migration issues.
2) *Career structure*: How many years should it take to train an anaesthetist after MBBS? It was currently taking 10 years before gaining specialist registration.
3) *Student selection process*: How can we get the best students? Should bright students be fast-tracked? Non-academic-based favouritism by Ministries of Health.
4) *New Programmes*: What are the needs? How are these determined? Do we have the training capacity?

    a) Generalists in Hospital/Emergency Medicine, General Practice
    b) Pathology, Radiology, Psychiatry
    c) Ophthalmology and other sub-speciality training (e.g. cardiology, oncology, ENT)

5) *Financial issues:*

    a) Payment of regional (non-Fiji) trainees for hospital work
    b) Tuition fees and FSMed costs

A particularly thorny issue was funding. The tuition fees for MMed students were FJ$9,000/year, but the cost to FSMed was closer to $20,000/year per student because for the small numbers per discipline and the heavy time commitment of specialist medical academic staff on high salaries. Of course, we could just dissolve these additional costs into the MBBS programme, since these same faculty also taught year 4-6 students. But a further issue was the fact that regional registrars (e.g. Samoa, Tonga, Solomon Island, etc) were not paid a salary by CWM Hospital, but were paid a scholarship by a donor agency like AusAID or by their government. This was essentially subsiding Fiji Ministry of Health with free labour, including after hours service. The issue was further complicated by longstanding underfunding of health in Fiji. So the Fiji Ministry of Health had no additional funding to spare, and the subsequent coup only made matters worse.

Unfortunately, due to the events of the coup that day, most of the donors did not attend and government employees were instructed to go home at noon, so the workshop only lasted 3 hours. There was agreement that Fiji had a regional responsibility to train more specialists, and that specialist training should be shortened to about 6-8 years after MBBS with earlier entry and recognition as a specialist upon completion of MMed (instead of after 2 years of further experience). As at other health forums, the PSC was criticised for inappropriate bureaucracy in recruitment of doctors. But—yet again—the political situation had prevented resolution of these key issues, which were further postponed. Fiji desperately needed to train more local and regional specialists, but until these issues were resolved, it would be difficult to do so.

Loss of Lautoka Clinical School

In September 2007, the Interim Minister announced on Fiji radio and by press release that the government supported a new medical school in Nadi by the University of Fiji and alleged that FSMed was at fault for allowing all their graduates to migrate. There was also mention of transferring the FJ$4m grant to the new school as well as Lautoka Hospital as a teaching hospital. The acting Interim Health Minister stated that "Fiji School of Medicine is not expected to be affected by the establishment of a second medical school." What was he thinking? How could the loss of our clinical school in Lautoka not affect us?

We had been aware of a proposed new medical school at the University of Fiji in March 2006 when former Prime Minister Qarase had officially opened the new university, predominantly for Indo-Fijian students. I had also met the Vice-Chancellor and a donor of A$1million to the university for a proposed new medical school. The donor was an Adelaide GP of Indo-Fijian origin, who had attended the School for a few years before transferring to Auckland.

This announcement of a new medical school, however, was a complete surprise. We had no prior discussions with the Interim Minister or Ministry of Health about these issues. Two weeks prior to this, I had requested a meeting with the Minister about threats to charge us rent for Hoodless House (we discovered their staff measuring our buildings), but he had refused to meet me, so I had met the Permanent Secretary, who was unaware of what was happening with either rent or the University of Fiji's proposed medical school. What was even more curious was that Lautoka Hospital and the Western Health Division were also unaware of the announced transfer of Lautoka hospital from FSMed to the University of Fiji.

The statements about funding and migration were also misleading. Of the $4 million Fiji government funding, only $2.6 million was block institutional funding, the remainder being student scholarships from the Public Services Commission and Fijian Affairs Board. This government funding was out of a total annual operating budget of $19 million per year and for a total of 1,050 students. We provided to the Ministry of Health—at no charge to them—the services of about 20 senior medical specialists who worked at CWM and Lautoka Hospitals. They spent at least 40% of their time (often much more) in clinical duties at the hospital, and also participated in on-call and after hours duties—all at the expense of FSMed with no MoH reimbursement. These specialist physicians and surgeons cost us over $1.5 million a year in salaries and on-costs, and we had great difficulty in recruiting these staff, just as the Ministry of Health did for its consultants. In addition, we paid over $70,000 in honorariums to clinical staff in the Ministry for supervising our students. We also paid over $200,000 in dental consumables for Ministry patients and supplied 12 regional specialist doctors as MMed trainees at no charge to CWM Hospital (except for some rental support). The Ministry did not seem to appreciate just how good a deal they were getting from FSMed. No Australian or NZ medical school had such an unfavourable financial arrangement with their teaching hospitals.

Migration of health workers is of course an international issue of great concern (chapter 13). In 2007, the School had 385 medical students (255 from Fiji) who were on full scholarships with bonding arrangements. The School does not have private fee-paying medical students, who might have been seen as getting a cheap medical degree in order to migrate. All medical students have a bonded obligation to remain in the region, which is the responsibility of the donor and Fiji government to enforce, not the School.

In 2008, Dr Jona Senilagakali, who had been the Minister for Health in the Interim Government of Bainimarama, made the following misleading statement:

> The government was short-sighted when it handed over ownership of the Fiji School of Medicine to a South Pacific regional institution in 1995—a move that transformed it into a centre that serves the whole region . . . When it was administrated by the Fiji government, every graduate had to work for government services and they were paid by the government. If that system had been maintained, Fiji would have had enough doctors and the health services and primary health care programmes would have achieved that 2000 target. Now the ministry of health has no power over the school and our nurses and doctors can go anywhere to work. Because of that decision, Fiji is still short of qualified doctors and nurses and will remain so in years to come.[378]

Senilagakali had occupied the roles over this time of Anatomy Tutor at the School, Permanent Secretary of Health, President of the Fiji Medical Association and Member of the School's Council, as well as being the father of one of the deans of the School. His statement is totally misleading. In fact, the exodus of doctors commenced in 1987 (Fig 29) when Fiji School of Medicine still came directly under the Ministry of Health, since autonomy was not granted until 1997. The Government of Fiji never handed over ownership of the School to USP in 1995, and it is exceedingly bad faith to blame regionalism for either the doctor shortage or failure of primary health care in Fiji. The School had been a more regional institution in Lambert's days than in 1995, and USP exercised almost no control over the School, other than granting its Bachelor and Masters degrees. In addition, there was strong evidence from regional countries such as Samoa, FSM and Palau that FSMed trained doctors were much less likely to migrate than those trained in Australia, NZ and the US, including for postgraduate studies. However, this diatribe does illustrate the anti-regionalism of the current Interim Government (2010).

FSMed had been discussing the issue of increasing the intake of medical students for over a year, and presented a proposal to its Council in April for a graduate entry stream (new 4-year course) to commence in 2008. The limitation of training doctors in Fiji is clinical supervision of year 4-6 students in hospital. Consequently, we were proposing an expansion of our campus in Lautoka Hospital and expansion of our training supervision to Labasa Hospital for final year students. This would have allowed us to increase from about 65 to over 90 graduates per year by 2012 (if we had gone ahead in 2008). Of course, with Lautoka hospital removed as a teaching hospital, we were now unable to expand the numbers of trainees. There is not enough capacity at Lautoka hospital to train both FSMed and University of Fiji students, and CWM Hospital was fully saturated already by FSMed students in years 4-5.

Upon his return, the Interim Minister of Health did give me a time to see him on September 18th. When I arrived, I discovered that without warning he had arranged a meeting which included three staff members of the University of Fiji, including, the new Dean, Dr Umanand Prasad (after whom the new school was named), and the Vice-Chancellor, Prof Rajesh Chandra (who is now VC of USP). The plan by the University of Fiji was to accept 40 students a year into a 6-year undergraduate MBBS course at a cost of FJ$12,000 /year for full fee-paying students commencing in 2008. This just undercut our cost of FJ$14,500, but all of our medical students were on scholarships, mostly from Fiji Government, AusAID and NZAID. Prior to the arrival of the University of Fiji staff, we had time for friendly discussion about the Minister's recent trip to South Korea and the unexpected death of a child at CWM Hospital after routine surgery for an arm fracture. The Minister's subsequent remarks on TV about this death were widely seen as callous and inappropriate.

Suddenly the tone of the conversation changed and the Minister told me that other Pacific Island Health Ministers at the Korea meeting had told him that they did not want me as Dean of FSMed. I replied that surely this was merely an expression of friendship to him as the father of the previous dean, but could he provide details of their concerns about me personally. He then went on a diatribe against Australia for the 'unfair' travel ban of Fijians associated with the coup government. I was rather taken aback by this attack as I had always had a very cordial relationship with Jona Senilagakali when he was on our Council and as President of the Fiji Medical Association. When the University of Fiji Faculty members arrived, the brief meeting established that they would have priority access to Lautoka Hospital, that the new medical school would be private with no government funding and that our funding would not be cut.

My discussions with the new Dean of the University of Fiji medical school did not reassure me. He had no academic experience and seemed to have little understanding of medical education, citing the reactionary ideas of Bruce Shepherd of the Australian Doctor's Fund on anatomy teaching. Although the new school was starting in a few months, he had not yet had any discussions with Lautoka Hospital and had only vague promises of teaching staff. It was widely understood that he had donated A$1 million to the University of Fiji, which strongly supported the new interim government through close links with the Permanent Secretary, Parmesh Chand, and the Minister of Finance, Mahendra Chaudhry.

I was concerned that the new medical school would cater to the children of wealthy Indo-Fijians who wanted a medical degree before migrating to Australia, NZ and North America. Dean Prasad's view on migration of doctors from Fiji was that it was a good thing, and they would return to Fiji after a successful career overseas, just as he had done. He was opposed to bonding of students, but his students would pay the full fees so there was no need of bonding. He repeatedly denied that there would be any harm to FSMed and claimed he only wanted to do what was good for Fiji. However, the loss of clinical training capacity to FSMed at Lautoka Hospital was a serious blow to our plans for expansion of medical student numbers, and the whole situation was rather demoralising.

Resignation

After careful consideration and with some reluctance, I decided to resign my position of Dean at Fiji School of Medicine while on leave for Christmas, so not return to Fiji for the 2008 academic year. I did not believe that this was leaving the School in the lurch because Eddie McCaig had acted in the position previously and during my absences. Moreover, my position as Dean would have been untenable under the circumstances if I were to have remained in the position after announcing my resignation, so I really saw no alternative but a sudden resignation.

The reasons for this rather precipitous resignation were not personal, as both my wife and I liked living in Fiji, but were entirely professional. In a word, the position of Dean for which I came to Fiji was **not** the job which I had been doing. I had hoped this would change over time, but saw by the end of 2007 that this was never going to change, and the union hostility and legal challenges would continue indefinitely. Life is too short to continue in a position which is 'a poisoned chalice'—excessively stressful, making me unhappy, and not allowing me to use either my clinical or educational skills. Although I could possibly have started to turn things around for the School, it would have taken another ten years at least, and it seemed just as likely that I would have been dismissed by forces hostile to change in the indigenous Fijian community.

I felt that I had rid the School of most of the dysfunctional elements, a task which probably only an expatriate could have done, but I did not expect gratitude for this thankless task. In a sense, I felt that as an expatriate Dean, the best role I could perform for the School was a 'clean-up' and then move on, such as happens in the corporate world. Another key factor was the military government which was intent on staying in power, was not addressing the vital economic issues facing Fiji and was committed to opening a new medical school at the University of Fiji to the detriment of FSMed.

I had come to Fiji School of Medicine with high hopes and believed that I had a lot to offer the School. What were my strengths? I had a good track record in clinical paediatrics, teaching, research, medical education and in managing a hospital department and academic institution. In particular, I had considerable expertise and experience in childhood malnutrition, diarrhoeal disease, acute respiratory disease, malaria, other infectious diseases, critical appraisal, evidence-based medicine, medical ethics, problem-based learning and academic assessment. Fiji was my fifth Pacific Island posting and 11th developing country appointment (Fig 1). I wanted nothing more than to be able to contribute in these areas to the academic activities of the School, and made this very clear on numerous occasions.

What had been my role at the School? Instead of an academic role, my position was CEO of a corporate sector with a weak management team which was not functioning as a team, largely because of the ethnic schism in Fiji. I found it difficult to delegate corporate tasks, so ended up spending my time on tasks which should have been delegated. So the tasks of the job seemed to relate mainly to managing human resources and finance, following the corporate review recommendations. We did manage to recruit some new corporate managers and turn the deficit around to a more favourable financial situation, so I was originally optimistic about the possibility of handing back much of the corporate responsibility so I could get on with academic activities in 2006. But a weak corporate director and finance manager, a conspiratorial QVS old boys' network and a malevolent Staff Association put paid to any chance of that, and in any case the Department of Medical Science did not want to allow me any academic role or make any changes. I was willing to supervise the management of the School, but had hardly spent all those years acquiring academic qualifications to waste all my time on administration alone.

Then there was the Staff Association (FSMEA). It seems to me that the union not only accomplished nothing, but harmed the interests of the School and its staff in my time as Dean. Could I have worked harder to have good relations with the union? I had an excellent working relationship with Rajendra Singh, who was FSMEA President for my first 6 months, which did not stop him from reneging on a decision which he had endorsed as a disciplinary committee member, and 'stabbing me in the back' at my first Council meeting. His replacement by a sacked staff member was a blow 'below the belt' for me, but even the subsequent Association President was one of his protégés, who continued to wage war on me with slanderous letters. What is the point of working hard to control budget expenditure when the union wastes our resources on legal fees? For several months in 2007, our legal fees exceeded my salary for the month with no end in sight.

In April 2007, the newly appointed Staff Association President had sent a libellous letter to Council members against me personally, which was subsequently withdrawn with an apology under pressure from other staff members. It is now clear that this apology was hypocritical as acknowledged in the December FSMEA letter to the Chair of Council, which constituted yet another personally insulting attack on my integrity behind my back. There is no place for such vicious personal attacks, and I had lost the desire to work in such a setting.

Another example was the rash of intemperate letters from staff members about their own or their children's failure to graduate. There had clearly been a practice of staff doing courses within the School at our expense for whom the rules were ignored. When Academic Office put a stop to this by insisting that academic transcripts justified the granting of qualifications, the outcry of 'injustice' was deafening. Clearly the principle of 'vested interest' had little meaning among many staff members. I was shocked by the credence given to these staff members complaints and the unfair opprobrium heaped upon Academic Office for ensuring that academic transcripts accurately reflected what qualifications were awarded without fear or favour.

One of the insistent demands of the Staff Association had been for a staff appraisal system. I had been reluctant to institute such a system because I feared it would be racially biased. However, the Council also insisted upon us implementing an appraisal system, and the new HR Manager had been appointed to implement such a system, but had failed to do so. Consequently, I took the bull by the horns and designed a 360° appraisal form, for which senior managers were obliged to nominate 12 appraisers. I was very concerned about confidentiality, so instituted a system which ensured security and also tried to educate staff about how the system worked. Although a few of the secretarial staff were too uncomfortable to evaluate senior managers, I was pleasantly surprised to find that nearly all of the other appraisers took the task very seriously, filling out perceptive comments as well as the scores.

Even more encouraging was the fact that there was no ethnic bias on analysis and the results strongly confirmed accepted views about poor performers. As the poor Indo-Fijian managers had all resigned, it meant that four indigenous Fijians were identified in the appraisal with low scores and negative comments. I met with each of the senior managers and gave then de-identified feedback. Despite the Staff Association having insisted on staff appraisal, they refused to accept the results. This resulted in the second letter of personal attacks on me sent to Council in December 2007and their meeting with the Chair of Council without so much as mentioning their concerns to me. Nevertheless, this episode did confirm that despite cultural constraints, the 360° appraisal system was highly effective in identifying poor performers.

The corporate review had called for a major shake-up in the corporate sector, which had been carried out. The School was bankrupt when I started and now has a reserve of at least $2 million in addition to new AusAID funding in the pipeline. Academic Office had been totally dysfunctional before I commenced, and had been greatly strengthened and probity ensured. Most of the other corporate sections had been improved. The prospect of fighting legal appeals, of negotiating with Ministry of Health and University of Fiji and of continuing battles with the Staff Association in 2008 was not appealing. Consequently, I decided to return to clinical paediatrics as an academic at James Cook University in Cairns in January 2008.

Conclusions

The Fiji School of Medicine celebrates its 120th anniversary in 2010. Although there have been brief articles on the history of the School, this book is the first attempt at a full history with the background of political and medical education developments which affected the School. The School has an interesting and distinguished history which is worth telling and of which it can be proud. In this final chapter, I have tried to summarise and draw lessons from the story of the School.

The last chapter comes across quite negatively about the School because it inevitably focuses upon the difficulties which I encountered. Nevertheless, there were some very **positive aspects** of my time as Dean. For example, the students' cultural evenings stick out as a highlight, with each cultural group proudly presenting dances from their islands as very entertaining and polished performances. One of our Samoan students won the contest for Mr Hibiscus at the annual festival, which was an unanticipated way of promoting the School's image. Our inaugural Open Day was another great public relations success. But by far the greatest asset of the School is its students, which were a very positive aspect of my experience as Dean. These are only a few of the many positive aspects of my experience at the School.

Above all, this is a story of **people**. MacGregor, Lambert and Hoodless were key players in the School's history, which would have been different without them. Cilento and Cumpston were influential Australian health bureaucrats who decided against sending Papua and New Guinea students to Central Medical School. If Gordon and Bavadra are the heroes and Rabuka and Speight the villains of the story, none had much to do directly with the School, illustrating the importance of background political factors to the School's history. Even the final chapter of the eventful 30 months of my deanship is fundamentally a personal story of how my weaknesses and strengths played out. Had I decided to play only the indigenous Fijian card and yield to those elements in the School, the story might well have turned out very differently. But, above all, the book tells some of the stories of the School's graduates. They are the ones who have made the School so successful.

But it is also a story of **key events**, which mostly happened outside of the School. The Suva Medical School was founded due to epidemics, doctor shortages and a paternalistic concern about native welfare. The Central Medical School followed on from Rockefeller Foundation philanthropy—a global health initiative—and its regional hookworm campaigns. The project almost floundered due to the Rockefeller's elitist view of medical education, but its ideology of academic scientific medicine (cf. Flexner and Osler) guaranteed a full-time tutor, a new focus on laboratory medicine and regional participation in the School. These were key innovations which greatly contributed to the success of Central Medical School.

The name change to Fiji School of Medicine corresponded to a decrease in the proportion of regional students, but a massive rise in total student numbers for which the school did not have the business expertise, structure or capacity to administer properly. The founding of the regional University of the South Pacific in 1968 meant that the medical course could be upgraded to degree-level (MBBS), but—unlike in PNG—the School missed the opportunity to become part of the regional university despite countless reports recommending it. Finally, the major events which impacted upon the School were again from outside, with the military coups, from which it has still not recovered.

The devastating **measles epidemic** of 1875 with some 40,000 deaths and a 28% mortality rate undoubtedly played an important role in the founding of the School a decade later. The first Chief Medical Officer, William MacGregor, arrived at the tail end of the epidemic, so would have seen its appalling consequences. The epidemic was directly attributable to quarantine failure, and the least one can say is it was an ominous start to British colonial rule, which had only commenced a few months earlier. By this time, Britain was a reluctant colonial power and Fiji was ceded—rather than conquered—by the Paramount Chief, Cakobau, mostly due to the threat of a rival Tongan chief, Ma'afa, and an unfairly imposed American debt. However, Fiji was most fortunate in the choice of Sir Arthur Gordon as Governor, since his connections with British aristocracy and politicians gave him the authority to institute a new form of colonialism which strongly favoured the indigenous population.

In order to appreciate the uniqueness of the **School's founding in 1885**, we need to look at comparable British colonies as isolated islands, such as in the Caribbean and Indian Ocean. Despite a longer colonial history in the West Indies and Mauritius, for example, medical schools were not established there until much later. The University of the West Indies was not founded until 1948 in Jamaica as a College of the University of London. In that year, 33 students from nine countries of the British West Indies were admitted to the new Faculty of Medicine, with the first students graduating with the MB BS degree in 1953. The first medical school in Mauritius only commenced in 1996 as an Indian off-shore school, which accepted some Mauritian students. Thus, in terms of training the local population as medical practitioners, one might conclude that the British Empire was much more concerned about the welfare of the indigenous populations of the Pacific than over former slaves or migrant labourers to its colonies.

Gordon's benign colonialism was a two-edged sword, however, since its paternalism towards indigenous Fijians contributed to the protection and undue prolongation of the almost-feudal social organisation in villages under the chiefly system, instead of modernising Fijian society so it could compete with the Indians both educationally and commercially. British colonial policy also permitted, and even encouraged, a virtual *apartheid* with little interaction between the two ethnic groups. When it was realised how far behind the Fijians had fallen, the imposition of positive discrimination, such as in scholarships, were seen as an injustice by Indo-Fijians, who were increasingly made to feel as strangers in their own country.

But the main cause of discord was the population explosion of Indo-Fijians which meant that they were in the majority by the end of the Second World War. It is easy to be judgemental after the event, but this was an impossible situation for both ethnic groups, not of their own making. Surely the language and/or religious differences in the two groups in Canada, Belgium or Ireland should have been much easier to deal with than the Fiji situation, yet they continue to cause considerable problems. So we do need to acknowledge that Fiji did manage to escape civil war and massacres in spite of its political difficulties.

Since the early colonial period, Britain had favoured the indigenous population over the indentured labourers, not just politically but also at a personal level. This may have been partly cultural, related to the British class system resembling the Fijian chiefly system, but the preference was quite overt in Gordon's time. By the advent of the two world wars, these attitudes were strengthened further as the loyal Fijians fought with the British whereas the troublesome Indo-Fijians refused to enlist and fomented strikes against the sugar industry, even letting the cane rot in the fields at a time when the Mother country was fighting a war of survival. With the transition from colony to independence, Britain found itself in the invidious position of having to compromise on the sacrosanct democratic principle of 'one-man one-vote'. Consequently, the opportunity to reach a workable compromise between the races for the future was lost, and the consequences were played out in the subsequent political instability and coups, which forced many Indo-Fijians to leave and seriously harmed the economy.

Returning to the School, however, there is no doubt that **Native Medical Practitioners** were highly successful, and the apprenticeship model of training worked well, at least in the early years. But this success was not just due to the institution; it was also related to the skills and dedication of the individual practitioners who graduated. This was amply illustrated in Chapter 9 with some evocative stories of NMPs. By the 1920s it was clear that after 35 years it was time for a change, partly to keep up with the new developments in medicine described in Chapter 10. These included the new emphasis on clinical skills from clinico-pathological correlations which had been led by the French, and the development of laboratory medicine such as bacteriology and clinical chemistry, which had been led by the Germans and Americans, and promoted by philanthropic organisations such as the Rockefeller Foundation.

In addition to improvements and expansion of infrastructure, the School used this occasion to consolidate its regional role in medical education. Sylvester Lambert accomplished this monumental task in the face of considerable resistance to the concept of Native Medical Practitioners by his employer, the Rockefeller Foundation. He formed an unusual alliance in this task with Aubrey Montague, unusual only in the sense that they were rather contrasting personalities.

Fig. 49: Staff & Student Numbers 1998-2007

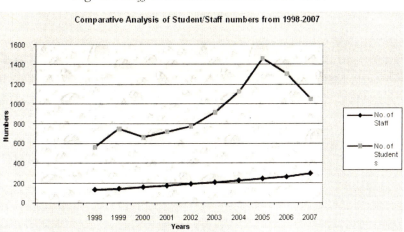

Although the term 'native' had become derogatory and unacceptable in most parts of the world, it was significant that the term Native Medical Practitioner was retained by the School until 1945, after which it was changed to Assistant Medical Practitioner. Although the initial training of an NMP was only 3-years, it was increased to 4-years from 1931-51 and to 5-years from 1952-81. By this time, the training and practice was becoming similar to a doctor, yet the School was slow to **upgrade to a degree** which only happened in 1982 when it became a 6-year course (Table 1).

Figures 31-2 and 49 show the **exponential increase in student numbers** since the 1990s which was mostly due to paramedical students from Fiji, especially part-time students in Public Health, although there was also an increase in medical student numbers. As often happens with small institutions with a long history, the school maintained the structure of a small institution, failing to adjust to the administrative structures required of a large institution with over a thousand students. Similarly, the corporate sector did not have the skills—particularly the financial and human resources expertise—to adequately manage such a large institution. This was not helped by the academic staff who resisted the necessary changes, preferring the feel of a small, friendly school which could respond flexibly to issues. During my time as Dean, hardly any of the academic staff had ever had an administrative role in a large university, so had little understanding of how they should function. There was little appreciation, for example, of the importance of enforcing admission policies and maintaining the rigour of examination procedures. So the School was still a small institution which had not adjusted administratively to being a large institution. This adjustment might have occurred earlier if the School had joined USP in the 1980s, as had been recommended in numerous reports.

The **failure to become a medical faculty** within the new regional university was another key event which was largely determined by USP and Fiji Government, rather than the School controlling its own destiny. There were a range of views within the School staff about this issue, but certainly during most of the last 30 years, a majority of staff have favoured this option, although still opposed by an influential minority. One reason for this was that USP salaries tended to be about 30% higher than the School's salaries, as documented by the Corporate Review in 2005. The donor agencies and regional organisations, such as AusAID, NZAID, SPC and the Forum also favoured FSMed joining the regional university, in order to strengthen regionalism. As we saw in chapter 11, the main reason for the failure of amalgamation in the 1980s was financial, that USP wanted additional funding whereas Fiji government was not prepared to adequately fund a new university medical school.

After the **1987 coup**, the issue largely fell off the agenda. During the 2003-5 Corporate Review of the School, Jimmie Rodgers put it very much back on the agenda, but the nationalistic Qarase government was not keen to hand over a Fijian institution—as they saw it—to a regional university. As Dean, I pushed the issue strongly initially, but soon got 'cold feet' due to concerns about the extravagant Australian USP Vice-Chancellor, who eventually resigned and was found to have approved excessive senior management salaries. My experience at the Northern Territory Clinical School in Darwin of the frustrations in dealing with a distant large university bureaucracy also made me wary of losing control of the School's affairs, so it would have required careful negotiation to join USP.

This was also overtaken by subsequent events, as the **2006 Bainimarama coup** led to an interim government that was hostile to regional interests, perhaps because it did not get support from the Pacific Forum. It did receive support from the University of Fiji, so not only acquiesced to its demand for a new medical school, but gave it access to Lautoka Hospital as its teaching hospital, which already had an Australian-funded FSMed campus for teaching final year medical students. The interim government also unfairly blamed the School for the migration of doctors. Migration is a complex issue, but evidence has showed that the political coups and dysfunction of the Ministry of Health were important 'push factors' for many of the doctors in Fiji who migrated.

The 2006 coup ended the School's expansion plans for an increase in medical students and meant that there were now not enough clinical placements at CWM Hospital for existing FSMed students due to the loss of the Lautoka teaching hospital. Under the circumstances, expanding clinical placements to Labasa seemed folly, so the School considered establishing a clinical school in Vanuatu or Solomon Islands. However, the interim government had other ideas and has established a National University of Fiji to include FSMed, Fiji School of Nursing and the new University of Fiji medical school. It also cut funding to USP, forcing it to downsize. This may mean the end of FSMed's regional credibility, but it remains to be seen what the response of regional governments will be in terms of sending medical students to a National University of Fiji in Suva.

What conclusions are to be drawn from **my experience as Dean**? I have called Chapter 15 'A Poisoned Chalice', implying that the dice were loaded against me. It tells a story of corruption and corporate incompetence, a hostile union, undermining by an old boys' network, resistance to change and a failure to be accepted as a colleague by senior clinical staff. While writing this book, I have spent a great deal of time reconsidering how I could have done things differently as Dean of FSMed. Even with the benefit of hindsight, I am convinced that it was essential for the institution to be rid of its destructive elements if it was to become once again an institution of integrity as in the past. As an expatriate, it was possible for me to do this, and was probably too difficult for my local predecessors. I certainly did not appreciate how difficult and personally stressful the backlash would be.

It was an issue of powerful individuals abusing the institution for their own ends, which were not consistent with the academic and financial goals of the School. It was not only senior staff as there were a number of less senior administrative staff doing much the same. I believe that I did the School a favour by getting rid of many of them, but one rarely gets gratitude for such actions, as with 'whistle-blowers'. I soon came to the view that the best I could offer the School was to rid it of the bad elements and then move on, as I did.

Many readers are probably convinced that my shortcomings as Dean were 'cultural', that as an expatriate I did not understand the local culture, or that only a local Dean could understand the cultural aspects of the problem and deal with it in a culturally sensitive way. I do not believe that this is true. Firstly, Fiji is multicultural and the School had faculty from all over the world, so the real issue was a Fijian tendency to reject multiculturalism and its dual ethnicity. Secondly, I made a deliberate effort to consult local staff and promote their interests over expatriates, provided they coincided with the overall interests of the School. Thirdly, the staff of the School were well educated and many had lived in or visited Australia or NZ, and were very familiar with dealing with expatriates, especially whites. Fourthly, sometimes it takes an outsider to deal with such issues because of cultural constraints imposed upon a local Dean. So the issues were more related to personalities, power and politics in an academic institution, with which I had already had considerable experience in a multicultural setting.

I had also known some of the key faculty members well over many years from working in other islands and as External Examiner at the School starting in 1998, so had formed friendly relationships which continued throughout my deanship, in spite of the difficulties encountered. It is also important to realise that I never had emotive arguments or hostile 'blow-ups' with individuals at the School, so continued with generally cordial relationships with all staff members. Even the unpleasantness of slanderous letters was never translated into angry exchanges. It was about politics rather than culture, which is why I have included 'Politics' in the title of the book, as it is central to the story.

Having read widely on the anthropology of Polynesia and Melanesia, including specifically for this book, I have found it has shed little light on my experience as Dean, so I have left most of it out of the book. This is, of course, not meant to deny the importance of traditional culture in Fiji. But the difficult issues that confronted me were fairly universal issues of academic institutions, rather than uniquely Fijian. I have spent my career living in many different cultures, so have surely acquired the requisite cultural sensitivity and perspective from experience. Having said that, a uniquely Fijian aspect of the problems at the School related to the denial by an influential indigenous Fijian minority of the multi-cultural nature of the School, specifically denying the rights of Fijians of Indian origin. Whatever one thinks of the 2006 coup, it cannot be denied that Bainimarama's interim government is motivated by a desire to address this issue in Fiji.

We are nearing the end, and by convention, the penultimate paragraph of the discussion section of medical journal articles discusses the **constraints** or limitations of the study, so I will attempt briefly to do the same here. There is no point in writing this story without being self-critical, so firstly, let me deal with my time as Dean of the School. I have already indicated that my qualifications and experience were appropriate for such a position and that even with hindsight I see no alternative to having rid the School of destructive elements, despite the difficulties it provoked. If—like Gordon—I had played the indigenous Fijian card to the hilt, I would undoubtedly have had an easier time of it at the School. Why did I refuse to do this? I had certainly developed a deep interest and attachment to the 'fa'a Samoa' and Melanesian cultures in my previous postings. The three main personal reasons I could not do this in Fiji were: an abhorrence of racism against Indians (after all, I do have a multi-racial family, including an Indian daughter), the poor performance of some key senior indigenous staff as managers, and the fact that I was in charge of the institution so could not ignore these issues.

It would have been much easier if I had been just a clinician. But therein lies another issue. I was probably not the right person for this job. My personality was too academic and introverted to make the position work; it would have been better to have had someone more outgoing and managerial, who could deal with difficult personalities and groups (e.g. the union) better than I—a better agent of change. Kim Oates of Sydney told me that paediatricians make good medical deans because we are good at dealing with difficult behavioural problems in children, which is good preparation for dealing with petty squabbles between academics. Perhaps he has a point, but behavioural problems were never my forte.

Secondly, let me deal briefly with the limitations of this book. As mentioned, the main strength is the extensive background information of developments which affected the School's history. However, I have not dealt with all of medical education, but have focused on doctors, largely ignoring nursing and paramedical disciplines. I have not consulted all of the primary sources of the School's history, particularly correspondence in archives in London, Canberra and New York. Nor have I detailed all the important events of the School's history in a systematic manner or used extensive oral histories of graduates of the School.

In addition, my background information is inevitably highly selective of influences which affected the School (e.g. Flexner via the Rockefeller Foundation and Problem-Based Learning via McMaster/Newcastle), rather than a comprehensive review of all trends in medical education. So there are gaps. In my defence, it would have required a much longer and less readable book to tell the story more comprehensively, so the decision to be selective was deliberate. Perhaps another limitation is that the book is not written in the elegant if slightly arcane English style of much of academic discourse. I am envious of the beautiful writing of much of the history and anthropology which I have read in researching the book, but there is also a lot of 'turgid prose' and jargon in postmodern academic writing. I have abided by the concise writing style of the medical literature with which I am familiar and which I hope is easier for readers. In spite of these constraints, I trust the book does make a modest contribution to the academic literature on the medical education and political history of the Pacific Islands, a relatively neglected area.

In conclusion, I have been quite critical of certain aspects of the history of the School. Some may see this as presumptuous—perhaps even offensive—but I can only tell my version, and others are encouraged to tell their different version of these events in reply. It is hard to deny that indigenous parochialism, political instability and mismanagement have been bad for the School. It is also hard to deny that certain individuals—both senior academic and junior administrative staff members—had become entrenched at the School, and were acting in their own interests with impunity and against the interests of the institution as a whole. Despite the uncertain future of the School, I am optimistic that the inherent resilience of the Fijians of both ethnicities will triumph over adversity and the School will once again play a key role in high quality training of health professionals for the region, which has been its legacy. This is my sincere hope in writing the book.

Annex 1

Heads of the School of Medicine in Fiji, 1885-2010

1885-1888
Sir William MacGregor, Chief Medical Officer (CMO) of Fiji

1888-1907
Hon Dr Bolton Glanville Corney, ISO; CMO

1907-1919
Hon Dr George William Augustus Lynch
MA, MB, BCh (Cantab), MRCS(Eng), LRCP (Lond); CMO

1919-1930
Dr Aubrey Montague
MB, BS(Lond), MRCS(Eng), LRCP(Lond); CMO

1930-1946
Dr David Win Hoodless, OBE
BSc (Lond), LMSSA, AKC; Tutor, Principal in 1936

1947-1953
Dr Alexander Smaill Frater, MBE
MB BS (Syd), DipTM (Syd); Principal

1954-1963
   Dr Archibald Roy Edmonds
   MB, BS(Melb); Principal

1963-1969
   Dr Kenneth James Gilchrist, OBE, OStJ
   MB, BS, LRCP(Lond), FRCS; Principal

1969-1974
   Dr Thomas Guy Hawley
   MB, ChB(NZ), DipPH(Eng), MFCM(UK); Principal

1974-1984
   Dr Bhupendra Pathik
   MB BS (Bombay), MRACP, MHPM (NSW); Principal

1984-1988
   Prof Harry Lander
   MB BS (Adel), FRACP, FAFPHM; Head of School

1988-1989
   Dr Brian Cameron; Acting Head of School

1989-1991
   Prof Ian Calder Lewis, AO
   MD (Edin), FRCP, FRACP, FAFPHM; Head of School

1991-1999
   Dr Jimi I Samisoni
   B Med Sci (Otago) MB BS, PhD (UQ); Dean

1999-2004
   Dr Wame Baravilala
   MBBS, MRCOG, FRANZCOG, FACTM; Dean

2005-2008
Prof David Brewster, AM
BA (Honours), MD (McMaster), MPH (Syd), FRACP, PhD (Newcastle); Dean 2008
Dr Eddie McCaig & Prof Rob Moulds: Acting Deans

2009-
Prof Ian Rouse
BSc (Hons), Grad Dip Hlth Sci, PhD; Dean

Annex 2

Chronology of the School

The medical school in Fiji was established 125 years ago, and has undergone three name changes: Suva Medical School (1885-1928), Central Medical School (1929-1960) and Fiji School of Medicine (FSMed since 1961). Its medical training programme has had five major course and curriculum changes: an original three year certificate (1885-1933), a four year certificate (1934-1981), a five year diploma (1952-1990), a seven year MBBS degree (1982-1990); and a six year MBBS degree (since 1991; see Table 1). The School also provides training in a number of the health science disciplines including dentistry, pharmacy, physiotherapy, radiography, laboratory technology, dietetics, public health and environmental health.

Major Timelines

1874 : Fiji ceded to Great Britain
1875 : Measles epidemic causes about 40,000 deaths
1877 : Manpower shortage relieved by 'blackbirding'
1879 : First group of indentured Indian labourers arrive in Fiji, quarantined due to smallpox and cholera on board
1885 : Ten Fijians commence training at Colonial Hospital as the start of the Suva Medical School
1888 : First three Fijians graduate as Native Practitioners
1912 : First Rotuman graduate

1916 : First two regional students graduate, both from Tokelau
1926 : First Indian graduates as Indian Medical Practitioner
1927 : First Samoan and Gilbert Island graduates
1928 : School renamed Central Medical School. Lambert secures Rockefeller Foundation funds to move the School to the Colonial War Memorial Hospital. David Hoodless appointed full-time Principal (initially Tutor).
1930 : First Solomon Islander graduate. Graduates now called Native Medical Practitioners (NMPs)
1931 : New 4-year syllabus. First Cook Island and Tongan graduates
1933 : 168 students graduated during the 46 years of the 3-year course
1938 : First graduates from Nauru and American Samoa
1943 : First graduate from the New Hebrides (Vanuatu).
1945 : Dental training commences with a 4-year course.
1946 : Assistant Laboratory Technicians Programme commences, later renamed Medical Laboratory Technology.
1950 : First medical graduate from Niue
1951 : NMPs renamed Assistant Medical Practitioners (AMPs). First medical graduates from Papua New Guinea and the US Trust Territories (transferred from Guam)
1952 : New 5-year course commenced. First women admitted to the medical course
1953 : Tamavua campus with facilities for teaching sciences, administration, research and dormitories. Opened on December 17th by Queen Elizabeth II
1955 : World Health Organization (WHO) provide lecturers in Biology and Physiology. Foundation programme commences for regional students
1956 : AMPs renamed Assistant Medical Officers (AMOs). 264 graduated during the 22 years (1934-1955) of the 4-year course.
1957 : Dental course shortened to 3 years
1959 : Department of Social and Preventive Medicine opened with funds from UK Nuffield Foundation

1960 : Certificate of Public Health (postgraduate 6 month course) commences
1961 : School renamed Fiji School of Medicine (FSMed). Assistant Health Inspector training commences
1964 : AMOs renamed Medical Officer (Fiji)
1966 : Opening of Department of Nutrition and Dietetics
1967 : Hoodless House built near CWM Hospital for clinical students
1968 : University of the South Pacific (USP) opens in Suva. Takes over 1st year of medical and dental students' training
1970 : USP Council commences investigation of taking over FSMed.
1973 : 195 medical students graduated during the 18 years (1956-1973) of the 5-year course
1975 : Extensions to Hoodless House. Three year Medical Assistants course commences
1978 : Further Hoodless House extensions (pathology laboratory, library)
1979 : Second Cole Report on USP-FSMed relationship
1980 : Conjoint Committee of USP, Health Ministry and FSMed formed for new MBBS programme
1981 : Memorandum of Understanding signed by USP and Health Ministry for an external MBBS degree awarded by USP
1982 : First group of 36 MBBS students enrol at FSMed after completing Foundation Year at USP. Physiology laboratory and anatomy museum renovated
1983 : The Hardy/Frank Report (University of Adelaide) for re-organisation of the School
1984 : Advisory Board replaced by new autonomous Council. Last group of Diploma of Surgery and Medicine (DSM) students graduate for a total of 250 over 17 years (1968-84) from 4-year DSM. Cessation of Diploma of Dental Surgery (DDS) but 2 dental students a year to be sent to Adelaide.
1985 : Centenary of School (overlooked at the time, celebrated in 1988). Total of 789 medical graduates over 100 years. Last graduation for Diploma in Dental Surgery (DDS)

for a total of 146 graduates over 35 years. New medical curriculum introduced for MBBS. Biddulph and Boelen reports on amalgamation with USP. Medical Officers Training programme for Micronesia commences.

1986 : WHO Master Plan for the School. Eleventh Regional Conference of Permanent Heads of Pacific Health Services endorse proposal to incorporate FSMed as a Faculty of USP. Recommend transferring dental training to the University of PNG

1987 : First group of 20 MBBS doctors graduate. Rabuka military coups cause crisis for School

1988 : Academic year delayed due to shortage of staff. WHO Western Pacific Regional Office helps with crisis

1989 : WHO Plan of Action recommends autonomy for School. Curriculum development consultants appointed by WHO to develop a new integrated problem-based learning curriculum

1991 : Commencement of Japanese–funded extension to CWM Hospital as the main clinical training facility

1992 : Start of new PCP/MBBS curriculum with first group of 32 Primary Care Practitioner (PCP) students enrolled

1993 : Autonomy postponed by new Minister for Health. Regional Director of WHO presents first 3-year Diplomas in Primary Health Care to 25 graduates. New Extension to CWM Hospital

1994 : Australian aid (AIDAB) consultancy on FSMed's institutional development

1996 : PCP curriculum ceases with graduation of first group of PCPs with MBBS

1997 : FSMed goes on the Internet

1998 : Autonomy from Ministry of Health

1999 : USP Council endorses the degrees Master of Medicine, Master of Public Health Practice, and the Bachelor of Environmental Health. FSMed Council approves 5-year capital development and staff professional training plan.
Fiji PM signs agreement with EU for a new campus

2005 : Corporate review commissioned by FSMed Council

2006 :   Official opening of Pasifika campus by Vice-President. Military coup by Bainimarama
2008 :   Commencement of University of Fiji medical school
2009 :   FSMed incorporated in new National University of Fiji

References

1. Burnham JC. How the idea of profession changed the writing of medical history. Med Hist Suppl.1998;18:1-10.
2. Kushner HI. Medical historians and the history of medicine. The Lancet 2008;372(9640):710-11.
3. Duffin J, editor. Clio in the Clinic: History in Medical Practice. Oxford: Oxford University Press, 2005.
4. Munro D. J.W. Davidson—the making of a participant historian. In: Lal BV, Hempenstall P, editors. Pacific Lives, Pacific Places: Bursting Boundaries in Pacific History. Canberra: The Journal of Pacific History, 2001:98-116.
5. Davison JW. Samoa Mo Samoa: The Emergence of the Independent State of Western Samoa. Melbourne: Melbourne University Press, 1967.
6. Wilcox RA, Whitham EM. The symbol of modern medicine: why one snake is more than two. Ann Intern Med 2003;138(8):673-7.
7. Froman CR, Skandalakis JE. One snake or two: the symbols of medicine. Am Surg 2008;74(4):330-4.
8. Lal BV, Pretes M. Coup : reflections on the political crisis in Fiji Canberra: ANU Press, 2001.
9. MacGregor W. Disease and its treatment. In: Rivers WHR, editor. Essays on the Population of Melanesia. Cambridge: Cambridge University Press, 1922:78-83.
10. Lange RT. Island ministers : indigenous leadership in nineteenth century Pacific Islands Christianity. Canberra: Pandanus Books, 2005.

11. Young J. Adventurous Spirits: Australian migrant society in pre-cession Fiji. St Lucia, Queensland: University of Queensland Press, 1984.
12. Stuart A. Parasites lost? The Rockefeller Foundation and the Expansion of Health Services in the Colonial South Pacific, 1916-1939 [PhD Thesis]. University of Canterbury, 2002.
13. Hoodless DW. Central Medical School. Suva: Medical Department, Government of Fiji, 1947:1-24.
14. Cumpston JHL. Health and Disease in Australia: A History. Canberra: AGPS Press, 1989 (written in 1928).
15. Anonymous. Bolton Glanvill Corney, ISO, MRCS. British Medical Journal 1924;2(3330):791.
16. Joyce RB. Sir William MacGregor. London: Oxford University Press, 1971.
17. Anonymous. Advertisement. Lancet 1891;April 11 issue:847.
18. Cook GC. Charles Wilberforce Daniels, FRCP (1862-1927): underrated pioneer of tropical medicine. Acta Trop. 2002; 81(3):237-50.
19. Lynch GWA. Medical report for the Year 1911 Fiji. Journal of Tropical Medicine & Hygiene 1914;June 15:85-102.
20. Lynch GWA. Colonial Medical Reports 1912 Fiji. Journal of Tropical Medicine & Hygiene 1916;Jan 1:1-25.
21. McArthur N. Island Populations of the Pacific. Canberra: ANU Press, 1967.
22. Barry JM. The Great Influenza : The epic story of the deadliest plague in history. New York: Viking (Kindle Edition), 2004.
23. Lander H, Miles V. The Fiji School of Medicine: a brief history and list of graduates. Sydney: Centre for South Pacific Studies, 1992.
24. Cliff AD, Haggett P. The Spread of Measles in Fiji and the Pacific: spatial components in the transmission fo epidemic waves through island communities. Canberra: Australian National University, 1985.

25. Thomson B. The Fijians. London: William Heinemann (Republished by Dawsons of Pall Mall,1968), 1908.
26. Morens DM, Taubenberger JK, Fauci AS. Predominant role of bacterial pneumonia as a cause of death in pandemic influenza: implications for pandemic influenza preparedness. J Infect. Dis. 2008;198(7):962-70.
27. Morens DM. Measles in Fiji, 1875: thoughts on the history of emerging infectious diseases. Pac. Health Dialog 1998;5:119-28.
28. Morley DC. Measles in the developing world. Proc.R.Soc.Med. 1974;67:1112-15.
29. Cliff A, Haggett P, Smallman-Raynor M. Measles: an historical geography of a major human viral disease from global expansion to local retreat, 1840-1990. Oxford: Blackwell Publishers, 1993.
29 b. Cliff AD, Haggett P. The Spread of Measles in Fiji and the Pacific: spatial components in the transmission for epidemic waves through island communities. Canberra: Australian National University, 1985.
30. Gravelle K. Fiji Times: A History of Fiji. Suva: Fiji Times & Herald Ltd, 1981.
31. Anonymous. Measles outbreak and response in Fiji, February-May 2006. Wkly Epidemiol Rec 2006;81(36):341-6.
32. Morens DM. Death in the "Cannibal Islands": An Emerging Infectious Disease Appearing in 1875. Historical Presentation: NIAID, NIH, Bethesda, Maryland, 2005.
33. Aaby P, Whittle H, Cisse B, Samb B, Jensen H, Simondon F. The frailty hypothesis revisited: mainly weak children die of measles. Vaccine 2001;20(5-6):949-53.
34. Whittle H, Hanlon P, O'Neill K, Hanlon L, Marsh V, Jupp E, Aaby P. Trial of high-dose Edmonston-Zagreb measles vaccine in the Gambia: antibody response and side-effects. The Lancet 1988;2(8615):811-14.
35. Aaby P. Is susceptibility to severe infection in low-income countries inherited or acquired? J Intern.Med. 2007;261(2):112-22.

36. Morgan G. What, if any, is the effect of malnutrition on immunological competence? The Lancet 1997;349(9066):1693-95.
37. Shaheen SO, Aaby P, Hall AJ, Barker DJ, Heyes CB, Shiell AW, Goudiaby A. Cell mediated immunity after measles in Guinea-Bissau: historical cohort study. BMJ 1996;313(7063):969-74.
38. Lucas KM, Sanders RC, Rongap A, Rongap T, Pinai S, Alpers MP. Subacute sclerosing panencephalitis (SSPE) in Papua New Guinea: a high incidence in young children. Epidemiol Infect 1992;108(3):547-53.
39. Kunitz SJ. Disease and Social Diversity: the European impact on the health of non-Europeans. Oxford: Oxford University Press, 1994.
40. Tomkins SM. The influenza epidemic of 1918-19 in Western Samoa. The Journal of Pacific History 1992;27(2):181-97.
41. Glanville Corney B. Medical Report 1903 Fiji. Journal of Tropical Medicine 1905;April 15:36-9.
42. Hermant P, Cilento R. Report of the Mission Entrusted with a Survey on Health Conditions in the Pacific Islands. Geneva: League of Nations Health Organisation, 1929:1-116.
43. Steer AC, Adams J, Carlin J, Nolan T, Shann F. Rheumatic heart disease in school children in Samoa. Archives of Disease in Childhood 1999;81(4):372.
44. Steer A, Colquhoun S, Noonan S, Kado J, Viale S, Carapetis J. Control of rheumatic heart disease in the Pacific region. Pac Health Dialog 2006;13(2):49-55.
45. Rallu JL. Pre—and Post-Contact Population in Island Polynesia. In: Kirch PV, Rallu JL, editors. The Growth and Collapse of Pacific Island Societies: Archaeological and Demographic Perspectives. Honololulu: University of Hawaii Press, 2007:15-34.
46. Stannard DE. American Holocaust: Columbus and the Conquest of the New World. Oxford: Oxford University Press, 1992.
47. Kirch PV, Rallu JL, editors. The Growth and Collapse of Pacific Island Societies: Archaeological and Demographic Perspectives. Honolulu: University of Hawaii Press, 2007.

48. Kirch PV, Rallu JL. Concluding Remarks: Methods, Measures and Models in Pacific Paleodemography. The Growth and Collapse of Pacific Island Societies: Archaeological and Demographic Perspectives. Honolulu: University of Hawaii Press, 2007:326-37.
49. Roberts SH. Population Problems of the Pacific. London: George Routledge & SOns, 1927.
50. Woodward A, Blakely T,. Mortality decline in the Pacific. In: Ohtsuka R, Ulijaszek SJ, editors. Health Change in the Asia-Pacific Region: Biocultural and Epidemiological Approaches. Cambridge: Cambridge University Press, 2007:234-353.
51. Glanville Corney B. Medical Report for the Year 1907 Fiji. Journal of Tropical Medicine & Hygiene 1909;March 1:19-23.
52. Rivers WHR, editor. Essays on the Population of Melanesia. Cambridge: Cambridge University Press, 1922.
53. MacGregor W. Some problems of tropical medicine. The Lancet 1900;13:1055-61.
54. Anonymous. Report of the Committee Appointed to Inquire into the Decrease of the Native Population. Suva, 1896:6-7.
55. Thomas N. Sanitation and Seeing: The Creation of State Power in Early Colonial Fiji. Comparative Studies in Society and History 1990;32(1):149-70.
56. McGregor R. The idea of racial degeneration: Baldwin Spencer and the Aborigines of the Northern Territory. In: MacLoed R, Denoon D, editors. Health and Healing in Tropical Australia and Papua New Guinea. Townsville: James Cook University, 1991:23-34.
57. Haddon AC, Bartlett FC, Fegan ES. 61. William Halse Rivers Rivers, M.D., F.R.S., President of the Royal Anthropological Institute, Born 1864, Died June 4th, 1922. Man 1922;22:97-104.
58. Petch A. Pitt Rivers: Technologies and Materials accessed Nov 11, 2009 *http://england.prm.ox.ac.uk/englishness-Pitt-Rivers-and-Technology-1.htm*

59. Pitt-Rivers GHL. The Clash of Cultures and the Contact of Races. London: George Routledge & Sons, 1927.
60. Brewster AB. The Hill Tribes of Fiji. London: JB Lippincott Company, 1922.
61. Sutton P. The Politics of Suffering: Indigenous Australia and the end of the liberal consensus. Melbourne: Melbourne University Press, 2009.
62. Keown M. Postcolonial Pacific Writing: Representations of the Body. Oxford: Routledge (Kindle edition), 2005.
63. Mead M. Coming of age in Samoa; a psychological study of primitive youth for western civilisation. New York,: W. Morrow & Company, 1928.
64. Wendt A. Three Faces of Samoa: Mead's, Freeman's and Wendt's. Pacific Islands Monthly, 1983:10-14.
65. Freeman D. Margaret Mead and Samoa : the making and unmaking of an anthropological myth. Cambridge, Mass.: Harvard University Press, 1983.
66. Cilento R. The Causes of the Depopulation of the Western Islands of the Territory of New Guinea. Canberra: Australian Government Printer, 1928.
67. Burkot TR, Taleo G, Toeaso V, Ichimori K. Progress towards, and challenges for, the elimination of filariasis from Pacific-island communities. Annals of Tropical Medicine and Parasitology 2002;96(Supplement 2):61-9.
68. McGusty VWT. The Decline and Recovery of the Fijian Race. Proceedings of the Seventh Pacific Science Association (held at Auckland and Christchurch, New Zealand, 2nd February to 4th March, 1949). Christchurch: Pegasus Press, 1953:51-61.
69. Scragg RFR. Depopulation in New Ireland: A Study of Demography and Fertility. Port Moresby: Territory of Papua and New Guinea, 1957.
70. Taylor R, Bampton D, Lopez AD. Contemporary patterns of Pacific Island mortality. International Journal of Epidemiology 2005;34(1):207-14.

71. Anonymous. Maori Carving Lecture accessed Nov 11, 2009 http://www.thebigidea.co.nz/grow/tips-tools/2009/may/56350-maori-carving-lecture
72. Anonymous. Epidemiology for All accessed Nov 11, 2009 http://www.events4you.co.nz/aea2009/keynote.html
73. Shlomowitz R. Infant mortality and Fiji's Indian migrants, 1879-1919. Indian Economic Social History Review 1986;23(3):289-302.
74. Stanner WEH. Postwar Fiji: The 1946 Census. PacificAffairs 1947;20(4):407-21.
75. Lal BV. Broken Waves: A history of the Fiji islands in the twentieth century. Honolulu: University of Hawaii Press, 1992.
76. Knaplund P. Gladstone-Gordon Correspondence, 1851-1896: Selections from the Private Correspondence of a British Prime Minister and a Colonial Governor. Transactions of the American Philosophical Society, New Series 1961;51(4):1-116.
77. Legge JD. Britain in Fiji 1858-1880. London: MacMillan & Co Ltd, 1958.
78. Chapman JK. The career of Arthur Hamilton Gordon, First Lord Stanmore, 1929-1912. Toronto: University of Toronto Press, 1964.
79. Heath I. Toward a reassessment of Gordon in Fiji. The Journal of Pacific History 1974;9(1):81-92.
80. France P. The Charter of the Land. Melbourne: Oxford University Press, 1969.
81. Moynagh M. Brown or White? a history of the Fiji sugar industry, 1873-1973. Canberra: ANU, 1981.
82. Nicholas T. Sanitation and Seeing: The Creation of State Power in Early Colonial Fiji. Comparative Studies in Society and History 1990;32(1):149-70.
83. Scarr D. John Bates Thurston: Grand Panjandrum of the Pacific. In: Scarr D, editor. More Pacific Island Portraits. Canberra: ANU Press, 1979:95-114.
84. Fanon F. Les damnés de la terre. [2. éd.] ed. Paris,: F. Maspero, 1961.
85. Robertson RT, Tamanisau A, editors. Fiji: Shattered coups. Sydney: Pluto Press, 1988.

86. Bain A. A protective labour policy? An alternative interpretation of early colonial labour policy in Fiji. The Journal of Pacific History 1988;23(2):119-36.
87. Stuart A. Contradictions and Complexities in an Indigenous Medical Service. Journal of Pacific History 2006;41(2):125-43.
88. Bynum WF. Science and the Practice of Medicine in the Nineteenth Century. Cambridge: Cambridge University Press, 1994.
89. Newman C. The Evolution of Medical Education in the Nineteenth Century. London: Oxford University Press, 1957.
90. Bonner TN. Becoming a Physician: Medical Education in Britain, France, Germany and the United States, 1750-1945. Baltimore: Johns Hopkins University Press, 1995.
91. Gelfand T. The history of the medical profession. In: Bynum WF, Porter R, editors. Companion Encyclopedia of the History of Medicine. London: Routledge, 1993:1119-50.
92. Rosner L. Medical Education in the Age of Improvement: Edinburgh students and apprentices, 1760-1826. Edinburgh: Edinburgh University Press, 1991.
93. French R. The Anatomic Tradition. In: Bynum WF, Porter R, editors. Companion Encyclopedia of Medical History. London: Routledge, 1993:81-101.
94. Calman KC. Medical Education: Past, Present and Future: Handing on Learning. Edinburgh: Churchill Livingstone, 2006.
95. Burnham JC. What is Medical History? Cambridge, UK: Polity Press, 2005.
96. Waddington K. Medical Education at St Bartholomew's Hospital, 1123-1995. Suffolk, UK: Boydell Press, 2003.
97. Porter D. Health, Civilisation and the State: A history of public health from ancient to modern times. London : New York: Routledge (Kindle edition), 1999.
98. Lawrence C. The shaping of things to come: Scottish medical education 1700–1939. Medical Education 2006;40(3):212-18.

99. Risse GB. Medical care. In: Bynum WF, Porter R, editors. Companion Encyclopedia of the History of Medicine. London: Routledge, 1993:45-77.
100. Nutton V. Humoralism. In: Bynum WF, Porter R, editors. Companion Encyclopedia of the History of Medicine. London: Routledge, 1993:281-91.
101. Osler W, McCrae T. The principles and practice of medicine; designed for the use of practitioners and students of medicine. 8th ed. New York and London,: D. Appleton and company, 1912.
102. Buchanan WW. Sir William Osler, M.D. (1849-1919) : his accomplishments and background, starting in Ontario, Canada. Toronto: Pro Familia Pub., 2006.
103. Lucas TP. Cries from Fiji. Melbourne: Dunn & Collins, 1885.
104. Saunders K. The pacific islander hospitals in colonial Queensland. The Journal of Pacific History 1976;11(1):28-50.
105. Siegel J. Origins of Pacific Islands labourers in Fiji. The Journal of Pacific History 1985;20(1):42-54.
106. Des Voeux GW. My Colonial Service. London: John Murray, 1903.
107. Moore C,. "Me Blind Drunk": Alcohol and Melanesians in the Mackay District, Queensland, 1867-1907. In: MacLoed R, Denoon D, editors. Health and Healing in Tropical Australia and Papua New Guinea. Townsville: James Cook University, 1991:103-22.
108. Robie D. Blood on their Banner. Sydney: Pluto Press Australia, 1989.
109. Cumpston IM. Indians Overseas in British Territories. Oxford: Oxford University Press, 1953.
110. Cumpston IM. Sir Arthur Gordon and the Introduction of Indians into the Pacific: The West Indian System in Fiji. The Pacific Historical Review 1956;25(4):369-88.
111. Lal BV, editor. The Encyclopedia of the Indian Diaspora. Singapore: Editions Didier Millet, 2006.
112. Kelly JD, Kaplan M, editors. Represented Communities: Fiji and world decolonization. Chicago: University of Chicago, 2001.

113. Farrell BH, Murphy PE. Ethnic Attitudes Towards Land in Fiji. Santa Cruz, USA: Center for Pacific Studies, University of California, 1978.
114. Kelly JD. Fiji Indians and "Commoditization of Labor". American Ethnologist 1992;19(1):97-120.
115. Spencer DM. Disease, Religion and Society in the Fiji Islands. Seattle: University of Washington Press, 1941.
116. Knapman B, editor. Fiji's Economic History, 1874-1939. Canberra: Australian National University, 1987.
117. Lawrence C. Rockefeller Money, The Laboratory, and Medicine in Edinburg 1919-1930: New science in an old country. Rochester: University of Rochester Press, 2005.
118. Birna A-E, Solorzano A. Public health policy paradoxes: science and politics in the Rockefeller Foundation's hookworm campaign in Mexico in the 1920s Social Science & Medicine 1999;49:1197-213.
119. Prociv P, Luke RA. The changing epidemiology of human hookworm infection in Australia. Med J Aust 1995;162(3):150-4.
120. Heiser V. An American Doctor's Odyssey: Adventures in 45 countries. New York: Grosset & Dunlap, 1936.
121. Lambert SM. A Doctor in Paradise. London: J.M. Dent & Sons, 1941.
122. Hall MC. Developments in Antihelminthic Medication. American Journal of Tropical Medicine 1926;6(4):247-60.
123. Lambert M. Carbon Tetrachlorid in the Treatment of Hookworm Disease: Observations on Fifty Thousand Cases. J Am Med Assoc 1923;80(8):526-28.
124. Lambert SM. Carbon tetrachloride in the treatment of hookworm disease. Observations in 20,000 cases". JAMA : the journal of the American Medical Association (0098-7484), 79, p. 2055. JAMA 1922;79:2055.
125. Lambert SM. Hookworm Disease in the South Pacific: ten years of tetrachlorides. JAMA 1933;100(4):247-48.

126. Meyer JR, Pessoa SB. A Study of the Toxicity of Carbon Tetrachloride. American Journal of Tropical Medicine 1923;3(3):177-97.
127. Manibusan MK, Odin M, Eastmond DA. Postulated carbon tetrachloride mode of action: a review. J. Environ. Sci. Health C. Environ. Carcinog. Ecotoxicol. Rev. 2007;25(3):185-209.
128. Kliks MM. Studies on the traditional herbal anthelmintic Chenopodium ambrosioides L.: ethnopharmacological evaluation and clinical field trials. Soc Sci Med 1985;21(8):879-86.
129. Anonymous. William Jenning Bryan. Wikopedia, 2009.
130. Fosdick R. The Story of the Rockefeller Foundation. New York: Harper & Brothers, 1951.
131. Anonymous. The Native Medical Practitioner 1930-41. The Native Medical Practitioner 1930;Vol 1 Nos 1-4; Vol 2, Nos 1-4; Vol 3 Nos 1-3(Nov 1930-Sept 1941).
132. Lambert SM. Yaws in the South Pacific. American Journal of Tropical Medicine 1929;1(6):429-37.
133. Lambert SM. A resurvey of hookworm disease in Fiji in 1935, ten years after mass treatment. J Trop.Med.Hyg. 1936;39:1-5.
134. Gillespie J. The Rockefeller Foundation, Hookworm Campaign and a National Health Policy in Australia, 1911-1930. In: MacLoed R, Denoon D, editors. Health and Healing in Tropical Australia and Papua New Guinea. Townsville: James Cook University, 1991:64-87.
135. Guthrie MW. Misi Utu: Dr David W Hoodless and the development of medical education in the South Pacific. Suva: Institute of Pacific Studies, USP, 1979.
136. Hawley TG. Medical education in the South Pacific. N.Z.Med. J. 1975;81(533):126-28.
137. Marshall BJ, Warren JR. Unidentified curved bacilli in the stomach of patients with gastritis and peptic ulceration. Lancet 1984;1(8390):1311-5.

138. Manson-Bahr P. Demonstration of colour film of filariasis in Fiji. Transactions of the Royal Society of Tropical Medicine and Hygiene 1951;45(2):154-6.
139. Waldron W. Lambert of Fiji. Harper's Monthly Magazine 1937(March):377-84.
140. Denoon D. Public Health in Papua New Guinea: Medical possibility and social contraint, 1884-1984. Cambridge: Cambridge University Press, 1989.
141. Burton-Bradley BGS. A History of Medicine in Papua New Guinea. Kingsgrove, NSW.: Australasian Medical Publishing Company, 1990.
142. Anderson W. The Collectors of Lost Souls: turning kuru scientists into whitemen. Baltimore: John Hopkins Press, 2008.
143. Taufa T, Bass C. Population, Family Health and Development: papers from the Waigani seminar. Port Moresby: UPNG Press, 1993.
144. Alpers MP. The First 50 Years of the Papua New Guinea Medical Journal: a celebration of its Golden Jubilee. PNG Med. J. 2005;48(1-2):2-26.
145. Amato D, Booth PB. Hereditary ovalocytosis in Melanesians. Papua New Guinea Medical Journal 1977;20:26-32.
146. Barnish G, Ashford RW. Strongyloides cf fuelleborni in Papua New Guinea: epidemiology in an isolated community, and results of an intervention study. Annals of Tropical Medicine & Parasitology 1989;83:499-506.
147. Biddulph J. Standard treatment regimens—a personal account of Papua New Guinea experience. Tropical Doctor 1989;19:126-30.
148. Murrell TG, Walker PD. The pigbel story of Papua New Guinea. Transactions of the Royal Society of Tropical Medicine & Hygiene 1991;85:119-22.
149. Shield JM, Hide RL, Harvey PW, Vrbova H, Tulloch J. Hookworm (Necator americanus) and Strongyloides fuelleborni-like prevalence and egg count with age in highlands fringe people

of Papua New Guinea. Papua New Guinea Medical Journal 1987;30:21-26.
150. Tefuarani N, Vince J, Hawker R, Nunn G, Lee R, Crawford M, Kevau IH. Operation Open Heart in PNG, 1993-2006. Heart Lung Circ. 2007;16(5):373-77.
151. Riley ID, Lehmann D. The Demography of Papua New Guinea. In: R. A, M. A, editors. Human Biology in Papua New Guinea: the small cosmos. Oxford: Oxford University Press, 1992:67-92.
152. Attenborough R, Alpers M, editors. Human Biology in Papua New Guinea: the small cosmos. Oxford: Oxford University Press, 1992.
153. Duke T. Inequity in child health: what are the sustainable Pacific solutions? Med J Aust 2004;181(11-12):612-4.
154. Duke T. Slow but steady progress in child health in Papua New Guinea. J Paediatr Child Health 2004;40(12):659-63.
155. Duke T. Decline in child health in rural Papua New Guinea. Lancet 1999;354(9186):1291-4.
156. Anonymous. Pacific Islands Monthly (PIM) April 1965 36 (4);26-7.
157. Howie-Willis I. A Thousand Graduates: Conflict in University Development in Papua New Guinea, 1961-1976. Canberra: ANU Press, 1980.
158. Werner D. Where there is no doctor : a village health care handbook. 1st English ed. Palo Alto, Calif.: Hesperian Foundation, 1978.
159. Griffin J. John Gunther and Medicine in Papua New Guinea. In: MacLoed R, Denoon D, editors. Health and Healing in Tropical Australia and Papua New Guinea. Townsville: James Cook University, 1991:88-102.
160. Yarwood AT. Sir Raphael Cilento and the white man in the tropics. In: MacLoed R, Denoon D, editors. Health and Healing in Tropical Australia and Papua New Guinea. Townsville: James Cook University, 1991:47-63.

161. Cilento R. The White Man in the Tropics. Melbourne: Commonwealth Department of Health Service, 1925.
162. Fisher FD. Raphael Cilento: a biography. Brisbane: University of Queensland Press, 1994.
163. Gordon D. Obituary: Sir Raphael West Cilento. Medical Journal of Australia 1985;143:260.
164. Lewis MJ. Editor's Introduction. In: Cumpston JHL, Lewis MJ, editors. Health and Disease in Australia: A History. Canberra: AGPS Press, 1989:1-31.
165. Bashford A. Medicine at the Border: Disease, Globalization and Security, 1850 to the Present. Basingstoke, UK: Palgrave MacMillan, 2006.
166. Denoon D, MacLoed R. The idea of tropical medicine and its influence on Papua New Guinea. Health and Healing in Tropical Australia and Papua New Guinea. Townsville: James Cook University, 1991:12-22.
167. Mikloucho-Maclay NN, Tumarkin D. Travels to New Guinea: diaries, letters, documents. Moscow, 1982.
168. Mikloucho-Maclay NN. New Guinea Diaries 1871-1883. Madang: Kristen Press, 1975.
169. Gilpin CM, Simpson G, Vincent S, O'Brien TP, Knight TA, Globan M, Coulter C, Konstantinos A. Evidence of primary transmission of multidrug-resistant tuberculosis in the Western Province of Papua New Guinea. Med J Aust 2008;188(3):148-52.
170. Zigas V. Laughing Death: the untold story of Kuru. Clifton, NJ, USA: The Humana Press, 1990 (republished).
171. Attenborough R. Health changes in Papua New Guinea: from adaptation to double jeopardy? In: Ohtsuka R, Ulijaszek SJ, editors. Health Change in the Asia-Pacific Region: Biocultural and Epidemiological Approaches. Cambridge: Cambridge University Press, 2007:254-302.
172. Foot SHC. Sir Hugh Foot Report. NY: United Nations Visiting Mission, 1962.

173. Currie SGC. Report on the Commission on Higher Education in Papua and New Guinea. Canberra, 1964.
174. Gunther JT. From Stone Age to Parliamentary Government in a Decade. In: Simpson C, editor. Plumes and Arrows: Inside New Guinea. Sydney: Angus & Robertson, 1962.
175. Crocombe R, Melesisea M, editors. Land Issues in the Pacific. Suva: USP, 1994.
176. Crocombe R. The South Pacific. Suva: USP, 2001.
177. Crocombe R. Asia in the Pacific Islands: Replacing the West. Suva: IPS Publications, USP, 2007.
178. Diaz A. The Health Crisis in the US Associated Pacific Islands: Moving Forward. Pacific Health Dialog 1998;4(1):116-28.
179. Miles V, Lander H. Curriculum for the External Degree of Bachelor of Medicine and Bachelor of Medicine of the University of the South Pacific. Suva: Fiji School of Medicine, 1987.
180. Dever G, Finau SA, Hunton R. The Pacific medical education model: introducing the process of innovation. Pacific Health Dialog 1997;4(1):177-90.
181. Flear JA. The Evolution of Community Health Training at PBMOTP. Pacific Health Dialog 1998;4(1):198-202.
182. Dever G, Finau S, Kuartei S, Durand AM, Rykken D, Yano V, Untalan P, Withy K, Tellei P, Baravilala W, Pierantozzi S, Tellei J. The Palau AHEC—academizing the public health work plan: capacity development and innovation in Micronesia. Pac Health Dialog 2005;12(1):110-7.
183. Shaw M. Proposing continuing medical education for the Pacific. Pac Health Dialog 2000;7(2):86-7.
184. Anonymous. Oceania Medical University accessed Nov 2009 *http://www.oceaniamed.org/*
185. Cheema S, McKimm J. Oceania University of Medicine: The New Face of Innovative Medical Education & Research in Samoa and the South Pacific Samoan Medical Journal 2009;1(1):30-33.
186. Anonymous. Foreign Medical Schools accessed Nov 2009 *www.escapeartist.com/studying_abroad/Foreign_Medical_Schools*

187. Hoodless DW. Medical Education and Employment of Native Doctors and Nurses. Proceedings of the Seventh Pacific Science Association (held at Auckland and Christchurch, New Zealand, 2nd February to 4th March, 1949). Christchurch: Pegasus Press, 1953:44-50.
188. Cochrane G. Big Men and Cargo Cults. Oxford: Clarendon Press, 1970.
189. Racule RK. Doctor in the Fijian islands: F. B. Vulaono 1924-76. In: Chapman M, Prothero RM, editors. Circulation in Population Movement: substance and concepts from the Melanesian case. London: Routledge & Kegan Paul, 1985:149-72.
190. De Boissiere R. Filariasis and Yaws in Fiji. Journal of Tropical Medicine 1904;June 15:179-81.
191. Finucane M. On Yaws as Observed in Fiji. Journal of Tropical Medicine 1901;April 15:129-32.
192. Montague AA. Tertiary Yaws. Journal of Tropical Medicine 1910;11(13):161-2.
193. Lynch GWA. Medical Report for the Year 1909 Fiji. Journal of Tropical Medicine & Hygiene 1913;May 15:37-41.
194. Robertson A. A Short Account of the Diseases of the Gilbert and Ellice Islands. Journal of Tropical Medicine & Hygiene 1908;2(11):17-21.
195. Bahr PH. Filariasis in Fiji. Journal of Tropical Medicine 1912; March 1:77-9.
196. Brunwin AD. Some Aspects of Filariasis in Fiji. Journal of Tropical Medicine & Hygiene 1901;24(12):365-71.
197. Amos DW. The Educational Programme on Filariasis in Fiji. Proceedings of the Seventh Pacific Science Association (held at Auckland and Christchurch, New Zealand, 2nd February to 4th March, 1949). Christchurch: Pegasus Press, 1953:230-38.
198. Griffiths PG. Tuberculosis in the Colony of Fiji. Proceedings of the Seventh Pacific Science Association (held at Auckland and Christchurch, New Zealand, 2nd February to 4th March, 1949). Christchurch: Pegasus Press, 1953:395-408.

199. Stella M. Makogai: Image of Hope. Suva: USP (Central Archives and WPHC, Fiji), 1971.
200. Buckingham J. The Pacific Leprosy Foundation Archive and Oral Histories of Leprosy in the South Pacific. The Journal of Pacific History 2006;41(1):81-6.
201. Hall F. Medical Report on the Treatment of Leprosy, Magokai. Journal of Tropical Medicine & Hygiene 1919;July 15:55-7.
202. Austin CJ. Leprosy in Fiji and the South Seas. Proceedings of the Seventh Pacific Science Association (held at Auckland and Christchurch, New Zealand, 2nd February to 4th March, 1949) Christchurch: Pegasus Press, 1953:279-91.
203. Harper P, Levine N, Liebow A. Notes on Age Incidences of Disease in the South Pacific. Proceedings of the Seventh Pacific Science Association (held at Auckland and Christchurch, New Zealand, 2nd February to 4th March, 1949). Christchurch: Pegasus Press, 1953:375-80.
204. Anonymous. Health Manpower Planning and Development. London: Commonwealth Secretariat, 1986:1-59.
205. Miles JAR. Public Health Progress in the Pacific. Helmstedt, Germany: Geowissenschafliche Gesellschaft, 1984.
206. Buchanan JCR. A Guide to the Pacific Island Dietaries. Suva: South Pacific Board of Health, 1947.
207. Price AG. The White Man in the Tropics. Adelaide: Blennerhassett's Commercial Educational Society of Australasia, 1935.
208. Fry G. The South Pacific 'Experiment': Reflections on the Origins of Regional Identity. The Journal of Pacific History 1997;32(2):180-202.
209. Lawrence S. Medical education. In: Bynum WF, Porter R, editors. Companion Encyclopedia of the History of Medicine. London: Routledge, 1993:1151-79.
210. Harris MR. Five Counterrevolutionists in Higher Education. Corvallis: Oregon State University Press, 1970.
211. Flexner A, Carnegie Foundation for the Advancement of Teaching., Pritchett HS. Medical education in the United States and Canada;

a report to the Carnegie Foundation for the Advancement of Teaching. New York City: Carnegie Foundation, 1910.
212. Flexner A. Medical Education in Europe: A Report to the Carnegie Foundation for the Advancement of Teaching. New York: Merrymount Press Boston., 1912.
213. Edmonds AR. The Fiji School of Medicine. Journal of Medical Education 1962;37:478-80.
214. Bapty W. The Training of Health Workers in Fiji. Canadian Medical Association Journal 1962;86:1125.
215. Lander H. Medical Education in Fiji and the South Pacific. Aust NZ J Med 1986;16:304-8.
216. Lander H. Postgraduate Medical Training in Fiji. Fiji Med J 1986;14(5-6):161-65.
217. Bailey MC, Khaiyum E, Prasad VR. Fiji School of Medicine Diploma in Pharmacy graduates, ten year analysis—where are they now? Pac Health Dialog 2006;13(2):151-4.
218. Parke A. The Qawa Incident in 1968 and Other Cases of 'Spirit Possession: Religious Syncretism in Fiji. The Journal of Pacific History 1995;50(2):210-26.
219. Irvine ROH, Cruickshank EK, Palmer GR. Medical Education in the South Pacific: a report by an international mission. Suva: University of the South Pacific, 1971:1-98.
220. Boelen C. Report on a Field Visit to Fiji. Manila: WHO, 1985:1-14.
221. Anonymous. MBBS Degree Programme USP/FSM Affiliation Arrangements and Memorandum of Understanding. Suva: From RACP History of Medicine Library, Sydney, 1981.
222. Biddulph RAJ, Ibbertson HK, Wellington JS. Report of the Senate Review Team on the Award of the External MBBS Degree by the University of the South Pacific (Biddulph Report, 1985). Suva: USP, 1985:1-19.
223. Katonivualika J. Medical Education in the Republic of Fiji. Suva: FSMed, 1988.
224. Lander H. School of medicine's uncertain future. Br.Med.J.(Clin. Res.Ed) 1988;296(6622):620-24.

225. Maxwell W, Murphy W. Report to the Independent Commission of a Committee of Inquiry to the Public Service Commission on the Fiji School of Medicine. Suva: Fiji Government Printer, 1983.
226. Cole DS, Kean MR, Maddison DC. An Assessment of the Fiji School of Medicine (Second Cole Report). Suva: Office of the Representative of the South Pacific, WHO, 1979.
227. WHO. Declaration of Alma-Ata: International Conference on Primary Health Care, Alma-Ata, USSR, 6-12 September, 1978: WHO, 2008.
228. Beeves RG. An Analysis of the Annual Operating Costs of the Fiji School of Medicine. Suva: FSMed (mimeograph), 1987.
229. Anonymous. Cabinet gives approval for FSM modernisation. Fiji Times 1989 12th September issue.
230. Anonymous. Annual Report of the Fiji School of Medicine. Suva: FSMed (mimeograph), 1985.
231. Cole DS, Hubbard J, Barker RA. Report to the Ministry of Foreign Affairs on a visit to the Fiji School of Medicine (First Cole Report). Suva: Fiji School of Medicine, 1977.
232. Morley CJ, Thornton AJ, Cole TJ, Hewson PH, Fowler MA. Baby Check: a scoring system to grade the severity of acute systemic illness in babies under 6 months old. Archives of Disease in Childhood 1991;66:100-05.
233. Hardy D, Frank IB. Fiji School of Medicine Management Programme: Report to the Public Service Commission, Fiji on an Investigation into the Organisation of the Fiji School of Medicine. Suva: FSMed, 1983.
234. Stuart K. Roles of Medical Schools in National Health Developments and Commonwealth Policies and Programmes for Disabled People. London: Commonwealth Secretariat, 1986.
235. Coombe DG. A Review of the Administrative Aspects of the Management of Health Services in Fiji. Suva: Fiji Government Printer, 1982.

236. Malcolm LA, Wright LA, Sharma KD. A Report to the Minister of Health on an Investigation into Divisional Health Boards for Fiji. Suva: Governemnt of Fiji, 1986.
237. Brown MG, Lander H, Cameron BH. Political instability and loss of medical manpower: a case study of Fiji. FSMed, Suva: Unpublished Paper, 1988.
238. Connell J. The Global Health Care Chain: From the Pacific to the World. New York; London: Routledge (Kindle edition), 2009.
239. Voigt-Graf C. Fijian teachers on the move: Causes, implications and policies. Asia Pacific Viewpoint 2003;44(2):163-75.
240. Oman KM. Should I migrate or should I remain? Professional satisfaction and career decisions of doctors who have undertaken specialist training in Fiji. University of Queensland, 2007.
241. Lander H. A Review of the Health Sector in Fiji. (2 volumes with appendices). Canberra: Australian International Development Assistance Bureau, 1988:1-193.
242. Walsh C. Fiji: an encyclopaedic atlas. Suva: USP, 2006.
243. Cameron BH. Teaching in Fiji: Practising medicine, coping with coups. Canadian Medical Association Journal 1980;140 (April 1): 833-35.
244. Lander H. Fiji Health Sector Initiatives: Options for consideration by the Government of Australia. Canberra: Australian International Development Assistance Bureau, 1988:1-18.
245. The Fiji School of Medicine and its founder, William McGregor 1966. History, Heritage & Health: Proceedings of the Fourth Biennial Conference of the Australian Society of the History of Medicine.
246. Anonymous. CWM hospital 'overcrowded'. Fiji Times 1989 18th September issue.
247. Hill P, Samisoni J. Two models of primary health care training. Medical Education 1993;27(1):69-73.
248. Busserau I. New course realistic and relevant says doctor. Fiji Times 1989 Sept 1st issue.

249. Spaulding WB. The undergraduate medical curriculum (1969 model): McMaster university. Can Med Assoc J 1969;100(14):659-64.
250. Rodgers J, Schramm M, Waqatakirewa L, Litidamu N. Corporate Review of Fiji School of Medicine. Suva: Fiji School of Medicine, 2005.
251. Neufeld VR, Spaulding WB. Use of learning resources at McMaster University. Br Med J 1973;3(5871):99-101.
252. Barrows H. Problem-Based Learning in Medicine and Beyond: a brief overview. New Directions for Teaching and Learning 1996;68:3-12.
253. Knowles M. The Adult Learner: A Neglected Species. Houston, Texas: Gulf Publishing Company
254. Neville AJ, Norman GR. PBL in the undergraduate MD program at McMaster University: three iterations in three decades. Acad Med 2007;82(4):370-4.
255. Lyon ML. Epistemology, medical education and problem-based learning: introducing an epistemological dimension into the medical school curriculum. In: Brosnan C, Turner B, editors. Handbook of the Sociology of Medical Education. London; New York: Routledge (Kindle Edition), 2009.
256. Barrows H. The Tutorial Process. Springfield, Illinois: Southern Illinois University, 1988.
257. Norman G. Research in clinical reasoning: past history and current trends. Medical Education 2005;39(4):418-27.
258. Newble DI. Assessing clinical competence at the undergraduate level. Medical Education 1992;26:504-11.
259. Eva KW. What every teacher needs to know about clinical reasoning. Medical Education 2005;39(1):98-106.
260. Norman G. Research in clinical reasoning: past history and current trends. Med Educ 2005;39(4):418-27.
261. Norman GR, Eva KW, Schmidt HG. Implications of psychology-type theories for full curriculum interventions. Medical Education 2005;39(3):247-49.

262. Neville AJ. Problem-based learning and medical education forty years on. A review of its effects on knowledge and clinical performance. Med Princ Pract 2009;18(1):1-9.
263. Cunningham CE, Deal K, Neville A, Lohfeld L. Modeling the Problem-based Learning Preferences of McMaster University Undergraduate Medical Students Using Discrete Choice Conjoint Experiment. Advances in Health Sciences Education 2006;11:245-66.
264. Norman G. Research in medical education: three decades of progress. British Medical Journal 2002;324(7353):1560-62.
265. Patel VL, Groen GJ, Norman GR. Effects of conventional and problem-based medical curricula on problem solving. Academic Medicine 1991;66:380-89.
266. Heale J, Davis D, Norman G, Woodward C, Neufeld V, Dodd P. A randomized controlled trial assessing the impact of problem-based versus didactic teaching methods in CME. Res Med Educ 1988;27:72-7.
267. Norman GR. Problem-solving skills, solving problems and problem-based learning. Med Educ 1988;22(4):279-86.
268. Norman GR, Schmidt HG. The psychological basis of problem-based learning: a review of the evidence. Acad Med 1992;67(9):557-65.
269. Norman G. Problem-based learning makes a difference. But why? CMAJ 2008;178(1):61-2.
270. Stevens FCJ. Innovations in medical education: European convergence, politics and culture. In: Brosnan C, Turner B, editors. Handbook of the Sociology of Medical Education. London; New York: Routledge (Kindle Edition), 2009.
271. Bleakley A, Brice J, Bligh J. Thinking the post-colonial in medical education. Med Educ 2008;42(3):266-70.
272. Karle H, Christensen L, Gordon D, Nystrup J. Neo-colonialism versus sound globalization policy in medical education. Medical Education 2008;42(10):956-58.

273. Husserl E. The idea of phenomenology. The Hague,: Nijhoff, 1964.
274. Husserl E. Phenomenology and the crisis of philosophy: Philosophy as a rigorous science, and Philosophy and the crisis of European man. New York,: Harper & Row, 1965.
275. Marcuse H. One-dimensional man; studies in the ideology of advanced industrial society. Boston,: Beacon Press, 1964.
276. Sartre J-P. Existentialism and humanism. London: Eyre Methuen, 1973.
277. Woodward CA, McAuley RG. Can the academic background of medical graduates be detected during internship? Can Med Assoc J 1983;129(6):567-9.
278. Fraenkel GJ. Medical education. McMaster revisited. Br Med J 1978;2(6144):1072-6.
279. Hamilton JD. The McMaster curriculum: a critique. Br Med J 1976;1(6019):1191-6.
280. Norman GR, Vleuten C, Newble D, editors. International Handbook of Research in Medical Education. Dordrecht, Netherlands: Kluwer Academic, 2002.
281. Mayer RE. The Cambridge Handbook of Multimedia Learning. Cambridge, U.K. ; New York: Cambridge University Press, 2005.
282. Groopman J. Diagnosis: What Doctors Are Missing. NY Review of Books 2009;56(17):Nov 5.
283. Groopman J. How Doctors Think. Boston: Houghton Mifflen Company, 2007.
284. Redelmeier DA. Improving patient care. The cognitive psychology of missed diagnoses. Ann Intern Med 2005;142(2):115-20.
285. Redelmeier DA, Cialdini RB. Problems for clinical judgement: 5. Principles of influence in medical practice. CMAJ 2002;166(13):1680-4.
286. Tu JV, Schull MJ, Ferris LE, Hux JE, Redelmeier DA. Problems for clinical judgement: 4. Surviving in the report card era. CMAJ 2001;164(12):1709-12.

287. Schull MJ, Ferris LE, Tu JV, Hux JE, Redelmeier DA. Problems for clinical judgement: 3. Thinking clearly in an emergency. CMAJ 2001;164(8):1170-5.
288. Redelmeier DA, Tu JV, Schull MJ, Ferris LE, Hux JE. Problems for clinical judgement: 2. Obtaining a reliable past medical history. CMAJ 2001;164(6):809-13.
289. Redelmeier DA, Schull MJ, Hux JE, Tu JV, Ferris LE. Problems for clinical judgement: 1. Eliciting an insightful history of present illness. CMAJ 2001;164(5):647-51.
290. Redelmeier DA, Ferris LE, Tu JV, Hux JE, Schull MJ. Problems for clinical judgement: introducing cognitive psychology as one more basic science. CMAJ 2001;164(3):358-60.
291. Wilkinson TJ, Newble DI, Frampton CM. Standard setting in an objective structured clinical examination: use of global ratings of borderline performance to determine the passing score. Med Educ 2001;35(11):1043-9.
292. Roberts C, Newble D, Jolly B, Reed M, Hampton K. Assuring the quality of high-stakes undergraduate assessments of clinical competence. Med Teach 2006;28(6):535-43.
293. Miller GE. The assessment of clinical skills / competence / performance. Academic Medicine 1990;65(9):S63-67.
294. Hafferty FW, Castellani B. The hidden curriculum: a theory of medical education. In: Brosnan C, Turner B, editors. Handbook of the Sociology of Medical Education. London; New York: Routledge (Kindle Edition), 2009.
295. Lempp H. Medical school culture. In: Brosnan C, Turner B, editors. Handbook of the Sociology of Medical Education. London; New York: Routledge (Kindle Edition), 2009.
296. Brosnan C, Turner BS, editors. Handbook of the Sociology of Medical Education. London ; New York: Routledge (Kindle edition), 2009.
297. Atkinson P, Delamont S. From classification to integration: Bernstein and the sociology of medical education. In: Brosnan

C, Turner B, editors. Handbook of the Sociology of Medical Education. London; New York: Routledge (Kindle Edition), 2009.
298. Regan de Bere S, Peterson A. Crisis or renaissance? A sociology of anatomy in UK medical education. In: Brosnan C, Turner B, editors. Handbook of the Sociology of Medical Education. London; New York: Routledge (Kindle Edition), 2009.
299. Becker H, Geer B, Hughes E, Strauss A. Boys in White: student culture in medical school. Chicago: University of Chicago Press, 1961.
300. Merton R, Reader G, Kendall P, editors. The Student-Physician: Introductory studies in the sociology of medical education. Cambridge: Harvard University Press, 1957.
301. Cockerham WC. Medical education and the American healthcare system. In: Brosnan C, Turner B, editors. Handbook of the Sociology of Medical Education. London; New York: Routledge (Kindle Edition), 2009.
302. Hartzband P, Groopman J. Other voices. Should money drive everything? Hosp Health Netw 2009;83(2):12.
303. Hartzband P, Groopman J. Money and the changing culture of medicine. N Engl J Med 2009;360(2):101-3.
304. Illich I. Medical nemesis : the expropriation of health. London: Calder & Boyars, 1975.
305. Marmot M. Social determinants of health inequalities. Lancet 2005;365(9464):1099-104.
306. Sokal A, editor. The Sokal Hoax: The sham that shook the academy. Lingua Franca: University of Nebraska Press, 2000.
307. Beauchamp TL, Childress TF. Principles of Biomedical Ethics. 4th edition ed. New York: Oxford University Press, 1994.
308. Marcum JA. An Introductory Philosophy of Medicine: Humanizing Modern Medicine: Springer (Kindle Electronic), 2008.
309. Horton R. Medicine: the prosperity of virtue. Lancet 2005;366(Dec 10th):1985-7.
310. Eva KW, Reiter HI, Rosenfeld J, Norman GR. The ability of the multiple mini-interview to predict preclerkship performance

in medical school. Academic Medicine 2004;79(10 Suppl): S40-S42.
311. Hartzband P, Groopman J. Keeping the patient in the equation—humanism and health care reform. N Engl J Med 2009;361(6):554-5.
312. Sackett D. Evidence-Based Medicine: how to practice and teach EBM. Edinburgh: Churchill-Livingstone, 2000.
313. Mitchell PB. Winds of change: growing demands for transparency in the relationship between doctors and the pharmaceutical industry. MJA 2009;191(5):273-75.
314. Sackett DL, Haynes RB, Tugwell P. Clinical Epidemiology: a basic science for clinical medicine. Boston: Little, Brown and Company, 1985.
315. Norman GR. Examining the assumptions of evidence-based medicine. J Eval Clin Pract 1999;5(2):139-47.
316. Lowe M. Evidence-based medicine—the view from Fiji. The Lancet 2000;356(9235):1105-07.
317. Lowe M, Brewster DR. Evidence-based medicine and clinical practice. J Paediatr.Child Health 2003;39:145-46.
318. Timmermans S, Chawla N. Evidence-based medicine and medical education. In: Brosnan C, Turner B, editors. Handbook of the Sociology of Medical Education. London; New York: Routledge (Kindle Edition), 2009.
319. Bauer P. Foreign Aid: Mend it or end it. In: Bauer P, Siwatibau S, Kasper W, editors. Aid and Development in the South Pacific. St Leonards, NSW: Centre for Independent Studies, 1991:3-18.
320. Gounder R. Overseas Aid Motivations. Aldershot, UK: Avebury, Ashgate Publishing, 1995.
321. Ruger JP. The changing role of the World Bank in global health. Am J Public Health 2005;95(1):60-70.
322. Anonymous. Pearson Report (Partners in development). NY: Praeger, 1969.
323. Anonymous. Brandt Report (Independent Commission on International Development Issues). London: Pan Books, 1980.

324. Anonymous. World Development Report 1993: Investing in Health. Washington: World Bank, 1993.
325. Sridhar D. The Battle Against Hunger: Choice, Circumstances, and the World Bank. Oxford: Oxford University Press, 2008.
326. Anonymous. Paris Declaration on Aid Effectiveness: Ownership, Harmonisation, Alignment, Results and Mutual Accountability. Paris, 2005.
327. Sen A. Development as Freedom. Oxford: Oxford University Press, 1999.
328. Sachs J. The End of Poverty: Economic Possibilities for our Time. London: Penguin, 2005.
329. Ruger JP. Global health governance and the World Bank. Lancet 2007;370(9597):1471-4.
330. Moyo D. Dead Aid: Why aid is not working and how there is another way for Africa. London: Allen Lane (Penguin), 2009.
331. Easterly W. The White Man's Burden: why the West's effort to aid the rest have so much ill and so little good 2007.
332. Connell J, editor. The International Migration of Health Workers. New York; London: Routledge (Kindle edition), 2008.
333. WHO. World Health Report: Working Together for Health. Geneva: World Health Organization, 2006.
334. Bourgeault IL, Aylward J. The challenges to achieving self-sufficiency in Canadian medical education. In: Brosnan C, Turner B, editors. Handbook of the Sociology of Medical Education. London; New York: Routledge (Kindle Edition), 2009.
335. Brown RP, Connell J. The migration of doctors and nurses from South Pacific Island Nations. Social Science & Medicine 2004;58(11):2193-210.
336. Pfeiffer J, Johnson W, Fort M, Shakow A, Hagopian A, Gloyd S, Gimbel-Sherr K. Strengthening health systems in poor countries: a code of conduct for nongovernmental organizations. Am J Public Health 2008;98(12):2134-40.
337. Hagopian A, Ofosu A, Fatusi A, Biritwum R, Essel A, Gary Hart L, Watts C. The flight of physicians from West Africa: views of

African physicians and implications for policy. Soc Sci Med 2005;61(8):1750-60.
338. Hagopian A, Thompson MJ, Fordyce M, Johnson KE, Hart LG. The migration of physicians from sub-Saharan Africa to the United States of America: measures of the African brain drain. Hum Resour Health 2004;2(1):17.
339. Hagopian A, Ofosu A, Fatusi A, Biritwum R, Essel A, Gary Hart L, Watts C. The flight of physicians from West Africa: Views of African physicians and implications for policy. Social Science & Medicine 2005;61(8):1750-60.
340. Negin J. Australia and New Zealand's contribution to Pacific Island health worker brain drain. Aust N Z J Public Health 2008;32(6):507-11.
341. Rokoduru A. Globalisation and Governance in the Pacific Islands. Canberra: ANU E Press, 2006.
342. Oman K, Malani J, Moulds R. Postgraduate internal medicine teaching in the Pacific: a sustainable approach. Medical Education 2003;37(11):1041-42.
343. Reddy M, Mohanty M, Naidu V. Economic Cost of Human Capital Loss from Fiji: Implications for Sustainable Development. The International Migration Review 2004;38(38):1447-61.
344. Anonymous. Jackson Report (Committee of Review: The Australian Overseas Aid Program). Canberra: Australian Government Publishing Service, 1984.
345. Anonymous. The Australian Aid Program: Report on Proceedings of a Seminar, 31 July 1996, Canberra. Canberra: Commonwealth of Australia, 1996:1-81.
346. Anonymous. Report on Australia's International Health Programs. Canberra: Australian Government Publishing Service, 1993:1-113.
347. Macdonald B. Decolonisation and Good Governance: Precedents and Continuities. In: Denoon D, editor. Emerging from Empire? Decolonisation in the Pacific. Canberra: ANU, 1996:1-9.

348. Hughes H. Aid Has Failed the Pacific,. Issue Analysis 2003;Centre for Independent Studies(33):1-31.
349. Siwatibau S. Some Aspects of Development in the South Pacific: an insider's view. In: Bauer P, Siwatibau S, Kasper W, editors. Aid and Development in the South Pacific. St Leonards, NSW: Centre for Independent Studies, 1991:21-44.
350. Kasper W. The Economic and Politics of South Pacific Development: an outsider's view. In: Bauer P, Siwatibau S, Kasper W, editors. Aid and Development in the South Pacific. St Leonards, NSW: Centre for Independent Studies, 1991:47-81.
351. van Fossen A. South Pacific Futures: Oceania towards 2050. Brisbane: The Foundation for Development Cooperation, 2005.
352. Bertram G. The MIRAB model twelve years on. The Contemporary Pacific 1999;11(1):105-11.
353. Anonymous. Australia's Relations with the South Pacific. Canberra: Australian Government Publishing Service, 1989:1-277.
354. Mara K. The Pacific Way: a memoir. Honolulu, Hawaii: University of Hawaii Press, 1997.
355. Bain K. Treason at Ten: Fiji at the crossroads. London: Hodder & Stoughton, 1989.
356. Lal BV. The Decolonisation of Fiji: Debate on Constitutional Change, 1943-1963. In: Denoon D, editor. Emerging from Empire? Decolonisation in the Pacific. Canberra: ANU, 1996:26-39.
357. Norton R. Accommodating Indigenous Privilege: Britain's Dilemma in Decolonising Fiji. the Journal of Pacific History 2002;37(2):133-56.
358. Heartfield J. The Dark Races Against the Light? Official Reaction to the 1959 Fiji Riots. The Journal of Pacific History 2002;37(1):75-86.
359. Sutherland W, Akram-Lodhi AH. The problematics of reform and the Fijian question. Confronting Fiji Futures. Canberra: Asia Pacific Press (ANU), 2000:205-25.
360. Whitehead C. Education in Fiji since Independence. Wellington: NZ Council for Educational Research, 1986.

361. Campbell IC. Worlds Apart. Christchurch, NZ: Canterbury University Press, 2003.
362. West FJ. Problems of Political Advancement in Fiji. Pacific Affairs 1960;33(1):23-37.
363. Sharpham J. Rabuka of Fiji: The authorised biography of Major-General Sitiveni Rabuka. Rockhampton: Central Queensland University Press, 2000.
364. Robertson R. Retreat from exclusion? Identities in post-coup Fiji. In: Akram-Lodhi AH, editor. Confronting Fiji Futures. Canberra: Asia Pacific Press (ANU), 2000:269-93.
365. Knapman B. The Economic Consequences of the Coups In: Robertson RT, Tamanisau A, editors. Fiji: Shattered coups. Sydney: Pluto Press, 1988:157-89.
366. Bavadra TU, Bain A, Baba T. Bavadra: Prime Minister, Statesman, Man of the People. Nadi, Fiji: Sunrise Press, 1990.
367. Ramesh S. Fiji, 1987-2007: The Story of Four Coups: Sydney, 2007.
368. Davis T. Island Boy: an autobiography. Christchurch, NZ: University of Canterbury, 1992.
369. Tuimaleali'ifano M. Current Developments in the Pacific: Veiqati Vaka Viti and the Fiji Islands Elections in 1999. The Journal of Pacific History 2000;35(3):253-67.
370. Fraenkel J. The Clash of Dynasties and Rise of Demagogues; Fiji's Tauri Vakaukauwa of May 2000. The Journal of Pacific History 2000;35(3):295-308.
371. Halapua W. Militarism and the Moral Decay in Fiji. Fijian Studies 2003;1(1):105-27.
372. O'Leary FM, Hunjan JS, Bradbury R, Thanakrishnan G. Fatal leptospirosis presenting as musculoskeletal chest pain. Medical Journal of Australia 2004;180(1):29-31.
373. Tuisuva J, Morse Z. Training of oral health personnel in Fiji. Pac Health Dialog 2003;10(1):4-5.
374. Tuisuva J, von Doussa R, Dimmer A, Smyth J, Davies G. The sequential modular curriculum for oral health personnel: an

evaluation of the Fijian experience after five years. Community Dent Health 1999;16(2):97-101.
375. Davies GN, Atalifo SF, Tuisuva J, King T, Mucunabitu M, Nawawabalavu N, Singh V, Vukunisiga S. A new approach to the training and education of oral health personnel. N Z Dent J 1993;89(398):113-8.
376. Bailey MCE, Khaiyum E, Prasad VR. Fiji School of Medicine Diploma in Pharmacy Graduates, Ten Year Analysis—where are they now? Pacific Health Dialog 2006;13(2):151-54.
377. Larkins R. A battle we must not lose. Australian 2008;25.
378. Jerety J. Primary Health Care: Fiji's Broken Dreams. Bulletin of the World Health Organization 2008;86(3):166-7.

Index

A

Aaby: Peter 59
Aberdeen 38, 88, 108
Alma-Ata Declaration 222
AMPs: Assistant Medical
    Practitioners 28, 175, 197,
    225, 255
Anderson: Matron 36, 43
  Warrick 186
apothecaries 100, 101, 102, 103,
    104, 108, 109, 115
apprenticeship 31, 35, 43, 47, 102,
    104, 105, 158, 393
Asklepios 23, 24
Assessment 282, 283, 285
  360-degree 272, 285, 290, 388,
    389
AusAID 252, 257, 317, 318, 368,
    373, 374, 379, 380, 384, 389,
    395
Australian Institute of Tropical
    Health 177
Autonomy 257

B

Bain: 'Atu 96, 324
Bainimarama: Frank 315, 318,
    345, 346, 347, 348, 382, 395,
    398
Baravilala: Wame 257, 258, 259,
    350, 366, 396, 402
Barnes: CE 189
Barrows: Howard 267
Bavadra: Timoci 248, 320, 329,
    330, 331, 332, 333, 334, 336,
    337, 338, 339, 340, 341
Bernard: Claude 114, 217
Biddulph: John 237, 238
body-snatching 104, 107
Bradford Hill: Prof 234
Brandt: Chancellor Willy 300
Breinl: Anton 131, 177, 179, 182
Brewster: Sir David 217
Bryan: William Jennings 140
Bryant: Bronwen 367
Burnham: John 19

C

caduceus: symbol 22, 23, 24
Cakobau 17, 53, 54, 87, 321, 328, 345, 391
Calman: Sir Kenneth 115, 289
Cambridge 80, 88, 101, 103, 106, 171, 226, 266
Cameron: Brian 252, 257, 402
Centenary: School 246
Central Medical School 22, 24, 28, 98, 116, 133, 135, 136, 139, 141, 142, 143, 147, 149, 151, 153, 156, 158, 159, 160, 164, 165, 166, 172, 175, 187, 193, 197, 198, 199, 200, 204, 205, 209, 210, 212, 213, 214, 215, 221, 222, 235, 241, 315, 321, 330, 363, 390
Chandra: Rajesh 384
Cilento: Sir Raphael 77, 78, 79, 131, 133, 166, 167, 168, 170, 171, 172, 173, 174, 176, 177, 178, 179, 180, 181, 182, 183, 187, 390
CMO: Chief Medical Officer 31, 34, 35, 36, 39, 41, 43, 46, 50, 53, 56, 63, 79, 88, 132, 135, 141, 148, 149, 152, 153, 201, 205, 210, 211, 230, 401
cognitive errors 279
Cole Report 241
Colonial Medical Service 38, 42, 155
Commission: Depopulation 67, 68, 69, 71, 80
Connell: John 305
Cook: James 49, 50, 64, 66, 150, 206
Cook Islands 53, 135, 143, 147, 159, 172, 196, 247, 337
Coombe: David 245
Corney: BG 41, 43, 44, 50, 67, 69
Glanville 36, 215, 401
Council of Chiefs 90, 94, 122, 136, 148, 150, 154, 334, 338, 340, 342, 343, 344
coup 248, 249, 250, 251, 252, 253, 256, 258, 259, 264, 315, 317, 320, 327, 330, 332, 333, 334, 335, 336, 337, 338, 339, 340, 341, 343, 344, 345, 346, 347, 348, 350, 351, 353, 374, 379, 380, 384, 395, 398
Crocombe: Ron 190, 191
CROP: Council of Regional Organisations of the Pacific 260, 315, 316, 347
CSR: Colonial Sugar Refining Company 123
Cullen: William 110
Cumpston: John 120, 131, 167, 172, 174, 177, 180, 181, 183, 187, 210, 390
Currie: Sir George 188
CWM Hospital 157, 200, 227, 231, 244, 245, 246, 250, 254, 260, 317, 364, 380, 382, 383, 384, 396

D

Daniels: Charles Wilberforce 42
Davidson: James 22
　Lindsey 234
David Newble 237, 239
demography 61, 273
Denoon: Daniel 174, 175, 181, 182, 183
dental exam scam 366
Dental School: issues 363
Des Voeux 34, 88, 118
Dever: Greg 194
disciplinary committee 365
duodenal ulcer 157
dysentery 32, 33, 37, 42, 49, 50, 52, 55, 59, 62, 63, 67, 71, 86, 120, 134, 161, 166, 173, 184, 205, 282, 321

E

Easterly: William 304, 373
EBM: Evidence-Based Medicine 292, 293, 294, 351
Edinburgh 108, 110, 218
Edmonds: Archibald 199, 225, 228, 229, 402
Ellice: Island 134, 143, 148, 157, 159, 160, 162, 172, 197, 198, 199, 201, 206, 227
Engel: Charles 244

epidemics 18, 42, 49, 52, 55, 56, 58, 59, 60, 61, 63, 64, 67, 82, 85, 112, 199, 390

F

Fanon: Frantz 95
Fiji Times 248
filariasis 63, 77, 134, 161, 166, 205, 207, 214
Finau: Sitaleki 155, 194, 351, 371, 378
Flear: Joseph 194, 369, 375
Flexner: Abraham 146, 219, 220, 221, 222, 390, 399
France 93, 103, 105, 108, 113, 201, 213, 216, 217, 256, 272, 273, 276
Frater: Alexander 157, 199, 401
Freeman: Derek 77
FSMEA: Union 357, 362, 365, 366, 387
FSMed: Fiji School of Medicine 189, 190, 193, 194, 195, 213, 225, 226, 229, 230, 231, 232, 233, 234, 235, 236, 238, 239, 240, 241, 242, 243, 244, 245, 246, 249, 250, 252, 253, 254, 255, 256, 260, 261, 264, 294, 295, 316, 317, 347, 355, 359, 361, 365, 369, 370, 371, 372, 373, 374, 376, 378, 379, 380, 381, 382, 383, 384, 385, 386, 395, 396

G

Galen 112
Gandhi 123
Gilbert Islands 47, 134
Gilchrist: Kenneth 226, 227, 228, 229, 402
girmitiyas 121
Glasgow 38, 108, 215
Gordon: Sir Arthur 17, 31, 53, 76, 80, 82, 87, 88, 89, 90, 91, 92, 93, 94, 96, 98, 99, 117, 119, 120, 122, 123, 125, 174, 181, 320, 321, 322, 325, 390, 391, 392, 398
Gounder: Rukmani 297
Graduate Entry 373
Greg Dever 257, 369
Gris: Gabriel 176, 190, 192
Groopman: Jerome 280, 282
Guinea-Bissau 58, 59
Gunther: John 173, 174, 175, 186, 188, 189, 190

H

Hall: Maurice 133
Hamilton: John 265, 373
Hasluck: PMC 187
Hawaii 52, 65, 66, 76, 82, 193, 194, 238, 253, 349
Hawley: Thomas 231, 232, 233, 402
Heiser: Victor 129, 130, 131, 134, 141, 142, 143, 145, 147, 148, 153, 158, 161, 162, 164, 181, 208
Helicobacter pylori 157, 371
Hippocrates 112
Hoodless: David 36, 47, 56, 153, 154, 155, 156, 157, 159, 160, 197, 198, 210, 321, 363, 381, 390, 401
hookworm 62, 63, 78, 86, 128, 129, 130, 131, 132, 133, 134, 135, 136, 139, 141, 142, 143, 145, 147, 167, 172, 181, 183, 185, 201, 202, 205, 208, 390
Human Resources 358, 373
Human Rights Commission 362
Hume: David 100, 110
Hunt: John 64
Husserl: Edmund 272
hybridity 97

I

Illich: Ivan 288
India 31, 56, 82, 83, 88, 103, 117, 120, 121, 123, 124, 144, 195, 232, 249, 251, 302, 316, 339, 374
Indian indentured labour 119
indirect rule 76, 90, 91, 93, 94, 96, 99
infant mortality 83, 84, 135, 166, 205, 206
influenza 45, 46, 52, 53, 55, 60, 66, 67, 71, 86, 130, 134, 205

J

Jackson Report 309
Johns Hopkins: University 113, 144, 146, 148, 162, 221, 222
John A Burns School of Medicine Hawaii 193

K

Kadavu 33, 67
Kasper: Wolfgang 313
kava 68, 119, 234, 254
Kelly: John 126
Keown: Michelle 95
Kiribati 118, 247, 312
  aid project 370
Kunitz: Stephen 81, 82
Kuper: Geoffrey 200
Kuresa: Ielu 135, 143

L

labour trade 117
Laënnec: René 114
Lal: Brij 96, 124, 125, 326, 342
Lambert: Sylvester 23, 24, 62, 130, 131, 132, 133, 134, 135, 136, 139, 140, 141, 142, 143, 144, 145, 147, 149, 150, 151, 152, 153, 154, 156, 158, 160, 161, 162, 163, 164, 166, 167, 172, 181, 200, 201, 202, 206, 208, 209, 210, 211, 212, 215, 383, 390, 393

Lancet 20, 42, 67, 234, 254, 294
Lander: Harry 237, 241, 243, 247, 248, 250, 251, 252, 253, 348, 402
Lautoka 237, 250, 253, 259, 316, 317, 330, 375, 376, 379, 380, 381, 383, 384, 385, 395
League of Nations 166, 168, 210
lecture 111
Levuka 31, 32, 53, 54, 207
Lewis: Ian 222, 254, 256, 257, 265, 402
Locke: John 100, 110
Lynch: GWA 41, 43, 44, 401

M

MacGregor: Sir William 17, 31, 32, 33, 34, 36, 38, 39, 41, 48, 53, 88, 89, 90, 93, 99, 108, 120, 132, 174, 182, 215, 316, 390, 391
MacPherson: Duncan 162, 163, 210
Maddocks: Ian 189, 190
Madraiwiwi: Ratu 96, 148, 155, 362
Makogai: leprosarium 141, 147, 158, 207, 208, 209, 212, 214, 227
Malani: Joji 194, 251, 351, 369
malaria 39, 42, 59, 77, 79, 129, 132, 143, 146, 166, 173, 184, 185, 201, 202, 205, 208, 386

Malekula: Vanuatu 201, 202
Manson-Bahr 161, 176
Mara: Kamisese 251, 252, 256, 320, 321, 322, 324, 326, 327, 328, 329, 332, 333, 334, 335, 336, 337, 339, 340, 341, 342, 345, 346, 349
Marcum: James 292
Marcuse: Herbert 272
Mauritius 38, 88, 117, 303, 349, 391
MBBS: Medical Degree 28, 190, 195, 232, 235, 236, 237, 238, 239, 240, 241, 242, 243, 245, 249, 254, 255, 256, 258, 259, 260, 264, 350, 355, 364, 369, 374, 375, 376, 377, 379, 380, 384, 390
McArthur: Norma 45, 55, 64, 65
McCaig: Eddie 351, 352, 364, 365, 366, 385, 396, 403
McMaster 19, 265, 266, 267, 268, 270, 272, 273, 276, 293, 294, 373, 399
Mead: Margaret 76, 77
measles 17, 31, 33, 41, 45, 46, 49, 52, 53, 54, 55, 56, 57, 58, 59, 60, 61, 62, 64, 66, 67, 71, 86, 88, 120, 391

medical education 17, 18, 21, 22, 48, 100, 105, 107, 108, 109, 110, 113, 114, 115, 116, 128, 144, 145, 146, 164, 165, 166, 174, 192, 193, 195, 197, 215, 216, 218, 219, 220, 221, 222, 241, 242, 243, 255, 265, 266, 270, 274, 276, 279, 289, 291, 293, 294, 315, 371, 373, 384, 386, 389, 390, 393, 399
medical ethics 289, 386
medical historian 19, 116
Micronesia 25, 165, 193, 195, 196, 214, 225, 247, 368, 369
migrant labour 118
migration 18, 25, 83, 123, 133, 181, 192, 232, 250, 255, 264, 271, 305, 308, 317, 318, 325, 339, 341, 348, 361, 379, 381, 385, 395
Mikloucho-Maclay 184
miscegenation 73
missionaries 32, 52, 55, 63, 71, 73, 90, 94, 168, 184
Montague: Aubrey 41, 46, 56, 141, 144, 150, 151, 153, 158, 172, 181, 205, 206, 210, 211, 393, 401
Morens: David 57, 58
Moriss: Wayne 259
Mother Hubbard 74
Moulds: Rob 403
Moyo: Dambisa 303

N

NAB: arsenical injections 43, 134, 198, 199, 206, 207
Nandam: Satendra 250
National University of Fiji 317, 360, 396
Native Practitioner 28, 35
Nauru 134, 151, 159, 198, 199
NCD: Non-Communicable Diseases 262
Neville: Alan 266, 270
Newman: Charles 116
New Hebrides 50, 53, 66, 118, 119, 143, 148, 151, 152, 159, 160, 168, 171, 181, 199, 201, 202, 211, 247. *See* Vanuatu
Nicholas: Thomas 80
Nigeria 39, 93
NMPs: Native Medical Practitioners 28, 36, 43, 44, 45, 46, 47, 63, 86, 98, 119, 134, 135, 136, 141, 142, 143, 144, 147, 151, 152, 153, 158, 160, 161, 162, 163, 167, 168, 171, 172, 175, 197, 200, 201, 202, 203, 208, 209, 210, 212, 256, 363, 393, 394
Norman: Geoffrey 268, 294
Nuffield: Clinic 212, 231, 232, 315

NZ: New Zealand 32, 60, 66, 77, 82, 91, 96, 123, 144, 148, 151, 155, 157, 162, 195, 197, 213, 233, 241, 248, 249, 254, 259, 262, 300, 308, 318, 319, 321, 329, 337, 339, 342, 347, 371, 372, 378, 385, 397
NZAID: New Zealand aid 318, 371, 372, 379, 384, 395

O

obesity 25, 184, 262, 371
Oceania Medical University 195
ODA: Foreign Aid 299, 319
Off-Shore' Medical Schools 195
officiers de santé 105
OSCE: Objective Structured Clinical Examination 258, 268, 271, 283, 284, 285, 291, 377
Osler: Sir William 20, 113, 219, 221, 390
Oxford 103, 106, 113, 221, 262, 266, 322

P

Pacific Basin: Medical Officers Training Program 193
Pacific Islands 18, 22, 23, 24, 32, 49, 53, 61, 63, 74, 76, 95, 129, 144, 149, 150, 152, 159, 165, 181, 193, 194, 195, 196, 197, 205, 207, 209, 210, 294, 311, 314, 399

Pacific Island Monthly 166
Pacific Paradox 312, 318
Palau 193, 194, 195, 368, 369
Papua 39, 53, 73, 79, 131, 132, 133, 141, 143, 166, 167, 168, 170, 171, 174, 182, 183, 185, 187, 247, 390
Papuan Medical College 190
Pasifika: campus 363
Pathik: Bhupendra 233, 236, 240, 402
PBL: Problem-Based Learning 265, 266, 267, 270, 271, 275, 276, 294, 376
Pearce: AHB 41, 63, 153
 Richard (Rockefeller) 144, 145, 150, 221
Pearson: Lester B 299
philanthropy 18, 25, 98, 128, 136, 145, 164, 296, 299, 390
philosophy 19, 100, 112, 220, 242, 272, 273, 274, 291
PHRC: Pacific Health Research Council 372
physician 100, 101, 103, 113, 200, 293
Pitt-Rivers: George 73
PNG: Papua New Guinea 25, 57, 58, 60, 117, 119, 165, 166, 168, 170, 176, 186, 187, 188, 189, 190, 191, 192, 229, 235, 238, 239, 248, 254, 260, 307, 310, 313, 315, 336, 372
Polynesia 25, 65, 66, 77, 82, 184, 214, 247, 397

Port Moresby 58, 168, 176, 184, 188, 190, 192
Prasad: Umanand 384
Pretrick: E 193
Primary Care Practitioners 255
professionalism 245, 286, 287, 290, 292
Pryor: Jan 257, 261, 351, 365, 369, 371, 372
Puamau: NMP Sowane 47
Public Health 79, 146, 153, 167, 168, 169, 173, 174, 179, 188, 189, 190, 194, 195, 204, 212, 214, 230, 231, 261, 330, 350, 351, 368, 369, 370, 378, 394

Q

Qarase: Laisenia 346, 381, 395
quarantine 33, 53, 54, 56, 60, 120, 141, 167, 171, 180, 182, 185, 199, 210, 212, 391
Queensland 39, 91, 92, 117, 118, 119, 131, 141, 162, 167, 177, 178, 179, 181, 253, 263, 364
Queen Victoria School 148, 153, 154, 200, 203, 325, 330, 332, 348, 352

R

Rabuka: Sitiveni 251, 256, 315, 318, 320, 327, 330, 332, 333, 334, 335, 336, 337, 339, 340, 341, 342, 343, 345, 348, 390

Rallu: Jean-Louis 65
Redelmeier: Donald 281
research 21, 42, 59, 77, 132, 139, 142, 161, 162, 163, 177, 182, 184, 186, 205, 212, 213, 214, 216, 219, 221, 222, 238, 261, 262, 267, 271, 277, 289, 293, 312, 352, 353, 364, 365, 368, 370, 371, 372, 386
Rivers: William 71, 72, 73
Roberts: Stephen 74, 75, 76, 378
Robinson: Sir Hercules Robinson 53
Rockefeller 23, 98, 128, 129, 130, 133, 136, 139, 140, 142, 144, 145, 146, 147, 148, 149, 150, 152, 153, 161, 162, 163, 167, 172, 181, 183, 185, 206, 208, 211, 215, 217, 219, 221, 222, 299, 315, 390, 393, 399
Rodgers: Jimmie 260, 352, 354, 395
Rogers: Terrence 193
Ross: Ronald 39, 42
Royal College 36, 101, 102, 109

S

Sachs: Jeffrey 302
Sackett: David 293, 294
Samisoni: Jimi 194, 222, 230, 256, 257, 369, 402
Samoa 22, 50, 53, 60, 66, 76, 82, 95, 117, 135, 141, 143, 148, 151, 159, 162, 172, 186, 193, 194, 195, 197, 198, 199, 206, 208, 246, 307, 336, 380, 398

sanitation 33, 37, 78, 80, 84, 129, 131, 136, 167, 169, 180, 184, 199, 225, 232
Savenaca Narube 353
Savenaca Siwatibau 313
school fees 204, 360
Scotland 38, 100, 104, 107, 108, 221
Scragg: R 189
Scripps: San Diego 260
Second World War 49, 57, 125, 157, 164, 174, 179, 209, 299, 392
Senilagakali: Jona 233, 236, 346, 382, 383, 384
Seychelles 38
Shigella dysenteriae 42
Shlomowitz: Ralph 83
Singh: Vikash 364
Siwatibau: Savenaca 261, 313
Solomon Islands 42, 53, 69, 70, 72, 117, 118, 133, 143, 148, 152, 159, 160, 167, 168, 171, 172, 181, 186, 192, 199, 206, 228, 247, 259, 330, 351, 352, 380, 396
Spate: OHK 188
SPC: Secretariat of the Pacific Community 212, 213, 214, 239, 260, 263, 305, 316, 352, 368, 373, 379, 395
Speight: George 56, 258, 315, 318, 344, 345, 351
Sridhar: Devi 302

Staphylococcus 52, 55
Strong: William 132, 167, 168, 170, 171, 192
Stuart: Annie 97, 140, 149, 161, 162, 163, 200, 203, 210, 211, 290
St Bartholomew's (Barts): Hospital 105
surgery 34, 35, 36, 42, 102, 105, 107, 109, 110, 113, 147, 148, 151, 158, 185, 198, 216, 226, 244, 259, 377, 384
Swami: Niraj 359
Sweeney: George 265
Sydney 17, 35, 52, 53, 54, 168, 179, 180, 181, 182, 187, 214, 248, 250, 338, 352, 398

T

Tamanitoakula: NMP Asaeli 47
Tamavua: campus 207, 213, 230, 231, 232, 233, 234, 240, 315
Taukei: Movement 332, 334, 335, 341, 343, 344, 348
Taveta: Mesulame:Mesulame 160, 200, 201, 202, 203
TB: Tuberculosis 62, 63, 71, 142, 146, 173, 175, 185, 186, 198, 205, 207, 230
Thomson: Basil 36, 50
Thurston: John 64, 89, 90, 94, 96, 118
Tinea imbricata 51, 209

Tonga 49, 53, 66, 95, 117, 135, 141, 143, 147, 148, 150, 159, 162, 172, 197, 198, 199, 211, 247, 262, 307, 336, 380
Tukuitonga: Colin 248
tultuls 173
tutor 36, 156, 383, 401
typhoid 62, 63, 67, 86, 162, 205, 209

U

USP: University of the South Pacific 96, 189, 191, 192, 226, 234, 235, 236, 238, 239, 240, 241, 242, 243, 244, 245, 246, 250, 253, 254, 260, 261, 264, 313, 316, 318, 325, 340, 345, 347, 348, 352, 353, 356, 359, 361, 373, 378, 379, 383, 394, 395, 396

V

Vanuatu: New Hebrides 42, 66, 117, 118, 148, 196, 206, 256, 336, 350, 396
Van Fossen 314
Veisamasama: Malikai 134, 135, 141, 201
virgin soil: epidemics 52, 54, 55, 56, 64, 66
Vulaono: Filipe 203, 204

W

Walsh: Prof Laurie 364
Western Pacific High Commission 47, 92, 148, 210
WHO 212, 213, 222, 235, 241, 242, 244, 248, 254, 255, 305, 368, 370, 373, 379
  World Health Organization 262, 263
whooping cough 50, 52, 62, 66, 282
Wilkes 64
Williams: Thomas 64
World Bank 298, 299, 300, 304, 310, 311

Y

Yarwood: AT 179
Yaws 51, 52, 206
yaws 43, 45, 50, 51, 62, 63, 86, 132, 134, 135, 136, 139, 142, 143, 166, 170, 183, 184, 185, 198, 202, 205, 206, 231

Z

Zigas: Vincent 186
Zimbabwe 58, 59, 349

Get Published, Inc!
Thorofare, NJ 08086
20 January, 2010
BA2010020